Fat-Soluble Vitamins in Health and Disease

Fat-Soluble Vitamins in Health and Disease

Editor: Lucy Taylor

AMERICAN
MEDICAL PUBLISHERS
www.americanmedicalpublishers.com

AMERICAN
MEDICAL PUBLISHERS
www.americanmedicalpublishers.com

Cataloging-in-Publication Data

Fat-soluble vitamins in health and disease / edited by Lucy Taylor.
p. cm.
Includes bibliographical references and index.
ISBN 978-1-63927-669-1
1. Vitamins, Fat-soluble. 2. Vitamins, Fat-soluble--Therapeutic use. 3. Vitamins.
4. Vitamin therapy. 5. Therapeutics, Physiological. 6. Health. I. Taylor, Lucy.
QP772.F37 F38 2023
612.399--dc23

American Medical Publishers,
41 Flatbush Avenue,
1st Floor, New York,
NY 11217, USA

ISBN 978-1-63927-669-1 (Hardback)

Contents

Preface

Vitamins are the organic compounds essential for human health. They are classified as fat soluble vitamins which include vitamins A, D, E, and K, and water soluble vitamins which include vitamin C and all the B vitamins. Fat soluble vitamins are stored in the human body in the fatty tissue and liver. These vitamins can be stored in the body for days and in certain cases, reserves of these vitamins remain in the body for months. Dietary fats facilitate the absorption of fat soluble vitamins through the intestinal tract. Vitamin A is a fat soluble vitamin found in sources like broccoli, carrots, butter, sweet potatoes, kale, pumpkins, spinach, etc. The deficiency of vitamin A causes keratomalacia and night blindness. Vitamin D is another fat soluble vitamin important for the healthy mineralization of bones and its deficiency results in rickets and osteomalacia. The topics included in this book on fat-soluble vitamins are of utmost significance and bound to provide incredible insights to readers. Those in search of information to further their knowledge on the health impacts of fat soluble vitamins will be greatly assisted by it.

This book is a comprehensive compilation of works of different researchers from varied parts of the world. It includes valuable experiences of the researchers with the sole objective of providing the readers (learners) with a proper knowledge of the concerned field. This book will be beneficial in evoking inspiration and enhancing the knowledge of the interested readers.

In the end, I would like to extend my heartiest thanks to the authors who worked with great determination on their chapters. I also appreciate the publisher's support in the course of the book. I would also like to deeply acknowledge my family who stood by me as a source of inspiration during the project.

Editor

1

Vitamin D Supplementation Improves the Effects of the Rehabilitation Program on Balance and Pressure Distribution in Patients after Anterior Cervical Interbody Fusion-Randomized Control Trial

Wojciech Skrobot [1,*,†], Ewelina Perzanowska [1,†], Katarzyna Krasowska [1], Damian J. Flis [2], Katarzyna P. Dzik [2], Wojciech Kloc [3,4], Jan Jacek Kaczor [2] and Jędrzej Antosiewicz [5,*]

1 Department of Functional Diagnostics and Kinesiology, Gdansk University of Physical Education and Sport, 80-336 Gdansk, Poland; ewelinaliedtke@gmail.com (E.P.); katarzyna.krasowska@awf.gda.pl (K.K.)
2 Department of Physiology and Biochemistry, Gdansk University of Physical Education and Sport, 80-336 Gdansk, Poland; damian.flis@awf.gda.pl (D.J.F.); kasi.dzik@gmail.com (K.P.D.); jan.kaczor@awf.gda.pl (J.J.K.)
3 Department of Neurosurgery, Copernicus Hospital, 80-803 Gdansk, Poland; wk56rak@gmail.com
4 Department of Neurology and Neurosurgery, University of Warmia and Mazury in Olsztyn, 10-719 Olsztyn, Poland
5 Department of Bioenergetics and Physiology of Exercise, Medical University of Gdansk, 80-211 Gdansk, Poland
* Correspondence: wojciech.skrobot@awf.gda.pl (W.S.); jant@gumed.edu.pl (J.A.)
† These authors contributed equally to this work.

Abstract: Study Design: A double-blinded, randomized controlled trial. Background: Surgery is effective in reducing pain intensity in patients with cervical disc disease. However, functional measurements demonstrated that the results have been not satisfactory enough. Thus, rehabilitation programs combined with the supplementation of vitamin D could play an essential role. Methods. The study recruited 30 patients, aged 20 to 70 years, selected for anterior cervical interbody fusion (ACIF). The patients were randomly divided into the placebo (Pl) and vitamin D (3200 IU D3/day) supplemented groups. The functional tests limits of stability (LOS), risk of falls (RFT), postural stability (PST), Romberg test, and foot pressure distribution were performed before supplementation (BS—week 0), five weeks after supplementation (AS—week 5), four weeks after surgery (BSVR—week 9), and 10 weeks after supervising rehabilitation (ASVR—week 19). Results. The concentration of 25(OH)D3 in the serum, after five weeks of supplementation, was significantly increased, while the Pl group maintained the same. The RFT was significantly reduced after five weeks of vitamin D supplementation. Moreover, a further significant decrease was observed following rehabilitation. In the Pl group, no changes in the RFT were observed. The overall postural stability index (OSI), LOS, and the outcomes of the Romberg test significantly improved in both groups; however, the effects on the OSI were more pronounced in the D3 group at the end of the rehabilitation program. Conclusions. Our data suggest that vitamin D supplementation positively affected the rehabilitation program in patients implemented four weeks after ACIF by reducing the risk of falls and improving postural stability.

Keywords: vitamin D supplementation; ACIF; cervical stabilization; balance; Romberg test; postural stability; risk of falls; limits of stability

1. Introduction

Patients with cervical disc disease often present with symptoms that include pain, sensory loss, motor loss, and reflex impairment. The consequence of these is a physical disability and a significant drop in quality of life [1]. Anterior cervical interbody fusion (ACIF) is a standard procedure for such problems; however, the outcome is strongly dependent on postsurgery rehabilitation [2]. Postoperative rehabilitation to increase the effects of cervical spine surgery by encouraging safe physical activities, improving function and reducing the fear of pain. Surgery has been shown to be very effective in pain reduction; however, in functions like balance, postural control, foot pressure distribution, and endurance, the progress is less evident [3].

Still, rules do not exist, and any guidance of time to conduct them initiate after an ACIF operation. Recently, it has been demonstrated that a self-directed home exercise program implemented immediately after surgery is effective in a short-term outcome [4]. Therefore, a rehabilitation program applied after surgery is crucial and usually focused on the improvement of cervical muscle endurance, strength, and postural control [3].

Vitamin D is an endogenous hormone synthesized in the skin from 7-dehydrocholesterol or taken from food. This vitamin is then metabolized in the liver by vitamin D-25-hydroxylase to 25-hydroxy vitamin D3 (25(OH)D3). 25(OH)D3 is converted by 1α-hydroxylase to 1,25-dihydroxy vitamin D3 (1,25(OH)2D3), which is an active form. Conversely, the serum concentration of 25(OH)D3 is considered to be a respectable marker of vitamin D status. If the concentration is lower than 30 ng/mL (75 nmol/L), it is considered inadequate by many scientists [5]. The kidneys and many other cell types possess the activity of 1α-hydroxylase and ability to synthesize 1,25(OH)2D3, including the skin, the human brain, prostate, white blood cells, and some others. The active form of vitamin D acts throughout its receptor (VDR), which is a transcriptional factor regulating around 900 genes [6]. Interestingly, VDR is present in the brain, skeletal muscles, and in most of the cells in the human body [7]. In agreement with this, skeletal muscle strength is associated with vitamin D status [8]. The anti-inflammatory properties of vitamin D have been also demonstrated [9]. All these properties make this vitamin an attractive remedy for patients after orthopedic surgery. A vitamin D deficiency is highly prevalent, and it is now considered a pandemic [10]. Its inadequacy is particularly common among orthopedic patients and osteoporosis. Besides, several studies have demonstrated the association between vitamin D deficiency, the spine, and joint morbidities [11,12].

Consequently, in the present study, we investigated the effects of vitamin D supplementation combined with 10 weeks of a supervised rehabilitation program in patients after ACIF surgery.

2. Materials and Methods

2.1. Participants, Therapists, and Centers

The study was a double-blinded, randomized controlled trial (Figure 1).

At the beginning of the study, 42 patients were recruited and randomly selected to the vitamin D supplemented (D3) and placebo groups (Pl). After supplementation, 4 patients resigned in the D3 group and three in the P1 group.

In the further process after the operation, 3 people in group D3 resigned and, in group Pl, 2 people.

The reasons for resignation were very different; in three cases, it was due to the change of the type of spine surgery, as well as the presence of other diseases or colds at that time.

A total of 5 people withdrew after surgery before starting rehabilitation. It was mainly related to well-being and organizing rehabilitation closer to home (Figure 1).

Vitamin D supplementation 3200 IU daily for 5 weeks. The physiotherapists conducted the treatment of the patients in both groups. The independent physiotherapists performed functional tests.

Patients were all coded, and the researchers, physiotherapists performing and reporting the statistical analyses, were unaware of the patients' assignments.

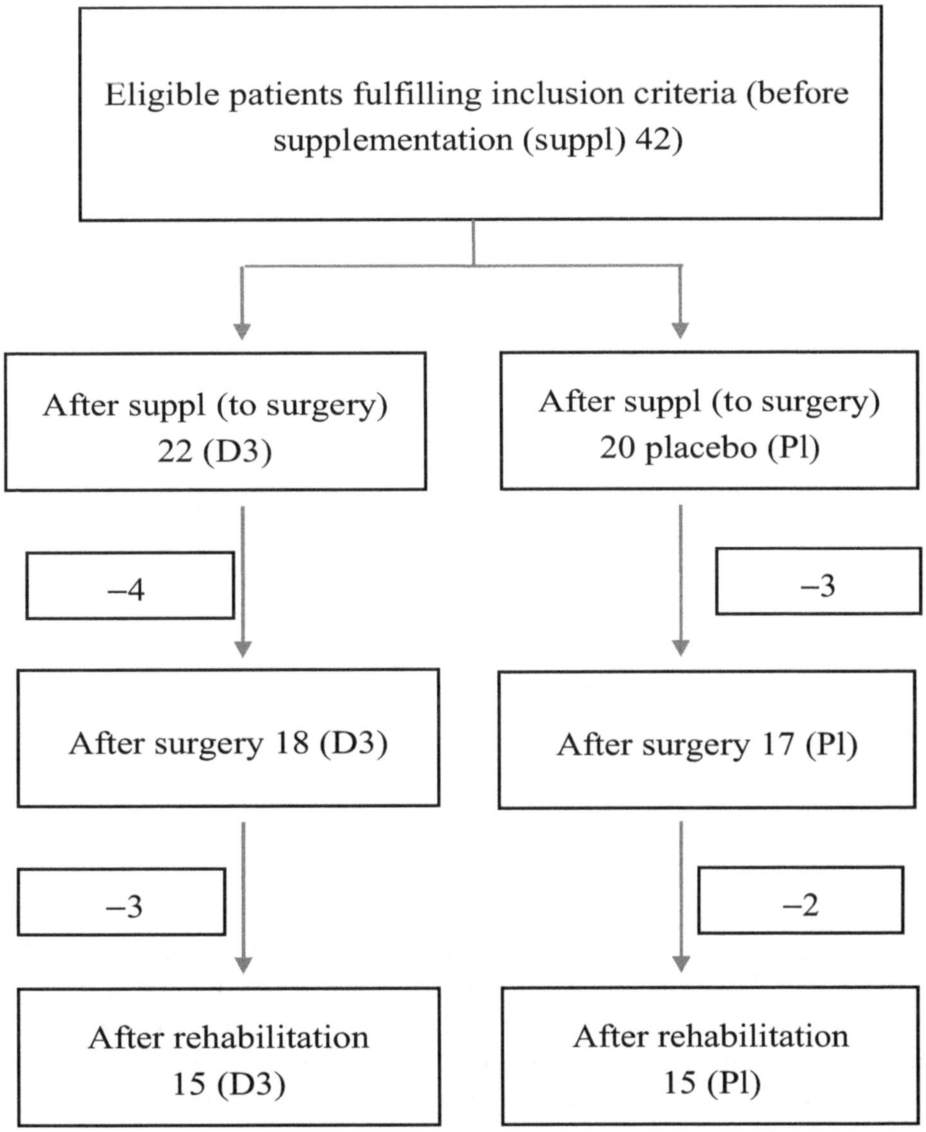

Figure 1. Participants flow diagram.

Patients did not know what kind of supplement they received. All the patients gave full written informed consent to participate in the study and could leave the study at any time.

Patients at COPERNICUS Hospital Neurosurgery Clinic in Gdansk, Poland were classified for ACIF surgery by a neurosurgeon clinical assessment and magnetic resonance imaging (MRI) scan.

The study group consisted of 30 people aged 31 to 68, 10 men and 20 women. Seventy-three percent of the respondents were people with secondary or vocational education, and 27% had higher education. Ten patients (5 women and 5 men) smoked cigarettes. The body mass index was 24.87 ± 5.83 and 25.67 ± 5.09 for the placebo and vitamin D groups, respectively.

2.1.1. Including Criteria

Ages between 20 and 70 years, neck pain, and/or upper limb neuropathy exceeding 12 months for which conservative treatment failed to improve a primary diagnosis of cervical spinal stenosis or degenerative disc disease, so the patient was selected for anterior cervical fusion with or without decompression.

2.1.2. Excluding Criteria

Previous cervical fusion cervical ankylosing spondylitis rheumatoid arthritis and worsening of existing or appearance of new symptoms.

2.2. Functional Tests

Postural stability test (PST), limits of stability test (LOS), and risk of falls test (RFT) were used to assess control of balance. Before testing on a Biodex Balance System (BBS), a familiarization was performed, as described before [13]. Additional Romberg test and distribution force of pressure was conducted on a treadmill. Tests were performed four times: before supplementation (BS)—vitamin D3 or placebo, 5 weeks after supplementation 2 or 1 days before surgery (AS), 4 weeks after surgery (BSVR), and 10 weeks after supervised rehabilitation (ASVR).

2.3. Sample Collection

Blood for biochemical research was collected four times: before supplementation (BS)—vitamin D3 or placebo, 5 weeks after supplementation 2 or 1 days before surgery ((AS), 4 weeks after surgery (BSVR), and 10 weeks after supervising rehabilitation (ASVR) in serum separation tubes (Becton Dickinson, Oxford, UK), The blood was collected at rest, while fasting, in the morning hours of 7:00–8:00 a.m. The samples for serum isolation were centrifuged at 2000× g and was stored at −80 °C until later analysis. Serum 25-OH Vitamin D3 was determined using the 25-OH Vitamin D total ELISA kit (DE1971, Demeditec Diagnostics, Kiel, Germany) according to the manufacturer's instructions. The intra-assay coefficients of variability (CVs) and inter-assay CVs reported by the manufacturer were 2–8% and 4–9%, respectively.

2.4. Postural Stability Test

The BBS (Biodex Medical System Inc., Shirley, NY, USA) allowed an objective evaluation of postural stability through three indexes: the Overall Stability Index (OSI), the Anterior-Posterior Stability Index (APSI), and the Medial-Lateral Stability Index (MLSI). During tests, the platform was stable. The participants were asked to step on the platform in a bipedal stance with bare feet and open eyes looking forward to the monitor (BSS monitor), while their hands are hanging by their sides (hand support was not permitted). They were asked to stand straight, not to change their feet position, and only sway their body when it was needed.

In these conditions, these indexes represent fluctuations around a zero point established before testing when the platform is stable [13]. Each measurement was taken on a static platform at intervals: 20 s of testing and 10-s breaks. Higher scores indicate poorer postural stability.

2.5. Risk of Falls Test

The risk of falls test measures the same properties as the postural stability test; however, this is performed on an unstable platform. RFT consisted of three measurements at intervals: 20 s of testing and 10-s breaks, as described in the Operation and Service Manual of Biodex Medical Systems. Bilateral assessment of the dynamic stance was done for assessing the risk of falls; levels 6 to 2 were used. Before the testing, a familiarization procedure was performed. In this test, only the Overall Stability Index was evaluated. This index was calculated through the degree of oscillation of the platform, where the lower-score indices indicated a lower risk of falls [14].

2.6. Limits of Stability Test

The patients performed three trials of the LOS test, which involved shifting their body weight while standing on the stable platform to move a cursor on the screen from a central target to a peripheral blinking target [15].

During the test, the best results are obtained by patients who can obtained the maximum angle of a body from vertical without losing one's balance. The Biodex Balance System provides scores for all eight directions, as well as an overall score. Higher scores indicated better performance. When the LOS is exceeded a fall, stumble, or step will ensue.

2.7. Romberg Test

In the current study, treadmill Zebris (the Zebris FDM-T system (Zebris® Medical GmbH, Isny im Allgäu, Germany) was used with sensors to measure the ground force of pressure. Patients were informed about the aim and methodological procedures of the test. The Romberg test served to assess balance and postural sway [16].

The subject kept a normal standing straight position, with his arms along his body and feet opened at an angle of 30 degrees to the front, heels 3 cm apart and narrow position [17].

The test was conducted with eyes closed (EC) during 30 s [18].

The outcomes of the Romberg test were gathered for the sway rate, center of pressure (CoP) path length, and ellipse sway area [19]. According to Kalron:

(1) the ellipse sway area (mm^2), defined as a 95% confidence ellipse area for the mean movements of the center of pressure (CoP) anterior, posterior, medial, and lateral coordinates.
(2) the sway rate (mm/s), defined as the mean speed of movement of the CoP throughout the testing period.
(3) the CoP path length (mm), defined as the absolute length of the CoP path movements throughout the testing period.
(4) the average pressure distribution of the left and right feet expressed in body weight (%). Additionally, the bilateral pressure distribution asymmetry score was calculated as the absolute difference in pressure distribution between the legs. In a perfect symmetrical stance, this variable is zero [20].

The study was approved by the local institutional Bioethical Committee in Gdansk, Poland (No. NKBBN/120/2012) and conformed to the Declaration of Helsinki guidelines and was registered as clinical trial NCT03417700.

2.8. Data Analysis

Statistical analysis was performed using Statistica 13.1 software (Statsoft, Tulsa, OK, USA). All values were expressed as the mean ± standard deviation (SD). The analysis of variance (ANOVA) in the repeated measures model, using the contrast method, was used for the analysis with $p < 0.05$. The study design was a two-arm randomized controlled trial with an allocation ratio of 1:1. An online software (https://www.graphpad.com/quickcalcs/randMenu/) was used to randomize the participants to the experimental group and, respectively, to the control group by the head of the project.

2.9. Rehabilitation Protocol

After recrution as a part of the preparation to surgery, the patients were instructed by a physiotherapist how to move ergonomically before and after the surgery. Besides that, the patients were motivated to start activity without pain as soon as possible after the operation.

The patients initiated a supervised rehabilitation protocol four weeks after ACIF surgery lasting 10 weeks (3 times a week). Physiotherapists were trained in rehabilitation protocols before the start of the exercises.

During the early postoperative phase, strengthening exercises were performed while keeping the cervical spine in a neutral position to minimize strain on the fused/adjacent segment and, thereafter, to avoid breakage of the fusion device (Table 1).

Table 1. The details of the rehabilitation protocol.

Week	Intervention
I	Instruction about ergonomics behavior during daily activities; instruction about keeping right position with correction of a head, shoulder, and pelvic girdle; and, also, deep trunk stabilization was led. Maintaining a neutral posture movement of the upper and lower limbs was performed.
II–III	The same exercise as above, but more difficulty was conducted. Exercises with a head's laser for control movement of the head was applied. Shoulder's girdle stabilization, with additional control of the key parts of the body, was carried out. Proprioception exercises were led with opened and closed eyes. Exercises in the closed chain on the wall in a standing position were performed, which were prepared with plank and balance exercises.
IV	Balancing exercises with sensorimotor discs with the control of body swaying were conducted. Learning tensions of the deep cervical flexors was managed.
V	Increasing the number of isometric contractions of stabilizing muscles exercises and changes in the sequence and time performed of the movement were applied.
VI–VII	At the beginning of the sixth week, independent head movements in the range to the threshold of pain in the cervical spines of patients were performed. In the next weeks, an increased intensity and difficulty of the exercises were applied.
VIII–X	From the eighth week, patients started plank exercises. After ten weeks of supervised rehabilitation, patients were encouraged to continue their activities at home.

3. Results

3.1. Vitamin D

The concentration of the serum 25(OH)D3 did not differ between the groups at the beginning of the study. After five weeks of vitamin D supplementation (3200 IU/day), it significantly increased serum 25(OH)D3 in group D3, while, in the Pl group, the changes were not significant (Figure 2). During the 14 weeks of the study, the higher concentrations of 25(OH)D3 were maintained in the D3 group as compared to the starting level.

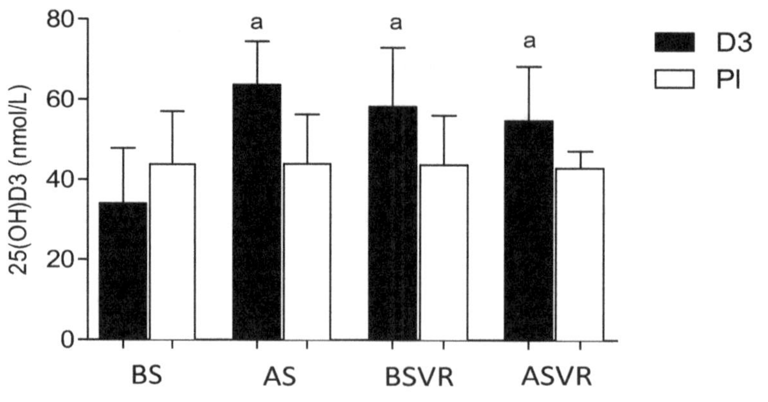

Figure 2. The concentration of 25(OH)D3 in the serum, after five weeks of supplementation, was significantly increased. Columns, mean; bars SD; and a, $p < 0.05$, significantly different compared with BS. BS—before supplementation, AS—5 weeks after supplementation, BSVR—4 weeks after surgery, and ASVR—10 weeks after supervised rehabilitation.

3.2. Risk of Falls

In patients who were supplemented with vitamin D during the five weeks, significant improvement in the RFT was observed before ACIF operation. In the Pl group, no changes were found. Besides, after the surgery and 10 weeks of supervised rehabilitation, improvement in the RFT was observed only in the D3 group. The rehabilitation program caused some improvement in the Pl group, but it did not reach statistical significance (Figure 3). At the end of the study, after supervised rehabilitation protocols, significant differences between the groups were observed.

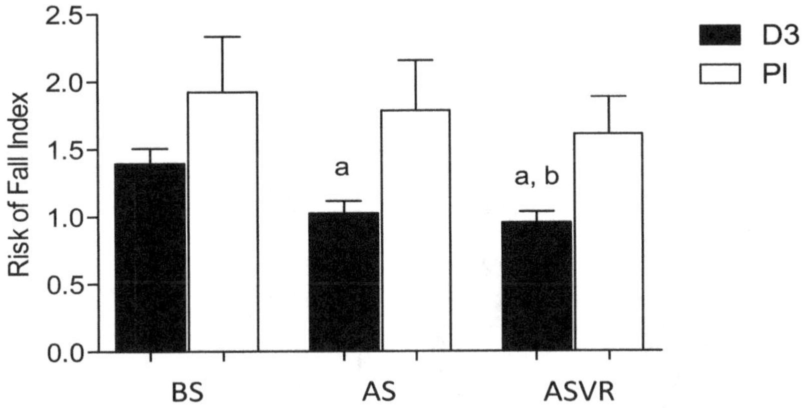

Figure 3. Vitamin D supplementation reduced the risk of falls of patients before anterior cervical interbody fusion (ACIF) surgery. The data are presented as the means and standard deviations (SDs). a, $p < 0.05$, significantly different compared with BS and b, $p < 0.05$, significantly different compared with Pl-ASVR.

3.3. *Postural Stability*

The Postural Stability Test consists of indices: Anterior-Posterior Stability Index (APSI), Medial-Lateral Stability Index (MLSI) and Overall Stability Index (OSI), which is the composite of the MLSI and APSI. The lower scores of these indices indicate the improvement in postural control. Vitamin D supplementation before the ACIF operation had no effects on the OSI (Figure 4); however, the index significantly decreased in the D3 group after 10 weeks of the rehabilitation. Besides, in the placebo group, the significant improvement was observed only in the APSI after 10 weeks of rehabilitation (not shown). Moreover, the OSI were significantly better in the D3 group as compared to the Pl group at the end of the study.

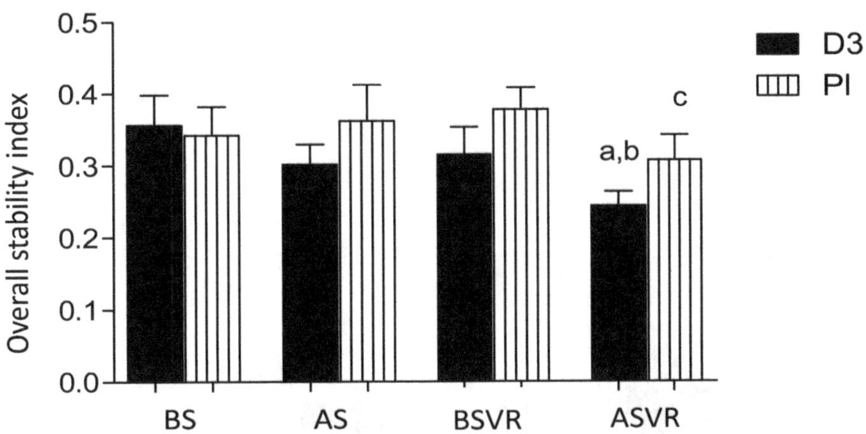

Figure 4. Vitamin D supplementation improves the effects of rehabilitation on the overall postural stability of patients after an anterior cervical interbody fusion surgery. Columns, mean and bars, standard deviations (SDs). a, $p < 0.05$, significantly different compared with the before supplementation (BS) control; b, $p < 0.05$, significantly different compared with the D3-BSVR group by one-way ANOVA; and c, $p < 0.05$, significantly different compared with the Pl-BSVR group.

3.4. *Limits of Stability*

Five weeks of vitamin D supplementation had no effects on the limits of stability. Ten weeks of supervised rehabilitation significantly improved the LOS in both the D3 and Pl groups, and there were no differences between the groups (Figure 5).

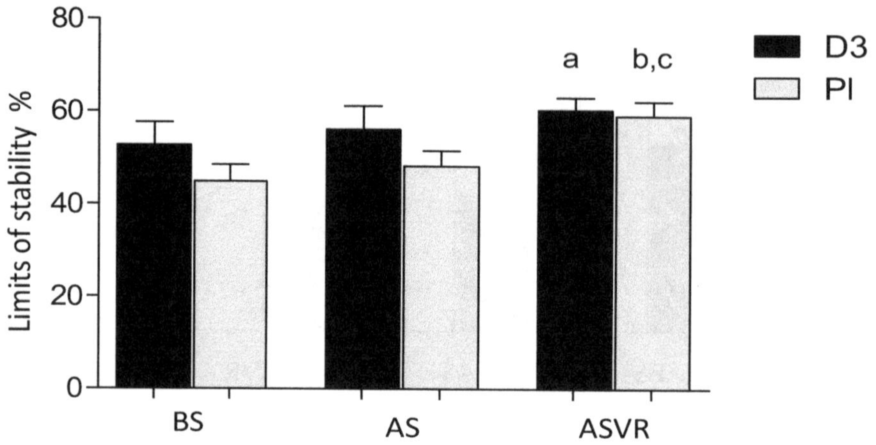

Figure 5. Vitamin D supplementation had no effects on the rehabilitation-induced improvement on the limits of stability of patients after anterior cervical interbody fusion surgery. Columns, mean and bars, standard deviations (SDs). a, $p < 0.05$, significantly different compared with the D3-BS; b, $p < 0.05$, significantly different compared with the Pl-BS; and c, $p < 0.05$, significantly different compared with and the Pl-after supplementation (AS) group, respectively by one-way ANOVA.

A higher score of the Limits Stability Test compared to the initial level showed an improvement of posture balance control. The limits of stability, both in the vitamin D and placebo groups compared to the level before supplementation, after rehabilitation was significantly increased—a and b, $p < 0.05$.

3.5. *Ellipse Sway Area*

The ellipse sway area (mm^2) is defined as a 95% confidence ellipse area for the mean movements of the CoP anterior, posterior, medial, and lateral coordinates. After supervisor rehabilitation, the level of this marker significantly decreased in both the D3 and placebo groups compared to the baseline values (Figure 6).

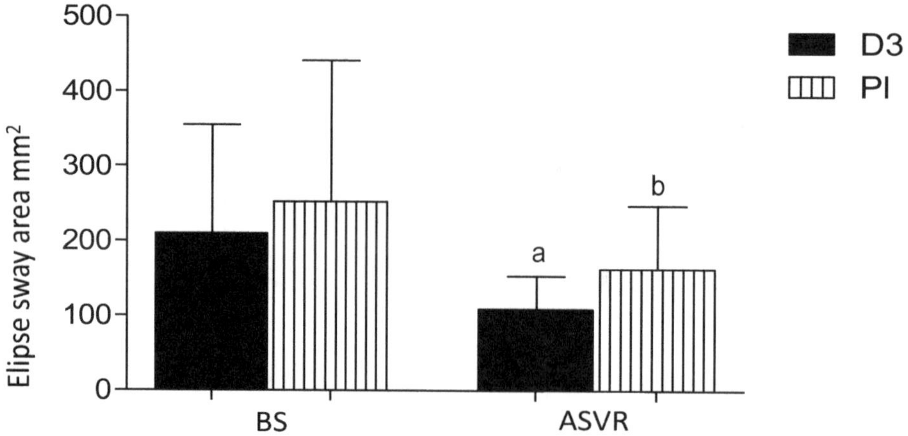

Figure 6. Vitamin D supplementation had no effects on the rehabilitation-induced improvement on the ellipse sway area (mm^2) of patients after anterior cervical interbody fusion surgery. Columns, mean and bars, standard deviations (SDs). a, $p < 0.05$, significantly different compared with D3-BS and b, $p < 0.05$, significantly different compared with Pl-BS by one-way ANOVA.

3.6. Sway Rate Center of Pressure (COP AV)

The sway rate (mm/s) COP AV is defined as the mean speed of movement of the CoP throughout the testing period. After supervisor rehabilitation, there was a significant difference between the groups being lower in the D3 group. As compared to the beginning of the study, the deterioration of the results of the placebo group to the vitamin D group was observed; a, $p < 0.005$ (Figure 7).

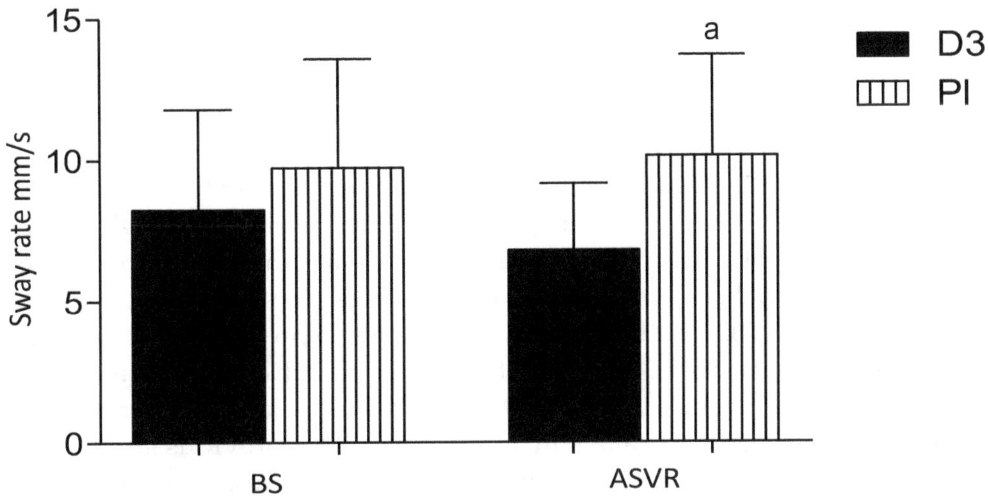

Figure 7. Vitamin D supplementation decrease sway rate (mm/s) in patients after anterior cervical interbody fusion surgery. Columns, mean and bars, standard deviations (SDs). a, $p < 0.05$, significantly different compared with ASVR D3 by one-way ANOVA.

3.7. CoP Path Length

The CoP path length (mm) is defined as the absolute length of the CoP path movements throughout the testing period. After supervisor rehabilitation, there was a significant difference between the groups being lower in the D3 group (Figure 8).

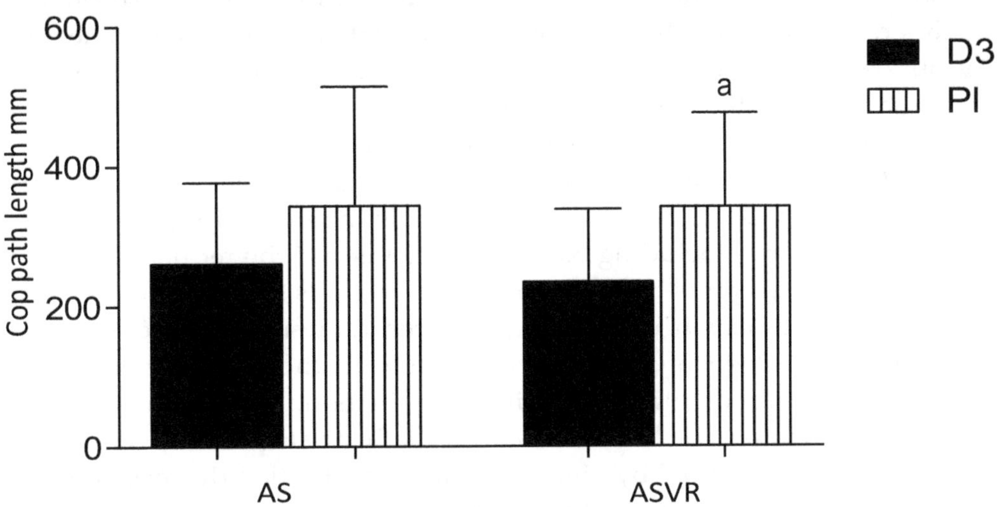

Figure 8. Vitamin D supplementation decreased the center of pressure (CoP) path length (mm) in patients after anterior cervical interbody fusion surgery. Columns, mean and bars, standard deviations (SDs). a, $p < 0.05$, significantly different compared with ASVR D3 by one-way ANOVA.

The average pressure distribution of the left and right feet expressed in body weight (%) was also evaluated in the patients; however, the changes were not significant.

4. Discussion

In the present study, we demonstrated that the vitamin D supplementation significantly improved the outcome of supervising rehabilitation in the D3 group who underwent ACIF surgery. Vitamin D supplementation was shown to exert positive effects on many aspects of human health, and many orthopedic patients were demonstrated to be vitamin D-deficient [21,22]. Despite this, we are not aware of any study where the effects of vitamin D on supervising the rehabilitation of cervical spine patients have been evaluated. Recently, some beneficial effects of vitamin D supplementation were observed during the functional recovery of patients after hip fractures and posterior interbody fusions [23,24]. Vitamin D has a pleiotropic function in the human body, including anti-inflammatory, and protects from skeletal muscle atrophy, improves proprioception, and many others [25]. It is worth noting that the five-week supplementation significantly increases 25(OH)D3 in the serum. 25(OH)D3 is considered to be a good marker of vitamin D status, as high concentrations (usually higher than 32 ng/mL) ensure the proper synthesis of 1,25(OH)2D3 in the target tissue. The presence of 25(OH)D3-1α-hydroxylase, the enzyme that converts 25(OH)D3 into 1,25(OH)2D3 in skeletal muscles, has been demonstrated [25]. However, up to today, it has not been well-defined what is the exact source of 1,25(OH)2D3 for skeletal muscles. The effects of 25(OH)D3 on skeletal muscle genes expression and muscle function were distinct when compared to 1,25(OH)2D3 [26]. Unfortunately, 1,25(OH)2D3 was not measured in this study; despite this, we found that a rise in 25(OH)D3 was associated with a lower risk of falls in patients even before the surgery. This data is in agreement with a previous study that demonstrated that vitamin D reduced the risk of falls in elderly subjects [26]. Impaired proprioception is one of the main factors that weakens postural control. Interestingly, a vitamin D deficiency was associated with poorer postural control and body sways [27]. Our data are partially in agreement with these observations. We demonstrated that 10 weeks of supervised rehabilitation decreased the risk of falls only in vitamin D-supplemented patients. Conversely, data from the LOS test showed improvement in both the Pl and D3 groups, which indicates that vitamin D supplementation did not modify the effects of rehabilitation. The LOS test measures the ability to shift the center of gravity toward the limits of stability in all directions, so its improvement indicates that the risk of falls decreases and quality of life increases. It is difficult to explain the difference in the results between the RFT and the LOS test. There is a tendency for better results in the LOS test in patients of the D3 group, which may indicate some positive effects. Additionally, the directional control, which is also evaluated in the LOS test, showed no differences between the group of unstable patients compared to healthy subjects [27]. On the contrary, our data indicated that the rehabilitation program improved the outcome of this test, which confirms its diagnostic value in patients after ACIF surgery. Moreover, the limits of stability are also known to decrease with age [28], which can also influence the results.

As mentioned above, the presence of VDRs in the human neurons, glial cells, and cortex have been demonstrated. Vitamin D deficiency in older people may contribute to failure in the central and peripheral nervous systems, including balance problems and the reduction of nerve conduction velocity [29]. Cervical spine receptors have important connections to the vestibular system, the organ of sight, and several connections with the areas of the central nervous system (CNS). A vitamin D deficiency, in addition to neck disorders, may contribute to the dysfunction of the upper spine proprioceptors and affect neuromuscular control and coordination. Besides, many studies have shown that the cervical spine has an impact on human balance [30]. Our data partially support this assumption, as supervised rehabilitation supported by vitamin D supplementation decreased the risk of falls and increased the overall stability. Additionally, the presence of VDR has been confirmed in the vestibular system [31], which plays an important role in stability control.

The importance of the muscles stabilizing the cervical spine, emphasizing the high content of spindles in them, especially in suboccipital muscles, as well as the function of the deep flexors of the cervical spine, additionally increase due to the type of the improvement program used, with vitamin D3 supplementation strengthening its effects. This is reflected in the reduction of deflections and increased stability in relation to CoP—posturography parameters, such as COP AV, ellipse sway area, and CoP path length.

One of the important aspects of vitamin D action is the ability to increase muscle cell regeneration and decrease their apoptosis [32], which may play an important role in the healing process after ACIF surgery. Besides, as mentioned before, vitamin D has anti-inflammatory action. The reduction of proinflammatory cytokines in circulation was shown after vitamin D supplementation [29]. Moreover, a study in rats demonstrated that vitamin D ameliorates skeletal muscle inflammation induced by exercise, decreasing the MAP kinase activation and tumor necrosis factor level [33].

These data became even more interesting in light of a previously published study that showed that neck-specific functions were not improved in patients in a six-year follow-up after surgery [34].

Limitation of the Study

Certainly, the number of patients is a significant limitation of this study. Despite severe improvements in postural control in patients supplemented with vitamin D, we did not observe differences between the placebo and vitamin D groups at the end of the study in most of the studied parameters. Possibly with a higher number of patients, the differences could be revealed. Skeletal muscles have been shown to possess VDR and the ability to the synthesized the active form of vitamin D, but it is also possible that they may also depend on 1,25(OH)2D3 from the blood [35,36]. In support of this, skeletal muscle genes expression are correlated strongly with blood 1,25(OH)2D3 [26]. Moreover, it has been shown that circulating 1,25(OH)2D3 correlates better with skeletal muscle strength and muscle genes expression than 25(OH)D3 [26]. Remember that exercise-induced changes in vitamin D metabolism and formation of some metabolites with no classical vitamin D activity like antioxidant or anti-inflammatory can be expected [37]. Thus, knowing the blood concentration of 1,25(OH)2D3, 24,25(OH)2D3 and 3-epi-25(OH)D3, in addition to 25(OH)D3 in both groups, could help better to explain the effects of vitamin D supplementation on the outcome of the rehabilitation.

5. Conclusions

Our data suggest that preoperative supplementations with vitamin D positively affected the rehabilitation program in patients if implemented four weeks after ACIF surgery, reducing the risk of falls and improving postural stability. We assume that patients should be treated with vitamin D preoperatively, as well as after surgery, as a form of supporting the rehabilitation process, because of a better and faster recovery.

Author Contributions: Conceptualization, W.S., E.P. and J.A.; methodology, W.S., J.A., E.P. and J.J.K.; formal analysis, W.S., E.P. and J.J.K.; investigation, W.S., E.P., K.K., K.P.D. and D.J.F.; writing—original draft preparation, W.S., E.P., K.K., K.P.D., D.J.F., J.J.K., J.A. and W.K.; project administration, W.S., E.P., W.K., D.J.F. and J.J.K.; and writing—review and editing, W.S., E.P. and J.A. All authors have read and agreed to the published version of the manuscript.

Acknowledgments: The authors would like to thank all patients who participated in the study.

Abbreviations

ACIF	Anterior cervical interbody fusion
OSI	Overall postural stability index
Pl	Placebo
LOS	Limits of stability
RFT	Risk of falls
PST	Postural stability
BS	Before supplementation
AS	After supplementation

BSVR	After surgery—Before supervising rehabilitation
ASVR	After supervising rehabilitation
$25(OH)D_3$	25-hydroxy cholecalciferol
$1,25(OH)_2D_3$	1,25-dihydroxycholecalciferol
VDR	Vitamin D receptor
MRI	Magnetic resonance imaging
BBS	Biodex Balance System
CVs	Coefficients of variability
APSI	Anterior-Posterior Stability Index
MLSI	Medial-Lateral Stability Index
EC	Eyes closed
CoP	Center of pressure
SDs	Standard deviations
CNS	Central Nervous System

References

1. Meleger, A.L.; Krivickas, L.S. Neck and back pain: Musculoskeletal disorders. *Neurol. Clin.* **2007**, *25*, 419–438. [CrossRef] [PubMed]
2. Peolsson, A.; Oberg, B.; Wibault, J.; Dedering, A.; Zsigmond, P.; Bernfort, L.; Kammerlind, A.S.; Persson, L.C.G.; Lofgren, H. Outcome of physiotherapy after surgery for cervical disc disease: A prospective randomised multi-centre trial. *BMC Musculoskel. Dis.* **2014**, *15*. [CrossRef] [PubMed]
3. Peolsson, A.; Soderlund, A.; Engquist, M.; Lind, B.; Lofgren, H.; Vavruch, L.; Holtz, A.; Winstrom-Christersson, A.; Isaksson, I.; Oberg, B. Physical Function Outcome in Cervical Radiculopathy Patients After Physiotherapy Alone Compared with Anterior Surgery Followed by Physiotherapy A Prospective Randomized Study With a 2-Year Follow-up. *Spine* **2013**, *38*, 300–307. [CrossRef]
4. Coronado, R.A.; Devin, C.J.; Pennings, J.S.; Vanston, S.W.; Fenster, D.E.; Hills, J.M.; Aaronson, O.S.; Schwarz, J.P.; Stephens, B.F.; Archer, K.R. Early Self-directed Home Exercise Program after Anterior Cervical Discectomy and Fusion A Pilot Study. *Spine* **2020**, *45*, 217–225. [CrossRef]
5. Pludowski, P.; Grant, W.B.; Bhattoa, H.P.; Bayer, M.; Povoroznyuk, V.; Rudenka, E.; Ramanau, H.; Varbiro, S.; Rudenka, A.; Karczmarewicz, E.; et al. Vitamin d status in central europe. *Int. J. Endocrinol.* **2014**, *2014*, 589587. [CrossRef] [PubMed]
6. Wang, T.T.; Tavera-Mendoza, L.E.; Laperriere, D.; Libby, E.; MacLeod, N.B.; Nagai, Y.; Bourdeau, V.; Konstorum, A.; Lallemant, B.; Zhang, R.; et al. Large-scale in silico and microarray-based identification of direct 1,25-dihydroxyvitamin D3 target genes. *Mol. Endocrinol.* **2005**, *19*, 2685–2695. [CrossRef] [PubMed]
7. Bischoff, H.A.; Borchers, M.; Gudat, F.; Duermueller, U.; Theiler, R.; Stahelin, H.B.; Dick, W. In situ detection of 1,25-dihydroxyvitamin D-3 receptor in human skeletal muscle tissue. *Histochem. J.* **2001**, *33*, 19–24. [CrossRef]
8. Mieszkowski, J.; Niespodzinski, B.; Kochanowicz, A.; Gmiat, A.; Prusik, K.; Prusik, K.; Kortas, J.; Ziemann, E.; Antosiewicz, J. The Effect of Nordic Walking Training Combined with Vitamin D Supplementation on Postural Control and Muscle Strength in Elderly PeopleA Randomized Controlled Trial. *Int. J. Environ. Res. Public Health* **2018**, *15*, 1951. [CrossRef]
9. Rai, V.; Dietz, N.E.; Dilisio, M.F.; Radwan, M.M.; Agrawal, D.K. Vitamin D attenuates inflammation, fatty infiltration, and cartilage loss in the knee of hyperlipidemic microswine. *Arthritis Res. Ther.* **2016**, *18*, 203. [CrossRef]
10. Pludowski, P.; Ducki, C.; Konstantynowicz, J.; Jaworski, M. Vitamin D status in Poland. *Polskie Archiwum Medycyny Wewnętrznej* **2016**, *126*, 530–539. [CrossRef]
11. Stoker, G.E.; Buchowski, J.M.; Chen, C.T.; Kim, H.J.; Park, M.S.; Riew, K.D. Hypovitaminosis D and Cervical Disk Herniation among Adults Undergoing Spine Surgery. *Glob. Spine J.* **2013**, *3*, 231–236. [CrossRef]
12. Warner, S.J.; Garner, M.R.; Nguyen, J.T.; Lorich, D.G. Perioperative vitamin D levels correlate with clinical outcomes after ankle fracture fixation. *Arch. Orthop. Trauma Surg.* **2016**, *136*, 339–344. [CrossRef] [PubMed]
13. Arnold, B.L.; Schmitz, R.J. Examination of Balance Measures Produced by the Biodex Stability System. *J. Athl. Train.* **1998**, *33*, 323–327.
14. Siddiqi, F.A.; Masood, T. Training on Biodex balance system improves balance and mobility in the elderly. *J. Pak. Med. Assoc.* **2018**, *68*, 1655–1659.

15. Stephenson, J.; Zesiewicz, T.; Gooch, C.; Wecker, L.; Sullivan, K.; Jahan, I.; Kim, S.H. Gait and balance in adults with Friedreich's ataxia. *Gait Posture* **2015**, *41*, 603–607. [CrossRef]
16. Black, F.O.; Wall, C., 3rd; Rockette, H.E., Jr.; Kitch, R. Normal subject postural sway during the Romberg test. *Am. J. Otolaryngol.* **1982**, *3*, 309–318. [CrossRef]
17. Tjernstrom, F.; Bjorklund, M.; Malmstrom, E.M. Romberg ratio in quiet stance posturography–Test to retest reliability. *Gait Posture* **2015**, *42*, 27–31. [CrossRef]
18. Scoppa, F.; Capra, R.; Gallamini, M.; Shiffer, R. Clinical stabilometry standardization: Basic definitions–acquisition interval–sampling frequency. *Gait Posture* **2013**, *37*, 290–292. [CrossRef]
19. Kalron, A. The Romberg ratio in people with multiple sclerosis. *Gait Posture* **2017**, *54*, 209–213. [CrossRef]
20. Kalron, A.; Achiron, A. Postural control, falls and fear of falling in people with multiple sclerosis without mobility aids. *J. Neurol. Sci.* **2013**, *335*, 186–190. [CrossRef]
21. Maier, G.S.; Horas, K.; Seeger, J.B.; Roth, K.E.; Kurth, A.A.; Maus, U. Vitamin D insufficiency in the elderly orthopaedic patient: An epidemic phenomenon. *Int. Orthop.* **2015**, *39*, 787–792. [CrossRef] [PubMed]
22. Maier, G.S.; Seeger, J.B.; Horas, K.; Roth, K.E.; Kurth, A.A.; Maus, U. The prevalence of vitamin D deficiency in patients with vertebral fragility fractures. *Bone Joint J.* **2015**, *97*, 89–93. [CrossRef] [PubMed]
23. Stemmle, J.; Marzel, A.; Chocano-Bedoya, P.O.; Orav, E.J.; Dawson-Hughes, B.; Freystaetter, G.; Egli, A.; Theiler, R.; Staehelin, H.B.; Bischoff-Ferrari, H.A. Effect of 800 IU Versus 2000 IU Vitamin D3 With or Without a Simple Home Exercise Program on Functional Recovery After Hip Fracture: A Randomized Controlled Trial. *J. Am. Med. Dir. Assoc.* **2019**, *20*, 530–536 e531. [CrossRef] [PubMed]
24. Skrobot, W.; Liedtke, E.; Krasowska, K.; Dzik, K.P.; Flis, D.J.; Samoraj-Dereszkiewicz, A.; Libionka, W.; Kortas, J.; Kloc, W.; Antosiewicz, J.; et al. Early Rehabilitation Program and Vitamin D Supplementation Improves Sensitivity of Balance and the Postural Control in Patients after Posterior Lumbar Interbody Fusion: A Randomized Trial. *Nutrients* **2019**, *11*, 2202. [CrossRef] [PubMed]
25. Krasowska, K.; Skrobot, W.; Liedtke, E.; Sawicki, P.; Flis, D.J.; Dzik, K.P.; Libionka, W.; Kloc, W.; Kaczor, J.J. The Preoperative Supplementation With Vitamin D Attenuated Pain Intensity and Reduced the Level of Pro-inflammatory Markers in Patients After Posterior Lumbar Interbody Fusion. *Front. Pharmacol.* **2019**, *10*. [CrossRef]
26. Bischoff-Ferrari, H.A.; Conzelmann, M.; Dick, W.; Theiler, R.; Stahelin, H.B. Effect of vitamin D on muscle strength and relevance in regard to osteoporosis prevention. *Z. Rheumatol.* **2003**, *62*, 518–521. [CrossRef]
27. Dhesi, J.K.; Bearne, L.M.; Moniz, C.; Hurley, M.V.; Jackson, S.H.; Swift, C.G.; Allain, T.J. Neuromuscular and psychomotor function in elderly subjects who fall and the relationship with vitamin D status. *J. Bone Miner. Res.* **2002**, *17*, 891–897. [CrossRef]
28. Gill, J.; Allum, J.H.; Carpenter, M.G.; Held-Ziolkowska, M.; Adkin, A.L.; Honegger, F.; Pierchala, K. Trunk sway measures of postural stability during clinical balance tests: Effects of age. *J. Gerontol. A Biol. Sci. Med. Sci.* **2001**, *56*, M438–M447. [CrossRef]
29. Gmiat, A.; Jaworska, J.; Micielska, K.; Kortas, J.; Prusik, K.; Prusik, K.; Lipowski, M.; Radulska, A.; Szupryczynska, N.; Antosiewicz, J.; et al. Improvement of cognitive functions in response to a regular Nordic walking training in elderly women—A change dependent on the training experience. *Exp. Gerontol.* **2018**, *104*, 105–112. [CrossRef]
30. Treleaven, J. Sensorimotor disturbances in neck disorders affecting postural stability, head and eye movement control. *Man. Ther.* **2008**, *13*, 2–11. [CrossRef]
31. Minasyan, A.; Keisala, T.; Zou, J.; Zhang, Y.; Toppila, E.; Syvala, H.; Lou, Y.R.; Kalueff, A.V.; Pyykko, I.; Tuohimaa, P. Vestibular dysfunction in vitamin D receptor mutant mice. *J. Steroid Biochem. Mol. Biol.* **2009**, *114*, 161–166. [CrossRef] [PubMed]
32. Barker, T.; Henriksen, V.T.; Martins, T.B.; Hill, H.R.; Kjeldsberg, C.R.; Schneider, E.D.; Dixon, B.M.; Weaver, L.K. Higher serum 25-hydroxyvitamin D concentrations associate with a faster recovery of skeletal muscle strength after muscular injury. *Nutrients* **2013**, *5*, 1253–1275. [CrossRef] [PubMed]
33. Choi, M.; Park, H.; Cho, S.; Lee, M. Vitamin D3 supplementation modulates inflammatory responses from the muscle damage induced by high-intensity exercise in SD rats. *Cytokine* **2013**, *63*, 27–35. [CrossRef] [PubMed]
34. Peolsson, A.; Vavruch, L.; Hedlund, R. Long-term randomised comparison between a carbon fibre cage and the Cloward procedure in the cervical spine. *Eur. Spine J.* **2007**, *16*, 173–178. [CrossRef] [PubMed]

35. Hassan-Smith, Z.K.; Jenkinson, C.; Smith, D.J.; Hernandez, I.; Morgan, S.A.; Crabtree, N.J.; Gittoes, N.J.; Keevil, B.G.; Stewart, P.M.; Hewison, M. 25-hydroxyvitamin D3 and 1,25-dihydroxyvitamin D3 exert distinct effects on human skeletal muscle function and gene expression. *PLoS ONE* **2017**, *12*, e0170665. [CrossRef] [PubMed]
36. Girgis, C.M.; Mokbel, N.; Cha, K.M.; Houweling, P.J.; Abboud, M.; Fraser, D.R.; Mason, R.S.; Clifton-Bligh, R.J.; Gunton, J.E. The vitamin D receptor (VDR) is expressed in skeletal muscle of male mice and modulates 25-hydroxyvitamin D (25OHD) uptake in myofibers. *Endocrinology* **2014**, *155*, 3227–3237. [CrossRef]
37. Mieszkowski, J.; Stankiewicz, B.; Kochanowicz, A.; Niespodziński, B.; Kowalik, T.; Żmijewski, M.; Kowalski, K.; Rola, R.; Bieńkowski, T.; Antosiewicz, J. Ultra-Marathon-Induced Increase in Serum Levels of Vitamin D Metabolites: A Double-Blind Randomized Controlled Trial. *Nutrients* **2020**, *12*, 3629. [CrossRef]

2

Evaluation of Vitamin D Metabolism in Patients with Type 1 Diabetes Mellitus in the Setting of Cholecalciferol Treatment

Alexandra Povaliaeva *, Ekaterina Pigarova, Artem Zhukov, Viktor Bogdanov, Larisa Dzeranova, Olga Mel'nikova, Elena Pekareva, Natalya Malysheva, Vitaliy Ioutsi, Larisa Nikankina and Liudmila Rozhinskaya *

Endocrinology Research Centre, 117036 Moscow, Russia; pigarova.ekaterina@endocrincentr.ru (E.P.); jukov.artem@endocrincentr.ru (A.Z.); bogdanov.viktor@endocrincentr.ru (V.B.); dzeranova.larisa@endocrincentr.ru (L.D.); melnikova.olga@endocrincentr.ru (O.M.); pekareva.elena@endocrincentr.ru (E.P.); malysheva.natalya@endocrincentr.ru (N.M.); ioutsi.vitalij@endocrincentr.ru (V.I.); nikankina.larisa@endocrincentr.ru (L.N.)

* Correspondence: povalyaeva.alexandra@endocrincentr.ru (A.P.); rozhinskaya.ludmila@endocrincentr.ru (L.R.)

Abstract: In this prospective controlled study, we examined 25 adults with adequately controlled (HbA1c level < 8.0%) type 1 diabetes mellitus (T1DM) and 49 conditionally healthy adults, intending to reveal the diversity of vitamin D metabolism in the setting of cholecalciferol intake at a therapeutic dose. All patients received a single dose (150,000 IU) of cholecalciferol aqueous solution orally. Laboratory assessments including serum vitamin D metabolites (25(OH)D_3, 25(OH)$D^{2\prime}$ 1,25(OH)$_2$$D_3$, 3-epi-25(OH)$D_3$ and 24,25(OH)$_2$$D_3$), free 25(OH)D, vitamin D-binding protein (DBP) and parathyroid hormone (PTH) as well as serum and urine biochemical parameters were performed before the intake and on Days 1, 3 and 7 after the administration. The studied groups had no significant differences in baseline parameters except that the patients with diabetes showed higher baseline levels of free 25(OH)D ($p < 0.05$). They also lacked a correlation between the measured and calculated free 25(OH)D in contrast to the patients from the control group (r = 0.41, $p > 0.05$ vs. r = 0.88, $p < 0.05$), possibly due to the glycosylation of binding proteins, which affects the affinity constant for 25(OH)D. The elevation of vitamin D levels after the administration of cholecalciferol was comparable in both groups, with slightly higher 25(OH)D_3 levels observed in the diabetes group throughout the study since Day 1 ($p < 0.05$). Overall, our data indicate that in patients with adequately controlled T1DM 25(OH)D_3 levels and the therapeutic response to cholecalciferol is similar to that in healthy individuals.

Keywords: vitamin D; type 1 diabetes mellitus; cholecalciferol; vitamin D-binding protein

1. Introduction

Sources of vitamin D for humans include exposure to sunlight, food and supplements. Vitamin D_3 (cholecalciferol) is produced in the skin as a result of exposure to UV radiation. Plant food and some supplements may contain vitamin D in the form of vitamin D_2 (ergocalciferol). Both of these forms (vitamin D_3 and D_2) are conjunctively referred to as vitamin D. In order to gain biological activity, vitamin D further undergoes two stages of hydroxylation: the first one in the C25 position, which takes place in the liver with the formation of 25-hydroxyvitamin D (25(OH)D), and the next in the C1α position. The compound 25(OH)D is universally accepted as the main marker of vitamin D status [1]. The kidneys are the main source of the circulating active form of vitamin D—1,25-dihydroxyvitamin D

(1,25(OH)$_2$D). Since the discovery of the extrarenal expression of 1α-hydroxylase, the extraskeletal effects of vitamin D due to the local synthesis of the active metabolite have been extensively studied [2,3]. The 24-hydroxylated metabolites of vitamin D are considered as lacking significant physiological roles. The 3-epimer of 25(OH)D is produced by 3-epimerase and is relatively inactive compared with 25(OH)D; however, 3-epi-25(OH)D may be as potent as 1,25(OH)$_2$D for parathyroid hormone (PTH) suppression, but there are fewer data on any other biological effects [4].

Vitamin D-binding protein (DBP) is the main transport protein for all vitamin D metabolites: under normal conditions, about 85% of the circulating metabolites are DBP-bound, while albumin binds almost 15% of the remaining metabolites. Less than 1% of the metabolites are found in the bloodstream in the unbound, or free, state [5]. Over the past 10 years, the "free hormone" hypothesis has been actively discussed, which suggests that it is unbound 25(OH)D that exerts many of the nonclassical effects of vitamin D [6].

Data indicating lower 25(OH)D levels in type 1 diabetes mellitus (T1DM) patients comes predominantly from case-control cross-sectional studies [7–9] and does not clarify a causal relationship. In this regard, both experimental and clinical prospective studies on the use of vitamin D supplements in T1DM are aimed exclusively at the investigation of the effect of this therapy on the course of the disease [10–20].

The loss of DBP-bound vitamin D in the presence of albuminuria could account for the lower levels of vitamin D in these patients. This is supported by the data of large cross-sectional analyses (NHANES III and NHANES 2001–2006), which showed an association of vitamin D deficiency with an increased rate of albumin excretion and the presence of albuminuria, respectively [21,22]. Urinary DBP levels [23] and vitamin D metabolites (25(OH)D and 1,25(OH)$_2$D) [24,25] were higher in individuals with T1DM compared to controls and showed a positive correlation with the duration of diabetes and severity of albuminuria.

The first studies, which were conducted to investigate disorders of vitamin D metabolism in the state of T1DM in the 1980s, proposed that insulin might have a stimulatory effect on enzymes involved in vitamin D metabolism, mostly 25- and 1α-hydroxylase. Hence, insulin deficiency could possibly reduce the activity of these enzymes, leading to decreased levels of some of the vitamin D metabolites [26–28]. This hypothesis was supported by more recent studies [29,30]. However, no prospective controlled studies in humans evaluating a broad spectrum of vitamin D metabolites and related biochemical parameters have been performed to date. Revealing the peculiarities of vitamin D metabolism in T1DM is of importance since it could contribute to the more effective compensation of vitamin D deficiency and, possibly, to the control of the underlying disease in these patients, as shown in several intervention studies [31–34].

The purpose of this study was to reveal distinctive features of cholecalciferol treatment in patients with adequately controlled T1DM compared to conventionally healthy individuals by the dynamic evaluation of serum vitamin D metabolites, free 25(OH)D, transport proteins, and other associated serum and urine biochemical parameters.

2. Materials and Methods

2.1. Study Population and Design

The study group included 25 adult patients with T1DM, and the control group included 49 conditionally healthy adult individuals. The inclusion criteria were an age from 18 to 60 and HbA1c level < 8.0% for the T1DM group. The exclusion criteria were vitamin D supplementation for 3 months prior to the study; severe obesity (a body mass index >35 kg/m^2); pregnancy; the presence of granulomatous disease, malabsorption syndrome, or liver failure; a decreased (less than 60 mL/min per 1.73 m^2); hypercalcemia; allergic reactions to vitamin D medications; and a 25(OH)D level more than 60 ng/mL (determined by immunochemiluminescence analysis). A few patients received therapy that is presumably associated with alterations in vitamin D metabolism within the 3 months preceding the study: antifungal drugs (4 people), oral contraceptives (7 people), anxiolytics (2 people) and antidepressants (3 people). All patients were recruited in the period from July 2019 to September 2020. The study was approved by the Ethics Committee of the Endocrinology Research Centre, Moscow, Russia, on 10 April 2019 (abstract of record No. 6); all patients provided signed informed consent to participate in the study.

All patients received 150,000 IU of an aqueous solution of cholecalciferol (Aquadetrim®, Medana Pharma S.A., Sieradz, Poland) orally as a single dose. We obtained blood and urine samples before the intake as well as on Days 1, 3 and 7 after administration. The assessment included serum biochemical parameters (total calcium, albumin, phosphorus, creatinine and magnesium), PTH, DBP, vitamin D metabolites (25(OH)D_3, 25(OH)D_2, 1,25$(OH)_2D_3$, 3-epi-25(OH)D_3 and 24,25$(OH)_2D_3$), free 25(OH)D and urine biochemical parameters (calcium–creatinine and phosphorus–creatinine ratios in spot urine).

2.2. *Sociodemographic and Anthropometric Data Collection*

At the baseline visit, patients completed a questionnaire aimed at assessing their lifestyles: the presence of unhealthy habits, the physical activity level, a balanced diet (the consumption of dairy products, meat, coffee and soft drinks) and exposure to solar radiation (traveling south and the number of daytime walks in sunny weather in the 3 months preceding study participation). Smoking status was classified as current smoker, former smoker and non-smoker; current and former smokers were collectively referred to as total smokers. A unit of alcohol was defined as a glass of wine, a bottle of beer or a shot of spirits, approximating 10–12 g of ethanol. A serving of dairy products was defined as 100 g of cottage cheese, 200 mL of milk, 125 g of yogurt or 30 g of cheese. Patients' weights were measured in light indoor clothing with a medical scale to the nearest 100 g, and their heights, with a wall-mounted stadiometer to the nearest centimeter. Body mass index was calculated as weight in kilograms divided by height in meters squared.

2.3. *Laboratory Measurements*

HbA1c levels (reference range, 4.0–6.0%) were measured by high-performance liquid chromatography using an automatic analyzer D10 (BioRad Laboratories, Hercules, CA, USA) and kits from the same manufacturer according to the standard method (certified according to the National Glycohemoglobin Standardization Program).

The total 25(OH)D levels (25(OH)D_2 +25(OH)D_3) at the baseline visit were determined by immunochemiluminescence analysis (Liaison, DiaSorin, Saluggia, Italy). PTH levels were evaluated by an electrochemiluminescence immunoassay (ELECSYS, Roche, Basel, Switzerland). Biochemical parameters of the blood serum and urine were assessed using an ARCHITECT c8000 analyzer (Abbott, Chicago, IL, USA) using reagents from the same manufacturer according to standard methods. Serum DBP and free 25(OH)D levels were measured by enzyme-linked immunosorbent assay (ELISA) using commercial kits. The assay used for free 25(OH)D level assessment (DIAsource, ImmunoAssays S.A., Louvain-la-Neuve, Belgium) has <6.2% intra- and inter-assay coefficients of variation (CVs) at levels of 5.8–9.6 pg/mL. The assay used for DBP level assessment (Assaypro, St. Charles, MO, USA) has a 4.0% average intra-assay CV and 9.2% average inter-assay CV.

The levels of vitamin D metabolites (25(OH)D_3, 25(OH)D_2, 1,25(OH)2D_3, 3-epi-25(OH)D_3 and 24,25$(OH)_2D_3$) in the serum were determined by ultra-high-performance liquid chromatography in combination with tandem mass spectrometry (UPLC-MS/MS) using an in-house-developed method broadly based on the ones published earlier by other research groups [35,36]. A detailed description of the experimental procedure is provided in the Supporting Information (SI). With this technique, the laboratory participates in DEQAS quality assurance program (lab code 2388), and the results fall within the target range for the analysis of 25(OH)D and 1,25$(OH)_2D$ metabolites in human serum (SI, Figures S1 and S2). All the UPLC-MS/MS measurements were performed after the first successful completion (5/5 samples within the target range) of the DEQAS distributions for both analytes simultaneously. Each batch contained control samples (analytes in blank serum) with both high and low analyte concentrations. The samples were barcoded and randomized prior to the measurements to eliminate analyst-related errors.

The serum samples (3 aliquots) collected at each visit were either transferred directly to the laboratory for biochemical analyses and total 25(OH)D and PTH measurement (1 aliquot) or were stored at − 80 °C, avoiding repeated freeze–thaw cycles, for the measurement of DBP, free 25(OH)D and vitamin D metabolites (2 aliquots).

Baseline free 25(OH)D levels were also calculated using the formula introduced by Bikle et al. [37,38] and repeatedly used in the work of various authors [39,40]. The affinity constant for 25(OH)D and albumin binding (Kalb) used for the calculation was equal to 6×10^5 M^{-1}, and the affinity constant for 25(OH)D and DBP binding (KDBP) was equal to 7×10^8 M^{-1}.

$$\text{Free 25(OH)D} = \frac{\text{total 25(OH)D}}{1 + \text{Kalb} * \text{albumin} + \text{KDBP} * \text{DBP}}$$

2.4. Statistical Analysis

Statistical analysis was performed using Statistica version 10.0 (StatSoft, Tulsa, OK, USA). All data were analyzed with non-parametric statistics and are expressed as median (interquartile range) unless otherwise specified. The Mann–Whitney U-test and Fisher's exact test were used for comparisons between two groups. Friedman ANOVA was performed to evaluate changes in indices throughout the study, and pairwise comparisons using the Wilcoxon test with adjustment for multiple comparisons (Bonferroni) were also conducted if the Friedman ANOVA was significant. The Spearman rank correlation method was used to obtain coefficients of correlation among indices. A *p*-value of less than 0.05 was considered statistically significant.

3. Results

The ages, sex ratios, body mass indices and total 25(OH)D levels determined by immunochemiluminescent analysis were equal between the groups (Table 1).

Table 1. General characteristics of the patients at the baseline visit. For a detailed description of the data format, please refer to Section 2.

	Diabetes Group ($n = 25$)	Control Group ($n = 49$)	p
Age, years	26.5 (22.7; 36.2)	26.3 (25; 33.5)	0.3
Sex (female, %)	84	80	0.76
Body mass index, kg/m^2	21.9 (20.7; 25.2)	22.2 (20.1; 26.1)	0.94
25(OH)D total, ng/mL	21.3 (15.9; 29.9)	18.4 (13.3; 25.2)	0.21

The features of the underlying disease course in the diabetes group are described in Table 2. The median duration of the disease in the diabetes group was 17 years (11; 19). The majority of the patients had intensive glycemic control at the time of participation in the study (median HbA1c level, 7.1% (6.5; 7.6)). All patients received therapy with insulin analogs: about 3/4 of patients received insulin pump therapy, whereas the rest were treated with a basal-bolus insulin regimen. Only two patients (8%) had moderately increased albuminuria, which corresponded to the A2 category; 40% of the patients had nonproliferative diabetic retinopathy, and about 2/3 of the patients had diabetic peripheral neuropathy.

Table 2. Characteristics of the patients with type 1 diabetes mellitus (T1DM) in terms of the underlying disease.

Parameter	Value
Median duration of T1DM, years	17 (11; 19)
HbA1c, %	7.1 (6.5; 7.6)
Treatment regimen	
Insulin pump (%)	76
Basal-bolus regimen (%)	24
Presence of diabetic complications	
Albuminuria (%)	8
Retinopathy (%)	40
Neuropathy (%)	68

The groups did not differ significantly in the reported levels of physical activity, the amounts of alcohol consumed and dietary habits (Table 3). There was a significantly higher total number of smokers in the control group (39% vs. 12%, $p = 0.03$), while the number of current smokers was comparable between the groups (22% vs. 8%, $p = 0.2$). The number of travelers to the south during the 3 months preceding the study also did not differ significantly (20% in the diabetes group vs. 16% in the control group, $p = 1.0$); however, the individuals in the diabetes group reported more walks in the daytime on a sunny day (9.5 (5; 30) vs. 5 (1; 10), $p = 0.04$).

Table 3. Questionnaire results.

	Diabetes Group	Control Group	*p*
Current smokers (%)	8	22	0.2
Total smokers (%)	12	39	0.03
Alcohol units, per week	1 (0; 2.5)	1 (0; 2)	0.2
Exercises lasting more than 30 min, per week	3 (2; 5.5)	3 (1.5; 5)	0.44
Dairy product consumption, servings per day	1.5 (1; 2)	1 (0.5; 2)	0.06
Meat dish consumption, portions per week	5 (2; 7)	4.5 (3; 6.5)	0.34
Coffee consumption, cups per week	7 (1; 8)	4.5 (2; 8)	0.61
Soft drinks, mL per week	0 (0; 300)	0 (0; 100)	0.3
Travelers to the south, %	20	16	1.0
Daytime walks in sunny weather, *n*	9.5 (5; 30)	5 (1; 10)	0.04

3.1. Baseline Laboratory Evaluation

The detailed results of the laboratory studies are presented in Tables 4 and 5.

Table 4. Changes in the levels of the biochemical parameters and parathyroid hormone (PTH) during the study.

Laboratory Parameter	Group	Day 0	Day 1	Day 3	Day 7	*p* (Friedman ANOVA)	*p* (Day 0–1)	*p* (Day 1–3)	*p* (Day 3–7)	Reference Range
Total calcium, mmol/L	Diabetes	2.37 (2.33; 2.46)	2.38 (2.33; 2.43)	2.41 (2.36; 2.48)	2.37 (2.31; 2.44)	0.53	-	-	-	2.15–2.55
	Control	2.38 (2.33; 2.45)	2.42 (2.36; 2.45)	2.40 (2.36; 2.46)	2.38 (2.36; 2.45)	0.17	-	-	-	
Albumin-adjusted calcium, mmol/L	Diabetes	2.28 (2.25; 2.32)	2.29 (2.24; 2.32)	2.32 (2.26; 2.36)	2.30 (2.24; 2.35)	0.25	-	-	-	2.15–2.55
	Control	2.26 (2.21; 2.31)	2.29 (2.25; 2.34)	2.30 (2.25; 2.35)	2.28 (2.25; 2.33)	0.007	0.003	0.49	0.17	
Phosphorus, mmol/L	Diabetes	1.19 (1.06; 1.32)	1.23 (1.14; 1.33)	1.27 (1.15; 1.43)	1.17 (1.05; 1.30)	0.001	0.22	0.2	0.001	0.74–1.52
	Control	1.15 (1.06; 1.23)	1.22 (1.10; 1.31)	1.23 (1.18; 1.35)	1.20 (1.12; 1.32)	0.002	0.006	0.21	0.05	
PTH, pg/mL	Diabetes	30.2 (23.5; 37.8)	32.1 (22.2; 38.6)	22.5 (20.9; 26.0) *	25.7 (20.1; 32.4)	0.0003	0.98	0.001	0.49	15–65
	Control	35.9 (28.6; 47.2)	34.3 (23.6; 46.7)	30.5 (21.8; 41.5)	28.6 (22.5; 39.2)	0.002	0.15	0.11	0.55	
Creatinine, µmol/L	Diabetes	71.0 (67.5; 80.2)	71.5 (66.8; 77.9)	73.8 (68.7; 76.6)	74.4 (66.6; 86.1)	0.86	-	-	-	Not applicable
	Control	70.0 (65.9; 74.1)	71.1 (65.7; 74.8)	69.6 (65.7; 73.2)	70.4 (65.5; 75.5)	0.25	-	-	-	
Albumin, g/L	Diabetes	45 (43; 47)	45 (43; 46)	45 (43; 47)	44 (42; 46)	0.65	-	-	-	35–50
	Control	46 (45; 48)	45 (44; 47)	45 (44; 47)	45 (44; 47)	0.66	-	-	-	
Magnesium, mmol/L	Diabetes	0.77 (0.74; 0.81)	0.78 (0.75; 0.83)	0.76 (0.72; 0.80)	0.79 (0.73; 0.82)	0.05	-	-	-	0.7–1.05
	Control	0.80 (0.77; 0.82)	0.79 (0.76; 0.84)	0.79 (0.75; 0.82)	0.79 (0.74; 0.84)	0.23	-	-	-	
Calcium–creatinine ratio, mmol/mmol	Diabetes	0.18 (0.14; 0.28)	0.25 (0.15; 0.31)	0.34 (0.18; 0.46)	0.29 (0.17; 0.46)	0.1	-	-	-	0.1–0.8
	Control	0.28 (0.13; 0.42)	0.31 (0.18; 0.44)	0.31 (0.19; 0.41)	0.30 (0.14; 0.46)	0.79	-	-	-	
Phosphorus–creatinine ratio, mmol/mmol	Diabetes	2.3 (1.8; 3.2)	2.3 (1.7; 3.2)	2.5 (1.9; 3.4) *	2.9 (2.1; 3.4) *	0.19	-	-	-	1.4–3.5
	Control	2.1 (1.3; 2.8)	2.2 (1.0; 2.6)	2.1 (1.4; 2.7)	2.0 (1.2; 2.6)	0.32	-	-	-	

* Significant difference in between-group comparison.

Table 5. Changes in the levels of free 25(OH)D, vitamin D-binding protein (DBP) and vitamin D metabolites during the study.

Laboratory Parameter	Group	Day 0	Day 1	Day 3	Day 7	*p* (Friedman ANOVA)	*p* (Day 0–1)	*p* (Day 1–3)	*p* (Day 3–7)	Reference Range
Free 25(OH)D, pg/mL	Diabetes	8.4 (6.9; 11.3) *	10.7 (8.2; 13.8)	14.1 (9.9; 15.9)	13.3 (10.6; 16.3)	0.02	0.09	0.02	0.72	2.4–35 [1]
	Control	5.9 (4.0; 7.5)	11.2 (8.3; 14.4)	14.0 (10.3; 17)	13.0 (10.0; 15.8)	<0.00001	<0.00001	<0.00001	0.003	
DBP, mg/L	Diabetes	280 (252; 308)	276 (232; 376)	261 (219; 311)	265 (214; 343)	0.03	0.19	0.03	0.65	176–623 [1]
	Control	255 (212; 289)	300 (246; 338)	259 (218; 287)	275 (240; 313)	0.001	0.001	0.007	0.04	
$25(OH)D_3$, ng/mL	Diabetes	22.3 (18.6; 28.1)	35.9 (29; 41.8) *	41.9 (33.4; 46.7) *	41.4 (35.0; 46.3) *	<0.00001	0.00001	0.00004	0.69	>30 [2]
	Control	20.5 (14.8; 24.6)	31.0 (26.8; 34.4)	34.5 (31.8; 43.1)	36.4 (32.8; 43.1)	<0.00001	<0.000001	<0.000001	0.004	
3-epi-$25(OH)D_3$, ng/mL	Diabetes	1.6 (1.3; 2.1)	3.7 (3.0; 4.5) *	4.9 (4.4; 5.8)	4.4 (3.8; 5.1)	<0.00001	0.00001	0.00003	0.00006	Not available
	Control	1.4 (0.9; 1.8)	3.0 (2.5; 3.9)	4.6 (3.9; 5.6)	4.3 (3.4; 5.2)	<0.00001	<0.000001	<0.000001	0.00003	
$1,25(OH)_2D_3$, pg/mL	Diabetes	35 (32; 41)	43 (38; 49)	42 (35; 53)	44 (39; 54)	0.001	0.002	0.33	0.15	25–66 [3]
	Control	39 (34; 45)	48 (39; 53)	46 (40; 53)	43 (38; 51)	0.001	<0.00001	0.98	0.28	
$24,25(OH)_2D_3$, ng/mL	Diabetes	1.8 (1.4; 3.0)	2.2 (1.6; 3.3)	3.3 (2.2; 4.5)	3.8 (2.6; 4.9)	<0.00001	0.00009	0.00002	0.00005	0.5–5.6 [3]
	Control	1.7 (0.9; 2.6)	1.9 (1.3; 2.7)	3.0 (2.1; 3.7)	3.5 (2.7; 4.6)	<0.00001	<0.000001	<0.000001	<0.000001	
$25(OH)D_3/24,25(OH)_2D_3$	Diabetes	12.5 (10.1; 16.0)	16.8 (13.3; 21.9)	11.7 (11.2; 16.0)	10.8 (9.8; 13.8)	<0.00001	0.00001	0.0002	0.00002	7–23 [3]
	Control	11.9 (9.6; 15.2)	17.0 (12.1; 20.5)	12.3 (10.1; 14.5)	10.4 (8.5; 12.3)	<0.00001	<0.000001	<0.000001	<0.000001	

* Significant difference in between-group comparison. [1] Reference ranges are specified according to kit manufacturers' recommendations. [2] Reference range is given for total 25(OH)D according to the clinical guidelines [1,41]; the $25(OH)D_2$ fraction is negligible (<0.5 ng/mL in absolute values) for the purposes of this study. [3] Reference ranges are given according to the literature data [42,43].

The studied groups had no significant differences in the baseline biochemical parameters of the blood and urine, PTH (Table 4), DBP and vitamin D metabolites (25(OH)D_3, 25(OH)D_2, 1,25$(OH)_2D_3$, 3-epi-25(OH)D_3 and 24,25$(OH)_2D_3$) (Table 5). The median 25(OH)D_3 levels were similar in both groups (22.3 (18.6; 28.1) ng/mL in the diabetes group vs. 20.5 (14.8; 24.6) ng/mL in the control group, $p = 0.12$) and corresponded to vitamin D insufficiency according to Endocrine Society and Russian Association of Endocrinologists guidelines [1,41]. Only five patients (20%) from the diabetes group and three patients (6%) from the control group had sufficient 25(OH)D_3 levels (more than 30 ng/mL); the proportions of people with sufficient 25(OH)D_3 levels did not differ significantly between the groups ($p = 0.11$). Four patients (8%) from the control group were diagnosed with secondary hyperparathyroidism; all participants in the diabetes group had PTH values within the reference interval.

The patients with diabetes showed significantly higher baseline levels of measured free 25(OH)D (8.4 (6.9; 11.3) vs. 5.9 (4.0; 7.5) pg/mL, $p = 0.0002$). The calculated free 25(OH)D levels had a prominent positive correlation with the measured free 25(OH)D levels in the control group ($r = 0.88$, $p < 0.05$), while in the diabetes group, there was only a tendency towards a moderate positive correlation, which did not reach statistical significance ($r = 0.41$, $p > 0.05$) (Figure 1). The measured free 25(OH)D correlated markedly with 25(OH)D_3 ($r = 0.92$, $p < 0.05$) and serum albumin ($r = -0.4$, $p < 0.05$) in the control group; in the diabetes group, there was no such relationship ($r = 0.42$ and 0, respectively, $p > 0.05$). A correlation between the baseline levels of free 25(OH)D and DBP was not observed in either group (Figure 2).

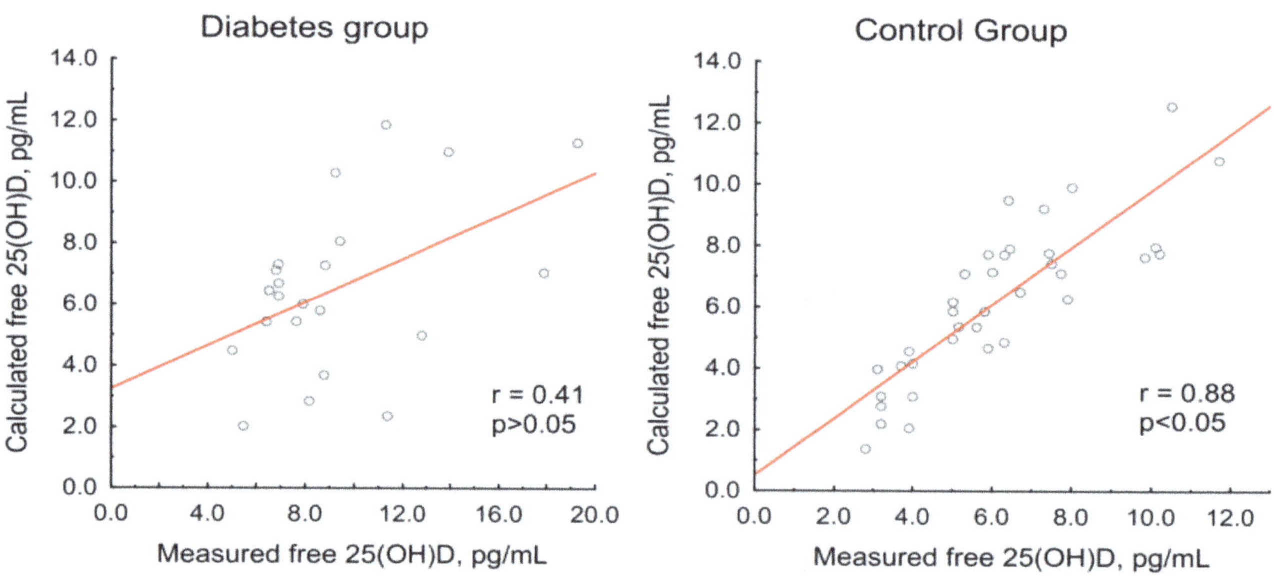

Figure 1. Relationship between measured and calculated free 25(OH)D in groups.

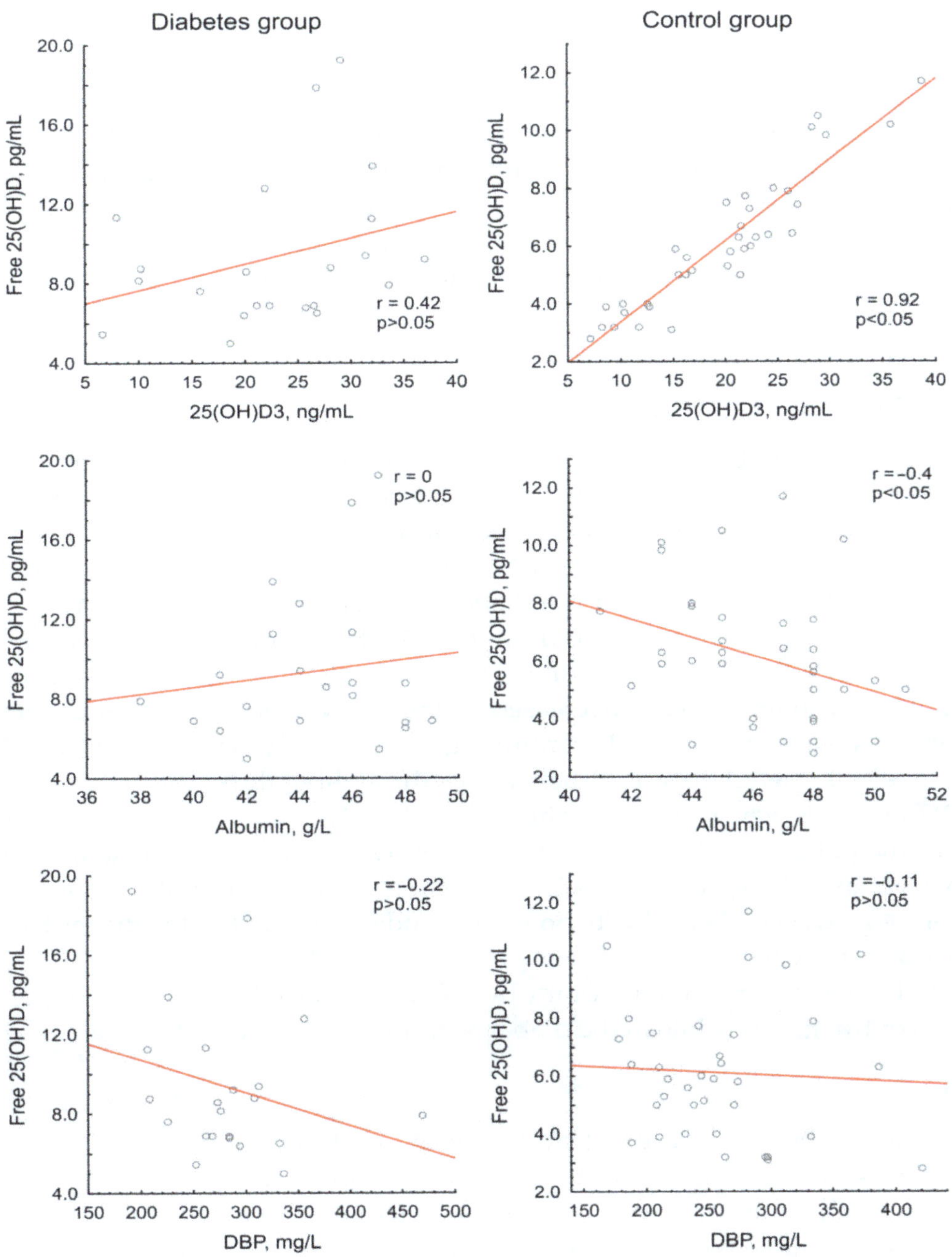

Figure 2. Interrelation of free 25(OH)D and 25(OH)D_3, transport proteins in groups.

When analyzing within the diabetes group, no differences were found between the studied parameters depending on the method of therapy received (pump or basal-bolus insulin therapy).

3.2. Laboratory Evaluation after Intake of Cholecalciferol

3.2.1. Biochemical Parameters, PTH and DBP

We observed a significant decrease in PTH levels from Day 1 to Day 3, as well as phosphorus levels from Day 3 to Day 7, in the patients with diabetes after they took the drug. A higher phosphorus–creatinine ratio was observed in the diabetes group on Days 3 and 7 compared with the control group.

In the control group, the albumin-corrected calcium and phosphorus levels increased by Day 1, as well as DBP levels, following which DBP decreased to its original values by Day 3. There was also a tendency towards a decrease in PTH by Day 7, of borderline statistical significance ($p = 0.008$). The degree of PTH decrease by Day 7 did not differ between the groups (−4.6 pg/mL in the diabetes group vs. −4.3 pg/mL in the control group, $p = 0.99$).

Only one out of the four patients with secondary hyperparathyroidism had their PTH level normalized by Day 7, which was associated with the normalization of the 25(OH)D_3 level (39.4 ng/mL on Day 7 vs. 7.1 ng/mL on Day 0). In two patients, an increase in PTH persisted, despite the achieved level of 25(OH)D_3 being above 30 ng/mL, and in one patient, the received cholecalciferol did not allow reaching the optimal level of vitamin D during the observation period.

One patient from the diabetes group had a transient increase in albumin-corrected calcium to 2.91 mmol/L on Day 1 after taking the drug; in all the other patients, the calcium levels did not exceed the reference range at any point of the study.

3.2.2. Vitamin D Metabolites and Free 25(OH)D

The changes in vitamin D metabolites were generally similar between the groups. The levels of 1,25$(OH)_2D_3$ increased by Day 1, after which they remained stable in both groups throughout the study. As for the other metabolites, we observed an increase in 25(OH)D_3, 3-epi-25(OH)D_3 and 24,25$(OH)_2D_3$ levels as well as in the 25(OH)D_3/24,25$(OH)_2D_3$ ratio by Day 1 in both groups (significantly higher levels of 3-epi-25(OH)D_3 were noted in the diabetes group on Day 1). By Day 3, the metabolite levels continued to increase, while the 25(OH)D_3/24,25$(OH)_2D_3$ ratio started decreasing. By Day 7, in both groups, the 24,25$(OH)_2D_3$ levels continued to increase, 3-epi-25(OH)D_3 levels started decreasing, and the 25(OH)D_3/24,25$(OH)_2D_3$ ratio decreased further. However, the level of 25(OH)D_3 remained stable in the patients with diabetes while continuing to increase in the control group. The 25(OH)D_2 levels did not exceed 0.5 ng/mL in any of the patients throughout the study.

The 25(OH)D_3 levels were significantly higher on Days 1, 3 and 7 in the diabetes group ($p < 0.05$). Overall, 92% of the patients with diabetes and 84% of the patients from the control group reached 25(OH)D_3 levels above 30 ng/mL on Day 7 after taking the drug. In both groups, the increase in 25(OH)D_3 levels negatively correlated with body mass index ($r = -0.41$ in the diabetes group; $r = -0.46$ in the control group; $p < 0.05$).

Free 25(OH)D levels increased significantly by Day 1, continued to increase to Day 3, and decreased by Day 7 in the control group, while in the diabetes group, they remained stable.

4. Discussion

The first major finding of the present study consists of the equivalent baseline 25(OH)D_3 levels between the groups. The patients with diabetes mellitus included in the study had intact kidney function despite a rather long course of the disease (median, 17 years); almost all of them had no albuminuria. Thus, we agree with previous researchers who regarded albuminuria as the principal contributor to the decreased vitamin D levels in patients with diabetes [44,45]. Furthermore, there was little difference in the reported lifestyles between the groups, although the patients with diabetes reported more walking, which may have worked towards a slight improvement in vitamin D status.

The elevation of vitamin D levels with the dose of cholecalciferol used was comparable in both groups, with slightly higher 25(OH)D_3 levels observed in the diabetes group throughout the study since Day 1. Nevertheless, a continuous increase in 25(OH)D_3 throughout the study period was observed in the control group and not in the diabetes group, which may suggest a faster plateau achievement in the diabetes group. The patients with diabetes showed a faster decrease in PTH (as early as Day 3, in contrast to a more gradual decrease throughout the observation period in the control group), which could have been due to higher 3-epi-25(OH)D_3 levels on Day 1 after taking the drug, as well as higher baseline levels of free 25(OH)D.

The second significant finding was that the patients with diabetes had higher baseline free 25(OH)D levels. As far as the authors are aware, to date, there have been no studies evaluating free 25(OH)D levels in patients with type 1 diabetes mellitus. This effect might be explained by a lower affinity of transport proteins for vitamin D metabolites in diabetes mellitus due to the glycosylation process. Our idea is consistent with the literature data on the altered affinity of glycosylated albumin for some ligands (e.g., several drugs [46,47] and zinc [48]). This hypothesis is also supported by the lack of correlation between the measured and calculated free 25(OH)D in the diabetes group in contrast with the control group. On the other hand, there was no correlation between free 25(OH)D levels and HbA1C or the duration of the disease, but it should be noted that most patients were in a relatively compensated state.

In the healthy individuals, a rapid increase in DBP levels was noted after taking cholecalciferol as early as Day 1, followed by a return to baseline values by Day 3. DBP is considered an acute-phase serum protein and increases during infections or minor injuries [49,50]. Given a high dose of cholecalciferol, a corresponding increase in free 25(OH)D levels is expected, so the observed increase in DBP levels is supposedly aimed at preventing vitamin D toxicity. This is supported by the negative correlation of free 25(OH)D and DBP levels on Days 3 and 7 of the study in the individuals from the control group ($r = -0.49$ and $r = -0.4$, $p < 0.05$, respectively). These changes were not observed in the patients with diabetes mellitus: there was no increase in free 25(OH)D or DBP levels, or a correlation between these parameters during the observation period. The foregoing facts could indicate a dysregulation of the mechanism for preventing vitamin D toxicity in patients with diabetes mellitus, and therefore, care should be taken when using high doses of vitamin D in such patients.

Our study had several limitations: the amount of dietary vitamin D and possible differences in DBP affinity to vitamin D metabolites due to genetic isoforms of DBP [51] were not taken into account. The modest sample size should also be noted. A few patients received therapy that might possibly alter vitamin D metabolism (oral contraceptives, antifungal treatments, antidepressants and anxiolytics).

5. Conclusions

Our study indicates that in patients with adequately controlled type 1 diabetes mellitus, in the absence of albuminuria and a corresponding progressive loss of vitamin D metabolites, total 25(OH)D levels and the therapeutic response to cholecalciferol are comparable to those in healthy individuals. The analysis of the vitamin D metabolite levels also suggests that for these patients, insulin deficiency alone does not significantly affect either the regulation of vitamin D metabolism or the activity of the enzymes involved. At the same time, the disturbed balance between the free and protein-bound 25(OH)D fractions observed in the patients with diabetes mellitus suggests that the careful use of high doses of cholecalciferol in the treatment of such patients is necessary. At present, the question remains unresolved regarding the optimal status of vitamin D and the most relevant marker for its assessment, especially under the conditions of various pathological processes. Additional studies are required to determine the constant of the affinity of transport proteins for vitamin D metabolites in diabetes mellitus, as well as the most appropriate marker for assessing the biological functions of vitamin D in this condition.

Author Contributions: Conceptualization, L.R., E.P. (Ekaterina Pigarova), A.P. and A.Z.; methodology, V.B., V.I. and L.N.; formal analysis, A.P. and V.B.; investigation, A.P., A.Z., O.M., E.P. (Elena Pekareva), V.B. and N.M.; resources, A.Z.; data curation, A.P. and V.B.; writing—original draft preparation, L.R.; writing—review and editing, A.P., A.Z., E.P. (Ekaterina Pigarova), L.D. and V.B.; visualization, A.P. and V.B.; supervision, L.D., E.P. (Ekaterina Pigarova) and L.R.; project administration, L.R.; funding acquisition, L.R. All authors have read and agreed to the published version of the manuscript.

References

1. Holick, M.F.; Binkley, N.C.; Bischoff-Ferrari, H.A.; Gordon, C.M.; Hanley, D.A.; Heaney, R.P.; Murad, M.H.; Weaver, C.M. Evaluation, treatment, and prevention of vitamin D deficiency: An Endocrine Society clinical practice guideline. *J. Clin. Endocrinol. Metab.* **2011** *96*, 1911–1930. [CrossRef] [PubMed]

2. Holick, M.F. Vitamin D: Extraskeletal Health. *Endocrinol. Metab. Clin. N. Am.* **2010**, *39*, 381–400. [CrossRef] [PubMed]
3. Rosen, C.J.; Adams, J.S.; Bikle, D.D.; Black, D.M.; Demay, M.B.; Manson, J.A.E.; Murad, M.H.; Kovacs, C.S. The nonskeletal effects of vitamin D: An Endocrine society scientific statement. *Endocr. Rev.* **2012**, *33*, 456–492. [CrossRef] [PubMed]
4. Bikle, D.D. Vitamin D metabolism, mechanism of action, and clinical applications. *Chem. Biol.* **2014**, *21*, 319–329. [CrossRef] [PubMed]
5. Speeckaert, M.; Huang, G.; Delanghe, J.R.; Taes, Y.E.S. Biological and clinical aspects of the vitamin D binding protein (Gc-globulin) and its polymorphism. *Clin. Chim Acta* **2006**, *372*, 33–42. [CrossRef] [PubMed]
6. Chun, R.F.; Peercy, B.E.; Orwoll, E.S.; Nielson, C.M.; Adams, J.S.; Hewison, M. Vitamin D and DBP: The free hormone hypothesis revisited. *J. Steroid Biochem. Mol. Biol.* **2014**, *144*, 132–137. [CrossRef] [PubMed]
7. Feng, R.; Li, Y.; Li, G.; Li, Z.; Zhang, Y.; Li, Q.; Sun, C. Lower serum 25(OH)D concentrations in type 1 diabetes: A meta-analysis. *Diabetes Res. Clin. Pract.* **2015**, *108*, e71–e75. [CrossRef]
8. Liu, C.; Lu, M.; Xia, X.; Wang, J.; Wan, Y.; He, L.; Li, M. Correlation of serum vitamin D level with type 1 diabetes mellitus in children: A meta-analysis. *Nutr. Hosp.* **2015**, *32*, 1591–1594. [CrossRef]
9. Shen, L.; Zhuang, Q.S.; Ji, H.F. Assessment of vitamin D levels in type 1 and type 2 diabetes patients: Results from metaanalysis. *Mol. Nutr. Food Res.* **2016**, *60*, 1059–1067. [CrossRef]
10. Gregoriou, E.; Mamais, I.; Tzanetakou, I.; Lavranos, G.; Chrysostomou, S. The effects of vitamin D supplementation in newly diagnosed type 1 diabetes patients: Systematic review of randomized controlled trials. *Rev. Diabet Stud.* **2017**, *14*, 260–268. [CrossRef]
11. Bogdanou, D.; Penna-Martinez, M.; Filmann, N.; Chung, T.L.; Moran-Auth, Y.; Wehrle, J.; Cappel, C.; Huenecke, S.; Herrmann, E.; Koehl, U.; et al. T-lymphocyte and glycemic status after vitamin D treatment in type 1 diabetes: A randomized controlled trial with sequential crossover. *Diabetes Metab. Res. Rev.* **2017**, *33*, e2865. [CrossRef] [PubMed]
12. Gabbay, M.A.; Sato, M.N.; Finazzo, C.; Duarte, A.J.S.; Dib, S.A. Effect of cholecalciferol as adjunctive therapy with insulin on protective immunologic profile and decline of residual b-cell function in new-onset type 1 diabetes mellitus. *Arch. Pediatr. Adolesc. Med.* **2012**, *166*, 601–607. [CrossRef] [PubMed]
13. Treiber, G.; Prietl, B.; Fröhlich-Reiterer, A.; Lechner, E.; Ribitsch, A.; Fritsch, M.; Rami-Merhar, B.; Steigleder-Schweiger, C.; Graninger, W.; Borkenstein, M.; et al. Cholecalciferol supplementation improves suppressive capacity of regulatory T-cells in young patients with new-onset type 1 diabetes mellitus—A randomized clinical trial. *Clin. Immunol.* **2015**, *161*, 217–224. [CrossRef] [PubMed]
14. Shih, E.M.; Mittelman, S.; Pitukcheewanont, P.; Azen, C.G.; Monzavi, R. Effects of vitamin D repletion on glycemic control and inflammatory cytokines in adolescents with type 1 diabetes. *Pediatr. Diabetes* **2016**, *17*, 36–43. [CrossRef]
15. Haller, M.J.; Wasserfall, C.H.; Hulme, M.A.; Cintron, M.; Brusko, T.M.; McGrail, K.M.; Wingard, J.R.; Theriaque, D.W.; Shuster, J.J.; Ferguson, R.J.; et al. Autologous Umbilical Cord Blood Infusion followed by Oral Docosahexaenoic Acid and Vitamin D Supplementation for C-Peptide Preservation in Children with Type 1 Diabetes. *Biol. Blood Marrow Transplant.* **2013**, *19*, 1126–1129. [CrossRef]
16. Walter, M.; Kaupper, T.; Adler, K.; Foersch, J.; Bonifacio, E.; Ziegler, A.E. No effect of the 1α,25-dihydroxyvitamin D3on β-cell residual function and insulin requirement in adults with new-onset type 1 diabetes. *Diabetes Care* **2010**, *33*, 1443–1448. [CrossRef]
17. Bizzarri, C.; Pitocco, D.; Napoli, N.; Di Stasio, E.; Maggi, D.; Manfrini, S.; Suraci, C.; Cavallo, M.G.; Cappa, M.; Ghirlanda, G.; et al. No protective effect of calcitriol on β-cell function in recent-onset type 1 diabetes: The IMDIAB XIII trial. *Diabetes Care* **2010**, *33*, 1962–1963. [CrossRef]
18. Pitocco, D.; Crinò, A.; Di Stasio, E.; Manfrini, S.; Guglielmi, C.; Spera, S.; Anguissola, G.B.; Visalli, N.; Suraci, C.; Matteoli, M.C.; et al. The effects of calcitriol and nicotinamide on residual pancreatic β-cell function in patients with recent-onset Type 1 diabetes (IMDIAB XI). *Diabet. Med.* **2006**, *23*, 920–923. [CrossRef]
19. Li, X.; Liao, L.; Yan, X.; Huang, G.; Lin, J.; Lei, M.; Wang, X.; Zhou, Z. Protective effects of 1- α -hydroxyvitamin D3 on residual β -cell function in patients with adult-onset latent autoimmune diabetes (LADA). *Diabetes Metab. Res. Rev.* **2009**, *25*, 411–416. [CrossRef]
20. Ataie-Jafari, A.; Loke, S.C.; Rahmat, A.B.; Larijani, B.; Abbasi, F.; Leow, M.C.S.; Yassin, Z. A randomized placebo-controlled trial of alphacalcidol on the preservation of beta cell function in children with recent onset type 1 diabetes. *Clin. Nutr.* **2013** *32*, 911–917. [CrossRef]

21. De Boer, I.H.; Ioannou, G.N.; Kestenbaum, B.; Brunzell, J.D.; Weiss, N.S. 25-hydroxyvitamin D levels and albuminuria in the Third National Health and Nutrition Examination Survey (NHANES III). *Am. J. Kidney Dis.* **2007**, *50*, 69–77. [CrossRef] [PubMed]
22. Diaz, V.A.; Mainous, A.G., 3rd; Carek, P.J.; Wessell, A.M.; Everett, C.J. The association of vitamin D deficiency and insufficiency with diabetic nephropathy: Implications for health disparities. *J. Am. Board Fam. Med.* **2009**, *22*, 521–527. [CrossRef] [PubMed]
23. Thrailkill, K.M.; Jo, C.H.; Cockrell, G.E.; Moreau, C.S.; Fowlkes, J.L. Enhanced excretion of vitamin D binding protein in type 1 diabetes: A role in vitamin D deficiency? *J. Clin. Endocrinol. Metab.* **2011**, *96*, 142–149. [CrossRef] [PubMed]
24. Fowlkes, J.L.; Bunn, R.C.; Cockrell, G.E.; Clark, L.M.; Wahl, E.C.; Lumpkin, C.K.; Thraikill, K.M. Dysregulation of the intrarenal vitamin D endocytic pathway in a nephropathy-prone mouse model of type 1 diabetes. *Exp. Diabetes Res.* **2011**, *2011*, 269378. [CrossRef]
25. Anderson, R.L.; Ternes, S.B.; Strand, K.A.; Rowling, M.J. Vitamin D homeostasis is compromised due to increased urinary excretion of the 25-hydroxycholecalciferol-vitamin D-binding protein complex in the Zucker diabetic fatty rat. *Am. J. Physiol. Endocrinol. Metab.* **2010**, *299*, E959–E967. [CrossRef]
26. Ikeda, K.; Matsumoto, T.; Morita, K.; Yamato, H.; Takahashi, H.; Ezawa, I.; Ogata, E. The role of insulin in the stimulation of renal 1,25-dihydroxyvitamin D synthesis by parathyroid hormone in rats. *Endocrinology* **1987**, *121*, 1721–1726. [CrossRef]
27. Colette, C.; Pares-Herbute, N.; Monnier, L.; Selam, J.L.; Thomas, N.; Mirouze, J. Effect of different insulin administration modalities on vitamin D metabolism of insulin-dependent diabetic patients. *Horm. Metab. Res.* **1989**, *21*, 37–41. [CrossRef]
28. Frazer, T.E.; White, N.H.; Hough, S.; Santiago, J.V.; McGee, B.R.; Bryce, G.; Mallon, J.; Avioli, L.V. Alterations in circulating vitamin D metabolites in the young insulin-dependent diabetic. *J. Clin. Endocrinol. Metab.* **1981**, *53*, 1154–1159. [CrossRef]
29. Mazanova, A.; Shymanskyi, I.; Lisakovska, O.; Hajiyeva, L.; Komisarenko, Y.; Veliky, M. Effects of Cholecalciferol on Key Components of Vitamin D-Endo/Para/Autocrine System in Experimental Type 1 Diabetes. *Int. J. Endocrinol.* **2018**, *2018*, 2494016:1–2494016:9. [CrossRef]
30. Pozzilli, P.; Manfrini, S.; Crinò, A.; Picardi, A.; Leomanni, C.; Cherubini, V.; Valente, L.; Khazrai, M.; Visalli, N.; IMDIAB Group. Low levels of 25-hydroxyvitamin D3 and 1,25-dihydroxyvitamin D3 in patients with newly diagnosed type 1 diabetes. *Horm. Metab. Res.* **2005**, *37*, 680–683. [CrossRef]
31. Aljabri, K.S.; Bokhari, S.A.; Khan, M.J. Glycemic changes after vitamin D supplementation in patients with type 1 diabetes mellitus and vitamin D deficiency. *Ann. Saudi Med.* **2010**, *30*, 454–458. [CrossRef] [PubMed]
32. Hafez, M.; Hassan, M.; Musa, N.; Atty, S.A.; Azim, S.A. Vitamin D status in Egyptian children with type 1 diabetes and the role of vitamin D replacement in glycemic control. *J. Pediatr. Endocrinol. Metab.* **2017**, *30*, 389–394. [CrossRef] [PubMed]
33. Panjiyar, R.P.; Dayal, D.; Attri, S.V.; Sachdeva, N.; Sharma, R.; Bhalla, A.K. Sustained serum 25-hydroxyvitamin D concentrations for one year with cholecalciferol supplementation improves glycaemic control and slows the decline of residual beta cell function in children with type 1 diabetes. *Pediatr. Endocrinol. Diabetes Metab.* **2018**, *2018*, 111–117. [CrossRef] [PubMed]
34. Ordooei, M.; Shojaoddiny-Ardekani, A.; Hoseinipoor, S.H.; Miroliai, M.; Zare-Zardini, H. Effect of vitamin D on HbA1c levels of children and adolescents with diabetes mellitus type 1. *Minerva Pediatr.* **2017**, *69*, 391–395. [CrossRef] [PubMed]
35. Wang, Z.; Senn, T.; Kalhorn, T.; Zheng, X.E.; Davis, C.L.; Hebert, M.F.; Lin, Y.S.; Thummel, K.S. Simultaneous measurement of plasma vitamin D3 metabolites, including 4β,25-dihydroxyvitamin D3, using liquid chromatography-tandem mass spectrometry. *Anal. Biochem.* **2011**, *418*, 126–133. [CrossRef] [PubMed]
36. Aronov, P.A.; Hall, L.M.; Dettmer, K.; Stephensen, C.B.; Hammock, B.D. Metabolic profiling of major vitamin D metabolites using Diels-Alder derivatization and ultra-performance liquid chromatography-tandem mass spectrometry. *Anal. Bioanal. Chem.* **2008**, *391*, 1917–1930. [CrossRef]
37. Bikle, D.D.; Siiteri, P.K.; Ryzen, E.; Haddad, J.G. Serum protein binding of 1,25-Dihydroxyvitamin D: A reevaluation by direct measurement of free metabolite levels. *J. Clin. Endocrinol. Metab.* **1985**, *61*, 969–975. [CrossRef]

38. Bikle, D.D.; Gee, E.; Halloran, B.; Kowalski, M.A.; Ryzen, E.; Haddad, J.G. Assessment of the Free Fraction of 25-Hydroxyvitamin D in Serum and Its Regulation by Albumin and the Vitamin D-Binding Protein. *J. Clin. Endocrinol. Metab.* **1986**, *63*, 954–959. [CrossRef]
39. Schwartz, J.B.; Lai, J.; Lizaola, B.; Kane, L.; Markova, S.; Weyland, P.; Terrault, N.A.; Stotland, N.; Bikle, D. A Comparison of Measured and Calculated Free 25(OH)Vitamin D Levels in Clinical Populations. *J. Clin. Endocrinol. Metab.* **2014**, *99*, 1631–1637. [CrossRef]
40. Powe, C.E.; Seely, E.W.; Rana, S.; Bhan, I.; Ecker, J.; Karumanchi, S.A.; Thadhani, R. First Trimester Vitamin D, Vitamin D Binding Protein, and Subsequent Preeclampsia. *Hypertension* **2013**, *56*, 758–763. [CrossRef]
41. Pigarova, E.A.; Rozhinskaya, L.Y.; Belaya, Z.E.; Dzeranova, L.K.; Karonova, T.L.; Ilyin, A.V.; Mel'nichenko, G.A.; Dedov, I.I. Russian Association of Endocrinologists recommendations for diagnosis, treatment and prevention of vitamin D deficiency in adults. *Probl. Endokrinol.* **2016**, *62*, 60–84. [CrossRef]
42. Dirks, N.F.; Martens, F.; Vanderschueren, D.; Billen, J.; Pauwels, S.; Ackermans, M.T.; Endert, E.; den Heijer, M.; Blankenstein, M.A.; Heijboer, A.C. Determination of human reference values for serum total 1,25-dihydroxyvitamin D using an extensively validated 2D ID-UPLC–MS/MS method. *J. Steroid Biochem. Mol. Biol.* **2016**, *164*, 127–133. [CrossRef] [PubMed]
43. Tang, J.C.Y.; Nicholls, H.; Piec, I.; Washbourne, C.J.; Dutton, J.J.; Jackson, S.; Greeves, J.; Fraser, W.D. Reference intervals for serum 24,25-dihydroxyvitamin D and the ratio with 25-hydroxyvitamin D established using a newly developed LC–MS/MS method. *J. Nutr. Biochem.* **2017**, *46*, 21–29. [CrossRef] [PubMed]
44. Storm, T.L.; Sørensen, O.H.; Lund, B.; Lund, B.; Christiansen, J.S.; Andersen, A.R.; Lumholtz, I.B.; Parving, H.H. Vitamin D metabolism in insulin-dependent diabetes mellitus. *Metab. Bone Dis. Relat. Res.* **1983**, *5*, 107–110. [CrossRef]
45. Kim, H.Y.; Lee, Y.A.; Jung, H.W.; Gu, M.J.; Kim, J.Y.; Lee, G.M.; Lee, J.; Yoon, J.Y.; Yang, S.W.; Shin, C.H. A lack of association between vitamin D-binding protein and 25-hydroxyvitamin D concentrations in pediatric type 1 diabetes without microalbuminuria. *Ann. Pediatr. Endocrinol. Metab.* **2017**, *22*, 247–252. [CrossRef] [PubMed]
46. Rondeau, P.; Bourdon, E. The glycation of albumin: Structural and functional impacts. *Biochimie* **2011**, *93*, 645–658. [CrossRef]
47. Soudahome, A.G.; Catan, A.; Giraud, P.; Kouao, S.A.; Guerin-Dubourg, A.; Debussche, X.; Le Moullec, N.; Bourdon, E.; Bravo, S.B.; Paradela-Dobarro, B.; et al. Glycation of human serum albumin impairs binding to the glucagon-like peptide-1 analogue liraglutide. *J. Biol. Chem.* **2018**, *293*, 4778–4791. [CrossRef]
48. Iqbal, S.; Qais, F.A.; Alam, M.; Naseem, I. Effect of glycation on human serum albumin–zinc interaction: A biophysical study. *J. Biol. Inorg. Chem.* **2018**, *23*, 447–458. [CrossRef]
49. Dahl, B.; Schiødt, F.V.; Rudolph, S.; Ott, P.; Kiaer, T.; Heslet, L. Trauma stimulates the synthesis of Gc-globulin. *Intensive Care Med.* **2001**, *27*, 394–399. [CrossRef]
50. Dahl, B.; Schiødt, F.V.; Gehrchen, P.M.; Ramlau, J.; Kiaer, T.; Ott, P. Gc-globulin is an acute phase reactant and an indicator of muscle injury after spinal surgery. *Inflamm. Res.* **2001**, *50*, 39–43. [CrossRef]
51. Arnaud, J.; Constans, J. Affinity differences for vitamin D metabolites associated with the genetic isoforms of the human serum carrier protein (DBP). *Hum. Genet.* **1993**, *92*, 183–188. [CrossRef] [PubMed]

3

The Effects of Vitamin D-Enriched Mushrooms and Vitamin D3 on Cognitive Performance and Mood in Healthy Elderly Adults

Ian T. Zajac [1,*], Mary Barnes [2], Paul Cavuoto [1], Gary Wittert [3,4] and Manny Noakes [1]

1 Commonwealth Scientific and Industrial Research Organisation—Health and Biosecurity, P.O. Box 10041, Adelaide 5000, Australia; cavuotop@gmail.com (P.C.); mannynoakes@icloud.com (M.N.)

2 Centre for Epidemiology and Biostatistics, Flinders University, Adelaide 5001, Australia; mary.barnes@flinders.edu.au

3 Freemasons Foundation Centre for Men's Health, North Terrace, Adelaide 5000, Australia; gary.wittert@adelaide.edu.au

4 Centre for Nutrition and Gastrointestinal Disease, South Australian Health and Medical Research Institute, Adelaide 5000, Australia

* Correspondence: ian.zajac@csiro.au

Abstract: Despite abundant cross-sectional evidence that low vitamin D status is associated with risk of cognitive decline in ageing, interventional evidence for benefits of vitamin D supplementation is lacking. This study was a 6 month randomised, double-blinded placebo-controlled clinical trial of the effects of vitamin D3 (D3), enhanced vitamin D2 in a mushroom matrix (D2M), standard mushroom (SM) and placebo (PL) on cognition and mood in $n = 436$ healthy older male (49%) and female volunteers aged ≥ 60 years. Primary end points were change in serum vitamin D metabolites (25-OH-D, 25-OH-D2 and 25-OH-D3), cognitive performance, and mood over 24 weeks. Levels of total 25-OH-D and 25-OH-D3 were maintained in the D3 arm but decreased significantly ($p < 0.05$) in the remaining arms (D2M, SM and PL). Analysis also revealed differential changes in these metabolites depending on total vitamin D status at baseline. There were no significant effects of treatment on any of the measures of cognitive function or mood. Overall, the results show that daily supplementation of ~600 IU of vitamin D3 was sufficient to maintain 25-OH-D throughout winter months, but in contrast to existing cross-sectional studies there was no support for benefit of vitamin D supplementation for mood or cognition in healthy elderly people.

Keywords: vitamin D; mushroom; cognitive function; mood

1. Introduction

Cognitive decline is observed throughout the ageing process. It is characterised by diminishing capacity in a variety of brain functions [1]. These age related declines in cognitive function are normal [2], even in the absence of underlying pathology [3] and they are most pronounced for tasks relying on information processing speed and executive functions [3,4]. Furthermore, this decline is not unexpected, with research showing that approximately 50% of older adults report concerns about memory function and that, for many, this is a most-dreaded component of ageing [5].

Vitamin D, by direct and indirect regulation of more than 200 genes, exerts bioactivity as a hormone and plays an important role in calcium absorption, tissue and immune cell growth, and inflammation [6]. The importance of vitamin D for brain health is supported by the presence of the enzyme that produces its active form—1α-hydroxylase—in cerebrospinal fluid [7]. Furthermore, the receptor for the active metabolite—1,25-dihydroxy vitamin D3—is found throughout the human brain [8]. Vitamin D has therefore been linked with neuron growth, differentiation and survival by its regulation of factors such as glutathione, growth factors, neurotrophins and neurotransmitters and to buffer calcium in the brain [9].

Humans obtain vitamin D from environmental and dietary sources. Vitamin D3 can be efficiently produced from sunlight (UV-B) exposure to human skin and moderate doses are available from consuming oily fish, egg yolk, meat and fortified foods [6]. However, these dietary sources provide <10% of the daily vitamin D requirement [10]. In comparison, vitamin D2, produced by UV conversion of ergosterol in fungi and plants, particularly mushrooms, represents a new, convenient and accessible source of dietary vitamin D2 [11]. The bioavailability of mushroom vitamin D2 and its capacity to contribute to vitamin D status has been substantiated with doses of 400 IU to 2000 IU/day, taken over 4 weeks to 3 months, producing increases in 25-OH-D2 and overall increases in total 25-OH-D [12–15].

Multiple systematic reviews and meta-analyses comparing cognitively normal with impaired, including Alzheimer Disease groups, have reported positive associations between vitamin D status and cognitive function in older adults [16–21]. For example, a recent meta-analysis of cross-sectional data demonstrated that low vitamin D status predicted executive dysfunctions including impaired mental shifting, information updating and processing speed [22]. However, like cognitive decline and dementia, vitamin D deficiency risk and deficiency per se is also related to ageing. Various age-related risk factors include inadequate dietary intake, inadequate exposure to sunlight, impaired transdermal and intestinal absorption, impaired metabolism in the liver and kidneys and medications that promote catabolism [23]. Therefore, the potential exists that the observed relationship between vitamin D and cognitive function is not causal but rather due to extraneous ageing-related variables.

To date, intervention studies exploring a causal link between vitamin D and cognitive function are lacking. Post-hoc analysis of data from the Women's Health Initiative study explored incidence of probable dementia and mild cognitive disorder in women aged >65 years who were dementia free at baseline, and treated with either placebo or daily doses of calcium (1000 mg of calcium carbonate) plus vitamin D3—400 IU [24]. Results of these analyses indicated no difference in onset of dementia between the treatments. Elsewhere, in relation to mood states, a recent systematic review of effects of vitamin D supplementation on depressive symptoms indicated that a moderate, statistically significant benefit was evident for improving mood but only in those with clinical depression at the outset [25].

This clinical trial sought to evaluate whether vitamin D supplementation delivered either as enhanced vitamin D2 (UV-exposed mushroom, D2M) or D3 (synthetic) is causally related to cognition and mood in a healthy, cognitively asymptomatic, elderly cohort. We hypothesised that consumption of either D2 or D3 treatments would lead to an elevation in vitamin D after 24 weeks compared to standard mushroom (SM) and placebo (PL) controls. Furthermore, we hypothesised that D2 and D3 supplementation would benefit cognitive function and mood after 6 months of intervention. This article reports on the primary outcomes of this trial.

2. Materials and Methods

2.1. Study Design

This was a single-centre, double-blinded, placebo-controlled, 4-armed parallel-group randomised clinical trial. This study (http://www.anzctr.org.au; ACTRN12613000891729) was conducted at the Commonwealth Scientific and Industrial Research Organization (CSIRO) Clinical Nutrition and Health Research Clinic, Adelaide, South Australia from April through to October in both 2014 and again in 2015 (two cohorts). This study was conducted according to the ethical guidelines of the National Health and Medical Research Council of Australia. Approval to undertake this study was obtained from the CSIRO Human Ethics Committee and written informed consent was obtained from all participants. The complete protocol for the current randomised controlled trial has been published previously [26].

2.2. *Participants and Screening*

Community dwelling healthy elderly participants were recruited through a variety of study advertisements including newsletters, volunteer databases and radio. For logistic reasons, participants were recruited in two separate cohorts in 2014 and 2015, respectively. A total of $n = 436$ participants were randomised to trial arms and a consort diagram showing progression through screening and recruitment is provided as Figure 1. Inclusion and exclusion criteria were assessed at screening through a variety of clinical measures including our standard medical questionnaire, the Centre for Epidemiological Studies-Depression Scale (CES-D), the Obstructive Sleep Apnoea 50 questionnaire (OSA−50) [27], and the Mini-Mental State Examination (MMSE) [28].

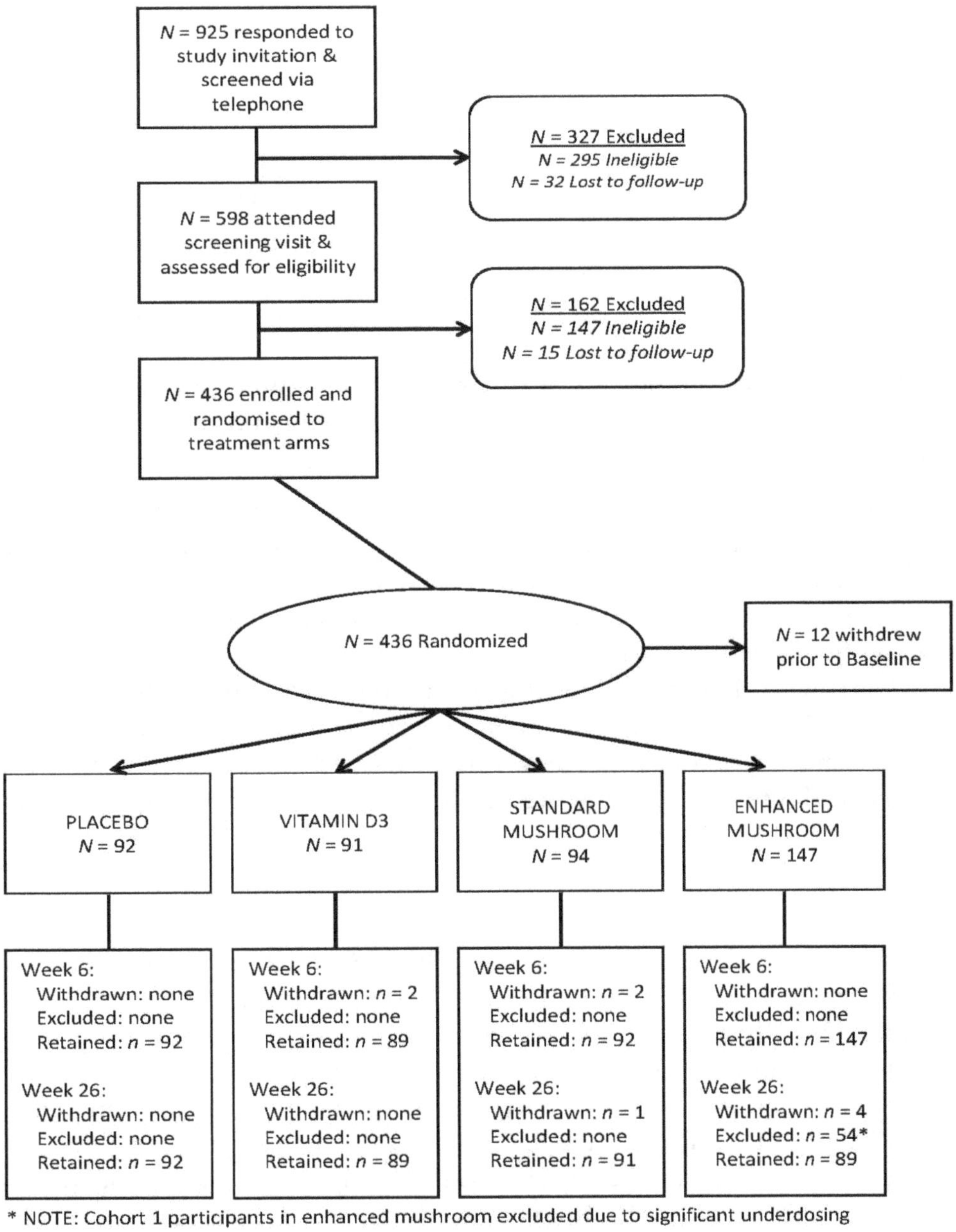

Figure 1. Flow of participants through the trial.

Inclusion criteria were: healthy males and females aged 60–90 years of age; fluent in the English language (for valid completion of the cognitive test battery); not taking any form of vitamin D supplementation for at least three months prior to this study and willing to refrain from additional supplementation during this study.

Exclusion criteria were: inability to swallow tablets; physical inability to attend our research clinic; poor cognitive function (score ≤ 24 on the MMSE); depression (scores ≥ 16 on the CES-D); diagnosis of intellectual disability, dementia, or neurological disorder including but not limited to cerebral vascular disease; previous head injury, stroke, or coronary artery bypass or neurosurgical procedure; history of smoking, alcohol or drug abuse; metabolic disease including diabetes; untreated asthma; shift workers; people who habitually sleep < 6 h per night; untreated but probable obstructive sleep apnoea (OSA−50 responses assessed by study medical doctor); abnormal thyroid function; abnormal vitamin B12 status; history of psychosis and/or taking anti-psychotic medication; or history of epilepsy and/or taking anti-epileptic medication; kidney disease or kidney function impairment, and/or a gastro-intestinal condition that interferes with nutrient absorption; sensitivity to or intolerance for consuming mushrooms. Figure 1 shows participant flow throughout this study.

2.3. Intervention

Participants were randomised by an independent statistician into four treatment groups using a computer-based minimization process to assist with balancing groups for sex and age: (1) vitamin D2-enriched mushroom (D2M); (2) vitamin D3 (D3); (3) standard mushroom (SM); or (4) placebo (PL). The four study arms were stratified with regards to age and gender. Participants attended the CSIRO clinic at 3 time points: baseline, 5 weeks and 24 weeks (~6 months). At each clinic visit, participants completed the cognitive assessment tasks, mood questionnaires and provided blood samples at baseline and end point. Participants were instructed to commence consumption of two capsules daily on the day following their baseline visit. Participants were able to consume the capsules at any time during the day and returned unused capsules at the end of the intervention period as a measure of compliance.

Capsules for all arms were provided to the research clinic in opaque containers marked with an allocation number to ensure blinding of research staff and also participants. The active intervention capsules were intended to provide a total daily dosage of 600 IU of either D2 (D2M) or D3 across two capsules. Mushroom powder for the D2M and SM groups was prepared as described previously [26]. Briefly, this involved freeze drying and grinding mushrooms to ensure suitable moisture (<5%) and water activity (<0.065) levels. In order to boost levels in the D2M arm, batches of mushroom powder were exposed to UV-B light, driving the conversion of ergosterol to vitamin D2, before vacuum sealing and storage at 4 °C, using a treatment process fully described elsewhere [26,29]. All capsules were manufactured with a shelf life of 2 years for storage at 4 °C and single batches of each treatment used for years 1 and 2 of the clinical study.

2.4. Cognition and Mood Measures

Cognitive function was assessed using the CSIRO Cognitive Assessment Battery (C-CAB) (Commonwealth Scientific and Industrial Research Organization, Adelaide, South Australia) as described previously [26]. Briefly, the C-CAB measures performance levels for a range of distinct cognitive abilities including processing speed, reaction time/attention, speed of reasoning, speed of memory scanning, verbal working memory, spatial working memory, recognition memory, and overall quality of memory. Abilities measured in the C-CAB are those considered most susceptible to change and which are commonly included in batteries designed to measure the impact of nutraceuticals on cognitive performance [30,31]. The methods and procedures underpinning the tasks have been used in previous studies conducted by current authors [32,33] and have been fully described previously in the published protocol [26]. Standardised questionnaires were used to assess mood and depressive symptoms at each of the three clinic visits. These measures included the Positive and Negative Affect Schedule (PANAS) [34], the 21 item Depression Anxiety and Stress Scales (DASS−21) [35], and the General Happiness Scale [36].

2.5. Vitamin D Metabolite and Serum Biomarkers

Vitamin D metabolite levels were analysed by an accredited pathology laboratory (SA Pathology, Adelaide, Australia). Levels of 25-hydroxy vitamin D2 and 25-hydroxy vitamin D3 were measured in blood sera by an accredited pathology laboratory (SA Pathology, Adelaide, Australia) using high throughput liquid chromatography tandem mass spectroscopy (LC-MSMS) [37]. As we have described elsewhere [32] this method involved precipitation of serum proteins with acetonitrile, with addition of internal standard (25- Hydroxyvitamin D3 26,26,26,27,27,27-d6, Medical Isotopes Inc, Pelham, NH, USA). Calibration was conducted using serum-based standards (Recipe Chemicals, Munich, Germany) traceable to NISTSRM972 (Gaithersburg, MD, USA). Chromatographic analysis was conducted using a Turboflow C18XL column (Thermo Scientific, Scoresby, Victoria, Australia) for on-line sample clean up, followed by an Accucore C18 analytical column (50 × 3 mm, Thermo Scientific) on a TLX4 multiplexed chromatography system (Thermo Scientific). Mass spectrometry detection utilised a TSQ Quantum Access MAX (Thermo Scientific) with APCI ionization in the positive mode and monitoring 3 MRM transitions per analyte. The limit of quantitation of the method was 5.2 and 5.0 nM for 25-OH vitamin D3 and 25-OH vitamin D2, respectively. Accuracy was assessed by running 20 samples from 4 cycles of the DEQAS external quality assurance program (Charing Cross Hospital, London, UK) for which the median value obtained by all LC-MS laboratories was between 90 and 109%, with a mean of 98%. The average coefficient of variation for these analysis was 7.5%.

2.6. Anthropometric and Covariate Measures

Height was measured using a stadiometer (SECA, Hamburg, Germany) and body weight using calibrated electronic digital scales (A & D Mercury HW-PW200 Platform Scales, A & D Australasia, Thomastown, Australasia). The contribution of environmental intakes of vitamin D3 was also assessed via a validated 7 day recall questionnaire completed by participants at each of the 3 clinic visits, in which both exposure time and skin type was recorded [38]. This survey was used to assess equivalence of the cohorts in terms of participant's exposure to an environmental source of vitamin D.

2.7. Power and Statistical Analysis

Power analyses were based on the Multivariate Repeated-Measures ANOVA (MANOVA) procedure and conducted using G*Power v3.1.7 (Heinrich Heine University, Düsseldorf, Germany). Recruitment of 100 participants per group was calculated to yield power of 95% to detect a small but statistically significant time × treatment effect size of f = 0.15. Accounting for a high drop-out rate of 25%, there would remain 80% power to detect an interaction effect size of f = 0.15. In the event of significant main or interaction effects, post-hoc pair-wise comparisons would be performed. With $n = 100$ per group, there would be 80% power to detect an effect size of 0.4 (Cohen's d) between any two groups. Allowing for attrition (~25%), there would remain 80% power to detect a medium effect size of ~0.45 (Cohen's d).

All statistical analysis was conducted using SPSS software version 23 (IBM Corporation, New York, USA). Univariate outliers of cognition and mood data (scores greater than 3.5 standard deviations (SD) from their respective means) were reduced to the next highest/lowest score within the main body of the distribution, in order to reduce their influence in analyses. Then, transformations of latency derived measures were undertaken to normalize distributions of the cognitive tasks; in line with previous studies (Danthiir, Wilhelm, Schulze, & Roberts, 2005) work rates representing the number of items correctly completed per second were calculated for all measures except for the overall quality of memory domain, which is a composite accuracy-only measure. These work rates were then weighted by accuracy (WR × % correct on respective task) to control for any speed–accuracy trade offs. Finally, domain scores were calculated by averaging performance across the relevant indicator tasks described previously [26].

Intention-to-treat analyses were undertaken and included all participants that attended for baseline, whether or not they withdrew before follow up, but excluding the 2014 cohort D2M participants who were underdosed (see explanation in results section below). For the measure of 25-OH-D2, participants were classified as ≥5 nM (no/yes) at each time point and, given the binary nature of this variable, it was modelled using Mixed-Effects Logistic Regression. Total 25-OH-D and 25-OH-D3 outcomes were modelled using Linear Mixed-Effects Regression (LMER) models. The repeated nature of the measurements were accounted for by permitting random slopes and intercepts for each participant and fixed effects (time, treatment and time × treatment) were specified. For cognitive and mood outcomes, a random slope for time was modelled enabling the comparison of rate of change on these measures over the three study visits. In the event of significant main and interaction effects, sub-groups defined by sex, and vitamin D adequacy at baseline (cut off of ≥75 nM [39]) were further examined by incorporating a three-way interaction (time × treatment × subgroup) and the significance of these were considered relative a conservatively modified $p \leq 0.025$ criterion to account for the multiple comparisons conducted herein. However, these subgroup analyses were not undertaken for the 25-OH-D2 groups because of low overall cell counts. An unstructured covariance matrix was specified for all random effects and all models controlled for age and BMI at baseline, sex and cohort, with the addition of MMSE screening scores and APOE-ε4 status (yes/no) for cognitive and mood models. The assumption of normally distributed residuals was assessed and was satisfied for all models.

3. Results

3.1. Capsule Composition, Compliance and Adverse Events

Compliance of all participants who attended the end-point visit exceeded 95%, with no serious adverse events reported. Analysis of vitamin D present in the intervention capsules was performed at the end of each cohort. Testing of the intervention product at the end of 2014 (Cohort 1) revealed that the D2M group had received a significantly lower dosage than intended due to a manufacturing error. Participants received only 114 IU per day (57 IU per capsule) as opposed to the target dosage of 600 IU. Therefore, the batch of capsules used in the second cohort was assessed prior to commencement of the 2015 cohort (500.2 IU per capsule) and again at the end point (500.2 IU per capsule) and was found to be stable and in excess of the daily target of 600 IU. Analysis of levels in the D3 arm for 2014 (367.2 IU per capsule) and 2015 (374.4 IU per capsule) were found to be acceptable and slightly higher than the target 600 IU daily dosage. Given the underdosing of D2M participants in 2014, they were excluded from the trial and all analyses.

3.2. Baseline Characteristics

Three-hundred and seventy remaining participants completed a baseline assessment and formed the intention-to-treat sample for main-effects analyses. Characteristics of these participants are presented in Table 1. The groups were relatively balanced although there was evidence of some differences for BMI: participants in the SM group had a lower BMI than in the D3 and PL groups (both $p < 0.02$). Analysis of exposure to environmental vitamin D using sun exposure scores controlling for sex, age and cohort, showed no statistically significant differences between the treatments groups over the three study visits in terms of their sun exposure ($p = 0.57$). However, as expected due to this study coinciding with winter months, the overall mean sun exposure was lower at visit two than baseline and end-point visits ($p < 0.05$).

Table 1. Characteristics of baseline participants by trial group.

VARIABLE	Vitamin D Enhanced Mushroom (n = 93)	Vitamin D3 (n = 91)	Standard Mushroom (n = 94)	Placebo (n = 92)
Female, %	51.6	53.8	51.1	51.1
APOE-ε4 0/1/2, n	72/21/0	72/17/2	76/18/0	72/18/2
Smoking Behaviour, n				
Smoker	0	1	0	0
Ex-Smoker	17	14	20	12
Never-Smoker	76	76	74	81
Alcohol Behaviour, n				
Regular	69	65	58	0
Rarely	7	2	2	67
Never	17	24	34	25
Mean Alcohol Consumption, L/week	1.5 (1.5)	1.2 (1.1)	1.1 (1.0)	1.3 (1.4)
Age in years	69.7 (6.6)	70.8 (6.4)	69.4 (6.7)	70.1 (5.7)
BMI *	27.5 (4.0)	28.0 (4.0)	26.6 (4.0)	28.2 (4.1)
MMSE Score	28.6 (1.3)	28.5 (1.4)	28.4 (1.5)	28.6 (1.4)
Mean Sun Exposure Score				
Week 0	21.4 (10.3)	21.6 (10.1)	21.0 (8.6)	21.5 (11.1)
+5 Weeks	15.4 (8.6)	16.4 (8.4)	16.0 (7.3)	17.8 (10.1)
+24 Weeks	20.1 (10.1)	22.9 (10.4)	20.0 (9.1)	22.8 (9.5)

Mean (SD), unless otherwise indicated. * One-way ANOVA (p = 0.03). APOE = Apolipoprotein E; n = number of participants; MMSE = Mini-Mental State Examination.

3.3. Vitamin D Outcomes

In individuals retained through to the final visit, average adherence to treatment was assessed on the basis of returned capsules. Adherence was high—89% (D2M), 89% (D3), 91% (SM) and 90% (PL)—and not different across treatment arms (one-way ANOVA, p = 0.48). Despite this, the models revealed significant time, treatment and interaction effects (see Table 2 and Figure 2). Overall, mean levels of total 25-OH-D declined over 24 weeks (all $p \leq 0.01$). However, the interaction effect showed that compared to PL, the decline in 25-OH-D in the D2M arm was less negative and slower (p = 0.047), whilst the change was actually positive for D3 ($p < 0.001$). Similarly, 25-OH-D3 levels declined overall and the interaction effect indicated that compared to placebo, the decline in D2M was more pronounced and faster ($p < 0.001$), whilst change was somewhat more positive in D3 ($p < 0.001$). The PL and SM treatments were not different for either of these measures. As shown in Table 2, levels of 25-OH-D2 were generally not detectable at baseline in any group. However, the number of individuals with detectable levels (>5.0 nM) increased with the interaction term, demonstrating that this was only apparent for the D2M arm ($p < 0.001$).

Table 2. Means (±SE) for 25-OH-D and 25-OH-D3 metabolite levels and proportion of 25-OH-D2 > 5.0 nM for treatment groups across study visits.

Measure	Visit	D2M		D3		SM		PL		Model p-Values
25-OH-D	Baseline +24 Weeks	74.64 66.76	±2.08 ±2.06	77.80 82.24	±1.94 ±1.90	77.95 64.91	±1.92 ±1.88	74.13 61.91	±1.94 ±1.89	T $p < 0.001$ Tr $p = 0.052$ T × Tr $p < 0.001$
25-OH-D3	Baseline +24 Weeks	74.30 47.02	±2.09 ±2.07	77.57 81.95	±1.95 ±1.92	77.91 64.71	±1.92 ±1.90	74.09 61.90	±1.95 ±1.90	T $p < 0.001$ Tr $p < 0.01$ T × Tr $p < 0.001$
25-OH-D2 > 5.0 nM	Baseline +24 Weeks	3 88	(3.2%) (94.6%)	3 4	(3.3%) (4.4%)	1 3	(1.1%) (3.2%)	1 3	(1.1%) (3.3%)	T $p < 0.001$ Tr $p < 0.001$ T × Tr $p < 0.001$

D2M (enhanced D2 mushroom), D3 (vitamin D3); SM (standard mushroom), and PL (placebo). Models controlled for baseline age, sex, BMI and cohort. p-value for time x treatment interaction term in mixed-effects regression models.

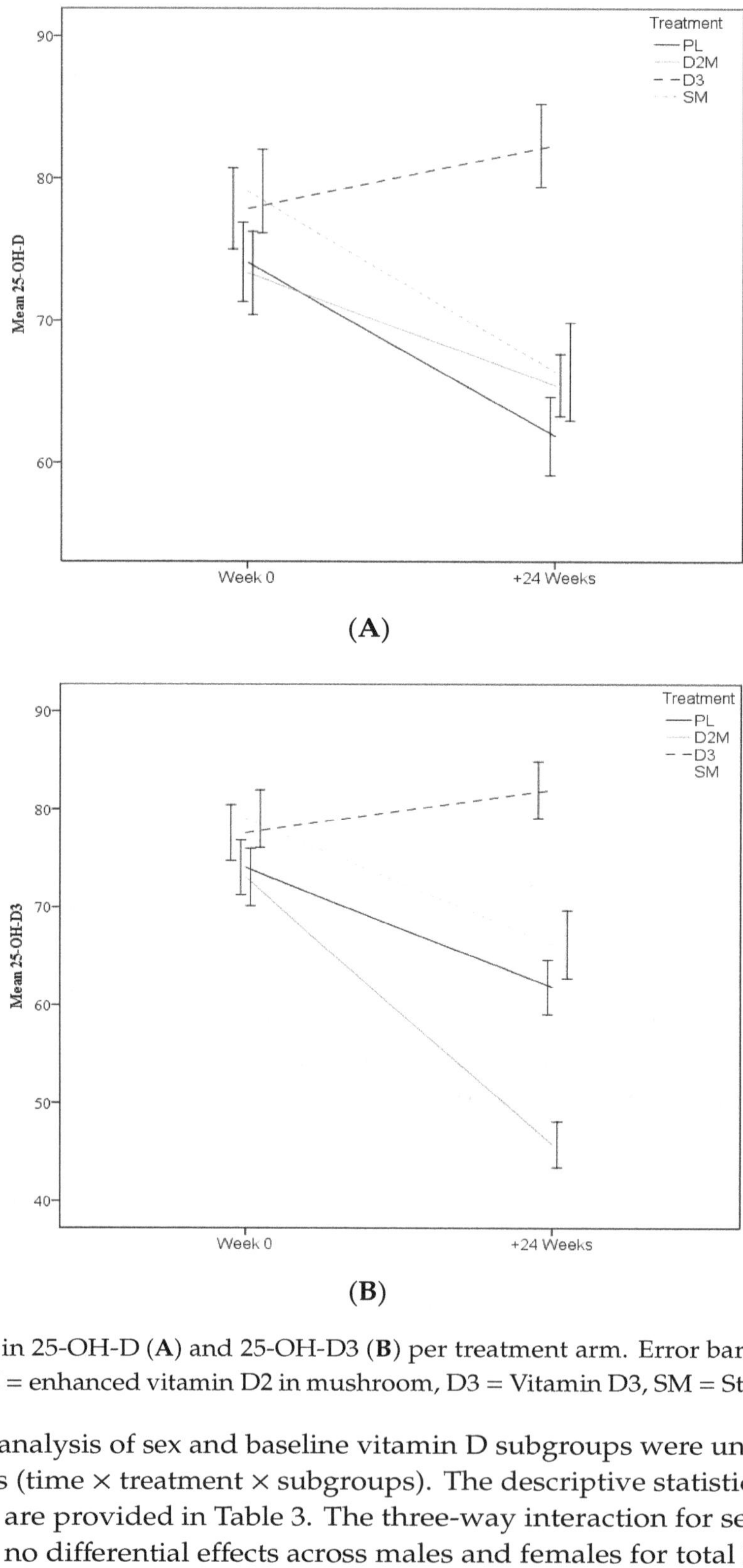

Figure 2. Changes in 25-OH-D (**A**) and 25-OH-D3 (**B**) per treatment arm. Error bars represent ±1.5 SE. PL = Placebo, D2M = enhanced vitamin D2 in mushroom, D3 = Vitamin D3, SM = Standard Mushroom.

Further planned analysis of sex and baseline vitamin D subgroups were undertaken by including three-way interactions (time × treatment × subgroups). The descriptive statistics for sex and baseline vitamin D subgroups are provided in Table 3. The three-way interaction for sex was not statistically significant indicating no differential effects across males and females for total 25-OH-D ($p = 0.66$) or 25-OH-D3 ($p = 0.52$). However, there was a three-way interaction with baseline vitamin D status for 25-OH-D ($p < 0.001$). Comparisons indicated that the degree of change differed between subgroups for each treatment level (all $p \leq 0.04$). As shown in Figure 3, 25-OH-D increased in the D3 arm but only in participants who were deficient at baseline (it remained relatively stable in sufficient individuals). The rate of 25-OH-D decline within the remaining treatments differed depending on baseline status with faster declines in the sufficient groups. The three-way interaction for 25-OH-D3 was also significant ($p < 0.001$) with comparisons indicating that degree of change differed between subgroups for D2M, D3 and PL treatments (all $p \leq 0.001$), but not for SM ($p = 0.07$). Quite different trajectories of change were apparent across the groups as shown in Figure 4, with faster rates of decline notable for the D2M treatment.

Table 3. Means (±SE) for 25-OH-D and 25-OH-D3 sex and vitamin D subgroups.

VARIABLE			D2M		D3		SM		CONTROL	
Male, *n*			*48*		*42*		*46*		*45*	
	25-OHD	Baseline	75.92	±2.53	79.12	±2.87	79.11	±2.85	72.87	±2.49
		+24 Weeks	66.38	±1.92	84.67	±2.85	67.67	±3.7	60.47	±2.45
	25-OHD3	Baseline	75.57	±2.55	78.73	±2.89	78.97	±2.88	72.7	±2.5
		+24 Weeks	48.95	±2.02	84.14	±2.81	67.46	±3.75	60.34	±2.47
Female, *n*			*45*		*49*		*48*		*47*	
	25-OHD	Baseline	70.6	±2.97	76.8	±2.54	79.08	±2.71	75.3	±2.76
		+24 Weeks	64.39	±2.26	80.26	±2.67	65.2	±2.75	63.26	±2.76
	25-OHD3	Baseline	70.42	±2.96	76.64	±2.55	79.1	±2.7	75.32	±2.76
		+24 Weeks	42.09	±2.31	80.11	±2.65	64.98	±2.76	63.28	±2.75
Deficient, *n*			*54*		*44*		*40*		*47*	
	25-OHD	Baseline	60.55	±1.52	62.45	±1.57	61.65	±1.67	60.38	±1.65
		+24 Weeks	58.57	±1.69	72.02	±2.26	50.71	±2.39	52.02	±1.85
	25-OHD3	Baseline	60.38	±1.54	62.27	±1.55	61.53	±1.67	60.2	±1.63
		+24 Weeks	38.36	±1.52	71.88	±2.23	50.28	±2.43	51.89	±1.83
Sufficient, *n*			*39*		*47*		*54*		*45*	
	25-OHD	Baseline	90.69	±1.97	91.77	±1.7	92.02	±1.66	88.75	±1.59
		+24 Weeks	74.71	±1.65	91.55	±2.42	77.68	±2.61	72.66	±2.42
	25-OHD3	Baseline	90.52	±1.95	91.42	±1.77	92	±1.67	88.79	±1.58
		+24 Weeks	55.77	±2.14	91.07	±2.39	77.62	±2.62	72.7	±2.41

D2M (enhanced D2 mushroom), D3 (vitamin D3), SM (standard mushroom). Classified as 25-OH-D deficient (<75 nM) or sufficient at baseline. n = number of participants.

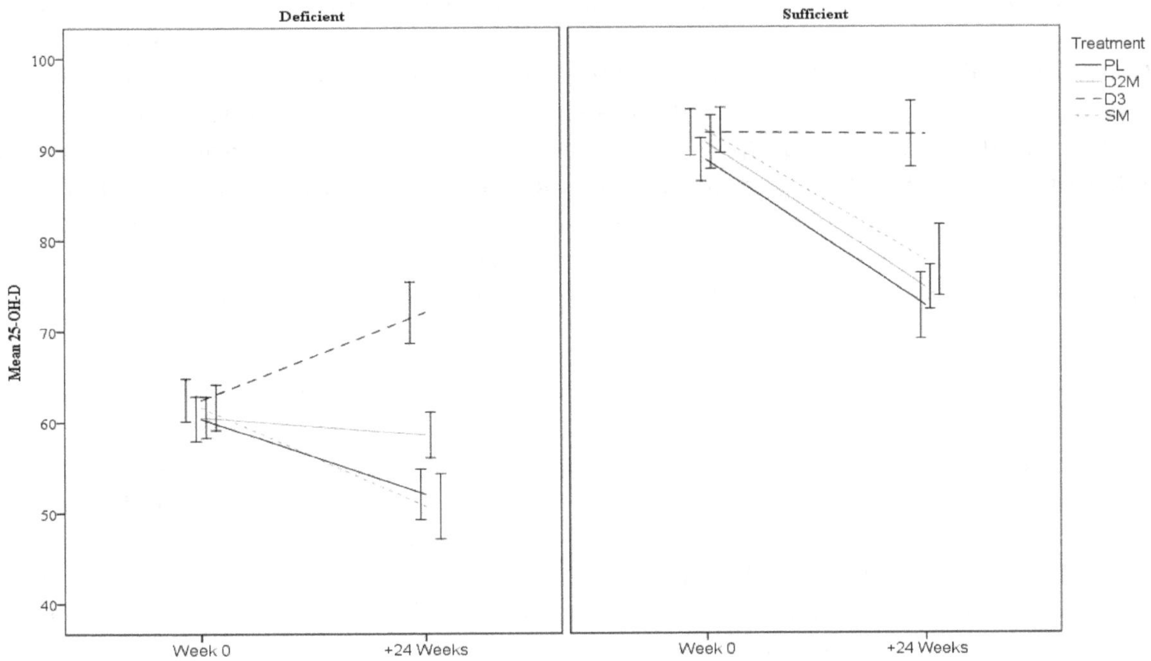

Figure 3. Changes in 25-OH-D per treatment arms for baseline total 25-OH-D-deficient (<75 nM) and -sufficient subgroups. Error bars represent ±1.5 SE. D2M (enhanced D2 mushroom), D3 (vitamin D3); SM (standard mushroom), and PL (placebo).

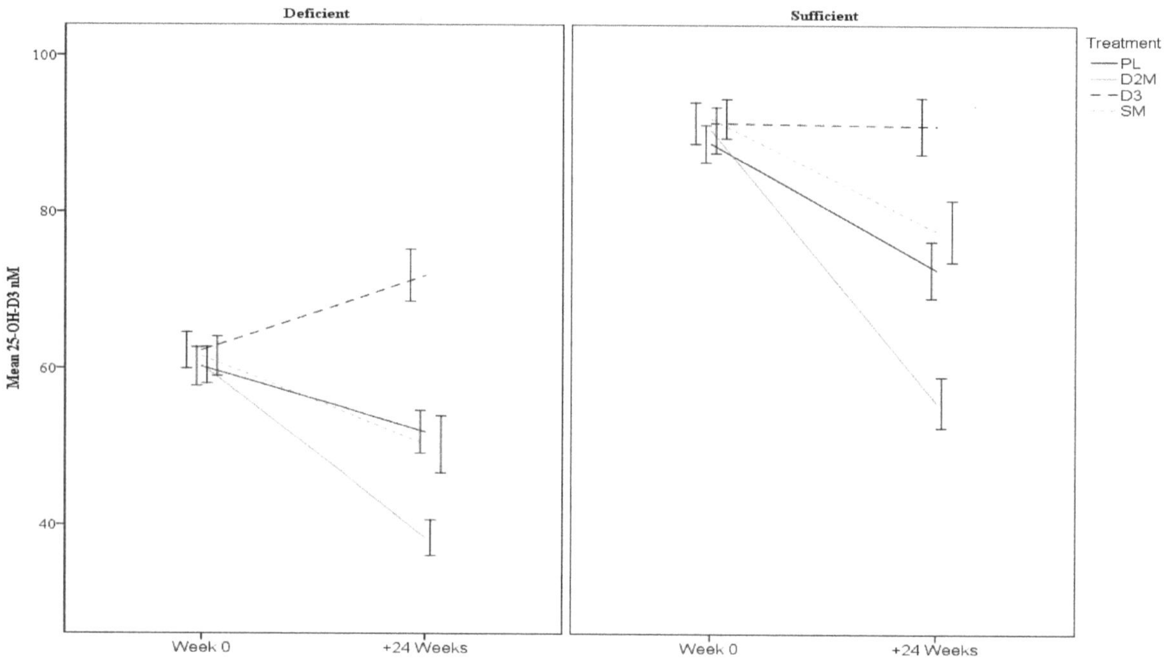

Figure 4. Changes in 25-OH-D3 per treatment arms for baseline total 25-OH-D-deficient (<75 nM) and -sufficient subgroups. Error bars represent ± 1.5 SE. D2M (enhanced D2 mushroom), D3 (vitamin D3); SM (standard mushroom), and PL (placebo).

3.4. Cognitive and Mood Outcomes

Results of models assessing cognitive outcomes are provided in Table 4. Overall time effects showed that for all but the quality of memory domain, participant's performance improved from baseline to end point, which is common across repeated cognitive assessments. There was only one interaction effect which was for the verbal working memory domain ($p = 0.04$). This showed that the slope of performance across the three visits was slightly negative for D3 and significantly different from the slope for the placebo group ($p = 0.009$), which was positive (i.e., performance improved over time). The slope for D2M and SM conditions was not different from PL, indicating that performance in these groups increased at a similar rate to PL and these increases are therefore not attributable to active intervention. None of the three-way interactions with sex and vitamin D subgroups exceed the adjusted criteria for significance (see statistical analysis section; descriptive data are not presented for brevity).

Results of models assessing mood outcomes are provided as Table 5. There were overall time effects for stress and negative affect showing decreases in these constructs over time in the combined sample. However, there were no significant treatment or time × treatment interaction effects for any mood outcome measures. Of all mood outcomes, only the three-way interaction of happiness with baseline vitamin D level exceeded criteria ($p = 0.009$). In this model, slopes were different between vitamin D-deficient and -sufficient subgroups for PL (increasing only in the deficient group, $p < 0.01$) and SM groups (decrease in the deficient yet increase in the sufficient group, $p = 0.03$); descriptive data for these models are not presented for brevity.

Table 4. Descriptive statistics (mean ± SE) for cognitive domain measures.

COGNITIVE MEASURE		D2M		D3		SM		PL		Model p
Reaction Time	Week 0	1.56	±0.03	1.55	±0.03	1.5	±0.03	1.55	±0.03	T $p < 0.001$
	+5 Weeks	1.58	±0.03	1.57	±0.04	1.57	±0.03	1.6	±0.03	Tr $p = 0.65$
	+24 Weeks	1.61	±0.03	1.61	±0.04	1.57	±0.03	1.59	±0.03	T x Tr $p = 0.82$
Speed of Processing	Week 0	0.49	±0.01	0.5	±0.01	0.47	±0.01	0.48	±0.01	T $p < 0.001$
	+5 Weeks	0.5	±0.01	0.51	±0.01	0.48	±0.01	0.5	±0.01	Tr $p = 0.10$
	+24 Weeks	0.5	±0.01	0.51	±0.01	0.48	±0.01	0.5	±0.01	T x Tr $p = 0.51$
Speed of Reasoning	Week 0	0.8	±0.02	0.79	±0.02	0.73	±0.02	0.79	±0.02	T $p < 0.001$
	+5 Weeks	0.85	±0.02	0.83	±0.03	0.77	±0.02	0.83	±0.02	Tr $p = 0.21$
	+24 Weeks	0.86	±0.03	0.86	±0.02	0.8	±0.02	0.83	±0.02	T x Tr $p = 0.77$
Speed of Memory Scanning	Week 0	0.75	±0.02	0.73	±0.02	0.7	±0.02	0.72	±0.02	T $p < 0.001$
	+5 Weeks	0.77	±0.02	0.75	±0.02	0.72	±0.02	0.75	±0.02	Tr $p = 0.39$
	+24 Weeks	0.77	±0.02	0.74	±0.02	0.74	±0.02	0.74	±0.02	T x Tr $p = 0.47$
Recognition Speed	Week 0	0.6	±0.02	0.61	±0.02	0.56	±0.01	0.59	±0.02	T $p < 0.001$
	+5 Weeks	0.6	±0.02	0.59	±0.02	0.56	±0.01	0.58	±0.02	Tr $p = 0.39$
	+24 Weeks	0.65	±0.02	0.63	±0.02	0.59	±0.02	0.63	±0.01	T x Tr $p = 0.43$
Verbal Working Memory	Week 0	0.79	±0.02	0.82	±0.02	0.74	±0.02	0.79	±0.02	T $p = 0.06$
	+5 Weeks	0.8	±0.02	0.83	±0.02	0.78	±0.02	0.83	±0.02	Tr $p = 0.05$
	+24 Weeks	0.82	±0.02	0.8	±0.02	0.76	±0.02	0.82	±0.02	T x Tr $p = 0.04$
Spatial Working Memory	Week 0	0.32	±0.02	0.29	±0.01	0.27	±0.01	0.3	±0.01	T $p < 0.001$
	+5 Weeks	0.29	±0.01	0.29	±0.01	0.28	±0.01	0.26	±0.01	Tr $p = 0.32$
	+24 Weeks	0.36	±0.02	0.33	±0.01	0.33	±0.01	0.33	±0.01	T x Tr $p = 0.59$
Overall Quality of Memory Performance	Week 0	0.79	±0.01	0.78	±0.01	0.76	±0.01	0.78	±0.01	T $p = 0.12$
	+5 Weeks	0.77	±0.01	0.76	±0.01	0.75	±0.01	0.75	±0.01	Tr $p = 0.13$
	+24 Weeks	0.8	±0.01	0.78	±0.01	0.77	±0.01	0.78	±0.01	T x Tr $p = 0.58$

D2M (enhanced D2 mushroom), D3 (vitamin D3), SM (standard mushroom), and PL (placebo). Models controlled for baseline age, sex, MMSE, BMI, cohort and APOE status. p-values arising from mixed-effects regression models. T = time; Tr = treatment.

Table 5. Descriptive statistics (mean ±SE) for mood measures.

		D2M		D3		SM		PL		Model p
ANXIETY	Week 0	2.52	±0.26	3.1	±0.39	3.04	±0.34	3.13	±0.4	T $p = 0.46$
	+5 Weeks	2.77	±0.27	2.94	±0.4	2.57	±0.33	2.91	±0.4	Tr $p = 0.86$
	+24 Weeks	2.63	±0.29	3.53	±0.47	3.08	±0.39	2.87	±0.44	T × Tr $p = 0.43$
DEPRESSION	Week 0	4.31	±0.42	4.52	±0.59	4.44	±0.55	3.91	±0.47	T $p = 0.17$
	+5 Weeks	3.7	±0.39	4.18	±0.45	4.07	±0.41	3.54	±0.44	Tr $p = 0.95$
	+24 Weeks	4.06	±0.48	4.29	±0.52	4.26	±0.51	3.39	±0.42	T × Tr $p = 0.97$
STRESS	Week 0	7.46	±0.6	6.58	±0.55	7.93	±0.58	8.15	±0.61	T $p = 0.04$
	+5 Weeks	7.75	±0.59	7.21	±0.67	7.43	±0.54	7.7	±0.77	Tr $p = 0.61$
	+24 Weeks	7.14	±0.62	6.25	±0.61	7.11	±0.56	7.52	±0.59	T × Tr $p = 0.92$
POSITIVE AFFECT	Week 0	33.16	±0.91	34.53	±0.93	31.18	±0.84	34.57	±0.71	T $p = 0.37$
	+5 Weeks	32.7	±0.79	33.58	±1	31.66	±0.85	33.89	±0.74	Tr $p = 0.12$
	+24 Weeks	33.56	±0.8	34.73	±0.92	31.8	±0.92	35.43	±0.73	T × Tr $p = 0.54$
NEGATIVE AFFECT	Week 0	12.18	±0.49	11.1	±0.21	11.21	±0.28	11.68	±0.39	T $p = 0.004$
	+5 Weeks	11.89	±0.48	11.01	±0.17	10.92	±0.2	11.24	±0.29	Tr $p = 0.06$
	+24 Weeks	10.82	±0.18	11.13	±0.31	10.65	±0.13	11.4	±0.31	T × Tr $p = 0.19$
HAPPINESS	Week 0	5.66	±0.1	6.19	±0.52	6.14	±0.44	5.52	±0.1	T $p = 0.29$
	+5 Weeks	5.94	±0.16	5.57	±0.1	5.68	±0.11	5.61	±0.09	Tr $p = 0.45$
	+24 Weeks	5.92	±0.18	5.7	±0.09	5.73	±0.1	5.7	±0.08	T × Tr $p = 0.45$

D2M (enhanced D2 mushroom), D3 (vitamin D3), SM (standard mushroom), and PL (placebo). Models controlled for baseline age, sex, MMSE, BMI, cohort and APOE status. p-values arising from mixed-effects regression models. T = time; Tr = treatment.

4. Discussion

This paper reports on the first randomised trial to explore a causative association between vitamin D supplementation and cognitive function in healthy community dwelling older adults. Participants in this trial received either vitamin D3 or enhanced D2 in a mushroom matrix for 24 weeks, with dosing levels approximating the recommended daily adult requirement of 600 to 800 IU [10]. The active interventions were shown to differentially impact vitamin D status through the winter months of this trial. Contrary to the hypothesis, neither the D2M nor D3 treatments resulted in elevated total vitamin D levels after 24 weeks. However, the D3 treatment was effective at maintaining vitamin D levels, with no significant declines observed for this group overall. Contrary to this, total vitamin D in participants receiving the D2 enhanced mushroom significantly declined. This decline was apparent despite the delivery of a notably higher (1000 IU) than anticipated (600 IU) dosage of D2, which exceeded the RDA [10] and was contrary to expectations. The present study is unable to glean the reasons for this but it may reflect either or both of physiological or analytical factors. Levels of 25-OH-D3 were also found to decline significantly faster in the D2M treatment compared to placebo (Figure 1).

Despite these main findings, differences were evident in rate of change of vitamin D according to baseline vitamin D status. In particular, it was noted that total 25-OH-D and 25-OH-D3 levels increased significantly in deficient individuals assigned to the D3 treatment, but these same measures remained stable in those sufficient at baseline. However, in the D2M arm, total 25-OH-D levels remained reasonably stable but only in individuals who were deficient at baseline. For 25-OH-D3, more rapid declines were evident in the D2 treatment than in the PL condition,.and arguably faster in individuals sufficient in D3. This finding supports previous reports of differentiated effects of vitamin D2 versus D3 on circulating 25-OH-D, which consistently show that supplementation with vitamin D2 induces downward adjustment of the level of 25-OH-D3 proportional to the increase in 25-OH-D2 [14,40,41].

Although previous evidence of a relationship between vitamin D and cognitive status is apparent in existing literature [16–21], with lower levels associated with poor functional state, this study has shown no evidence of benefit of vitamin D supplementation across a broad range of cognitive domains assessing speed, reasoning and memory throughout winter months. The time effects noted were present overall and were not due to treatment. Thus, they are interpreted as practice effects which are common in clinical trials with repeated cognitive assessments [42]. Although no effects of treatment with either D2M or D3 were found in terms of their affecting cognitive function, this result might not be considered unusual given that total vitamin D levels declined. Even in the D3 treatment, levels did not increase other than in deficient individuals. These results cannot discount the potential benefits of higher vitamin D doses and further research should consider the impact of different dosage levels for cognitive benefit.

In addition to cognitive function, we explored a range of mood outcomes including anxiety, stress, depression, positive and negative affect, and general happiness. Again, there were no results reflecting differential impacts of active treatments over time. These results are in contrast to some prior studies demonstrating efficacy of vitamin D for improving measures of depression in non-depressed [43] and depressed individuals [44]. The present study sample comprised of healthy adults free from depression. Therefore, their capacity to experience positive changes in mood is compromised. In line with a recent meta-analysis, these results support the conclusion that vitamin D supplementation is ineffective in non-depressed persons [25].

Study Limitations and Strengths

This study had several limitations. First, this was a single-centre study that utilised a relatively short treatment duration. It has been suggested that studies examining active interventions in terms of their exerting cognitive benefits should utilise durations as long as 5 years in otherwise healthy adults [45], whom formed the basis of the present study. It has been recommended therefore that future research might benefit from targeting individuals at risk of enhanced rates of decline [45], such as those exhibiting age-associated memory impairment in the absence of any underlying pathology [45]. Finding the right balance between conducting heavily controlled trials in healthy adults as opposed to studying those at greater risk, for whom myriad confounding factors are likely to exert influence, is a challenge for future cognitive interventions.

Second, this study did not control for vitamin D status at baseline and stratify randomisation accordingly. In the present case, this approach was adopted in order to avoid the necessity to refer-for-treatment individuals who were deficient in vitamin D but whom might benefit most from the active intervention. Nevertheless, it resulted in the presence of notable differences between the intervention arms in terms of overall vitamin D status which should be controlled for in future studies. The overall dosage used (~700 ID of D3, or 1000 IU of D2) might also be considered suboptimal for exerting benefits in otherwise healthy individuals. For example, studies that have shown benefits of vitamin D for improving mood have used as high as two-to-four times the dosage used in this trial [43,44].

Despite these limitations, there were distinct strengths to this study. This trial represents the first highly controlled randomised clinical trial assessing the efficacy of vitamin D supplementation for cognitive, mood and metabolic benefit in healthy community dwelling adults aged ≥60 years throughout winter months, when environmental vitamin D exposure is reduced. Participants were heavily screened to exclude a broad range of confounding factors including compromised cognitive function and depression. Furthermore, the cognitive assessments incorporated a robust battery of tests measuring distinct cognitive domains (e.g., reaction time and speed of processing). The strength of this methodology is that task-specific variance is removed from the cognitive data thus enabling the analysis of true underlying cognitive abilities [33]. The measurement of mood also comprised a broad range of standardised measures and mood constructs including both positive and negative states. Thus, these findings should be considered robust and generalisable to generally healthy community dwelling older adults. Authors should discuss the results and how they can be interpreted in perspective of previous studies and of the working hypotheses. The findings and their implications should be discussed in the broadest context possible. Future research directions may also be highlighted.

5. Conclusions

This is the first clinical evaluation of effects of supplementation of vitamin D2-enhanced mushroom on cognition and mood in a healthy elderly cohort. The four treatment arms compared vitamin D2 mushroom, vitamin D3, standard mushroom and placebo. D2M treatment resulted in a significant increase in 25-OH-D2 but an overall decline in total vitamin D, which was effectively maintained in the D3 condition only. Further, there was no benefit of vitamin D2-enhanced mushroom or D3 treatment for measures of cognitive function or mood. Based on the findings presented herein, it can be concluded that vitamin D supplementation in otherwise healthy, elderly populations free from depression and diminished cognitive capacity is ineffective at least in terms of helping improve either of these outcomes (mood or cognition), at the dosages used herein. It must be acknowledged that this result may not generalise to other populations such as those deficient in vitamin D, or those with objective cognitive impairments. Supplementation with ~600 IU daily of D3 does, however, appear sufficient for maintaining total vitamin D levels through winter. Future studies in healthy adults should seek to augment doses of vitamin D and longer durations to determine any long-term benefits during ageing.

Author Contributions: I.T.Z., P.C., M.N. and G.W. formulated the research question and overall methodology. I.T.Z. and P.C. were actively involved in the planning of the research described herein and managed the clinical team responsible for the collection of outcome data. M.B., I.T.Z. and P.C. analysed the data. P.C. and I.T.Z. compiled the first draft of the paper. All authors (I.T.Z., P.C., M.N., G.W. and M.B.) contributed to and reviewed the subsequent drafts and final publication. All authors have read and agreed to the published version of the manuscript.

References

1. Keller, J.N. Age-related neuropathology, cognitive decline, and Alzheimer's disease. *Ageing Res. Rev.* **2006**, *5*, 1–13. [CrossRef]
2. Deary, I.J.; Corley, J.; Gow, A.J.; Harris, S.E.; Houlihan, L.M.; Marioni, R.E.; Penke, L.; Rafnsson, S.B.; Starr, J.M. Age-associated cognitive decline. *Br. Med. Bull.* **2009**, *92*, 135–152. [CrossRef] [PubMed]
3. Salthouse, T.A. What and When of Cognitive Aging. *Curr. Dir. Psychol. Sci.* **2004**, *13*, 140–144. [CrossRef]
4. Salthouse, T.A. The processing-speed theory of adult age differences in cognition. *Psychol. Rev.* **1995**, *103*, 403–428. [CrossRef] [PubMed]
5. Dark-Freudeman, A.; West, R.L.; Viverito, K.M. Future Selves and Aging: Older Adults' Memory Fears. *Educ. Gerontol.* **2006**, *32*, 85–109. [CrossRef]
6. Holick, M.F. Vitamin D Deficiency. *N. Engl. J. Med.* **2007**, *357*, 266–281. [CrossRef]
7. McCann, J.C.; Ames, B.N. Is there convincing biological or behavioral evidence linking vitamin D deficiency to brain dysfunction? *FASEB J.* **2007**, *22*, 982–1001. [CrossRef]
8. Eyles, D.W.; Smith, S.; Kinobe, R.; Hewison, M.; McGrath, J.J. Distribution of the Vitamin D receptor and 1α-hydroxylase in human brain. *J. Chem. Neuroanat.* **2005**, *29*, 21–30. [CrossRef]
9. Brouwer-Brolsma, E.M.; De Groot, L.C.P.G.M.; Van De Rest, O. Vitamin D and the Association with Cognitive Performance, Cognitive Decline, and Dementia. In *Diet and Nutrition in Dementia and Cognitive Decline*; Elsevier: Amsterdam, The Netherlands, 2015; pp. 679–700.
10. A Nowson, C.; McGrath, J.J.; Ebeling, P.R.; Haikerwal, A.; Daly, R.M.; Sanders, K.M.; Seibel, M.J.; Mason, R.S. Vitamin D and health in adults in Australia and New Zealand: A position statement. *Med. J. Aust.* **2012**, *196*, 686–687. [CrossRef]
11. Tripkovic, L.; Lambert, H.; Hart, K.; Smith, C.P.; Bucca, G.; Penson, S.; Chope, G.; Hyppönen, E.; Berry, J.; Vieth, R.; et al. Comparison of vitamin D2 and vitamin D3 supplementation in raising serum 25-hydroxyvitamin D status: A systematic review and meta-analysis. *Am. J. Clin. Nutr.* **2012**, *95*, 1357–1364. [CrossRef]
12. Bogusz, J.; Pagonis, G.; Holick, M.F. Evaluation of the bioavailability of vitamin D2 in mushrooms in healthy adults. *FASEB J.* **2013**, *27*, 794.
13. Keegan, R.-J.H.; Lu, Z.; Bogusz, J.M.; Williams, J.E.; Holick, M.F. Photobiology of vitamin D in mushrooms and its bioavailability in humans. *Dermato-Endocrinology* **2013**, *5*, 165–176. [CrossRef] [PubMed]
14. Stepien, M.; O'Mahony, L.; O'Sullivan, A.; Collier, J.; Fraser, W.D.; Gibney, M.J.; Nugent, A.P.; Brennan, L. Effect of supplementation with vitamin D2-enhanced mushrooms on vitamin D status in healthy adults. *J. Nutr. Sci.* **2013**, *2*. [CrossRef] [PubMed]

15. Urbain, P.; Singler, F.; Ihorst, G.; Biesalski, H.K.; Bertz, H. Bioavailability of vitamin D(2) from UV-B-irradiated button mushrooms in healthy adults deficient in serum 25-hydroxyvitamin D: A randomized controlled trial. *Eur. J. Clin. Nutr.* **2011**, *65*, 965–971. [CrossRef]
16. Annweiler, C.; Llewellyn, D.J.; Beauchet, O. Low Serum Vitamin D Concentrations in Alzheimer's Disease: A Systematic Review and Meta-Analysis. *J. Alzheimer Dis.* **2013**, *33*, 659–674. [CrossRef]
17. Balion, C.; Griffith, L.E.; Strifler, L.; Henderson, M.; Patterson, C.; Heckman, G.; Llewellyn, D.J.; Raina, P. Vitamin D, cognition, and dementia: A systematic review and meta-analysis. *Neurology* **2012**, *79*, 1397–1405. [CrossRef]
18. Etgen, T.; Sander, D.; Bickel, H.; Sander, K.; Förstl, H. Vitamin D Deficiency, Cognitive Impairment and Dementia: A Systematic Review and Meta-Analysis. *Dement. Geriatr. Cogn. Disord.* **2012**, *33*, 297–305. [CrossRef]
19. Van Der Schaft, J.; Koek, H.; Dijkstra, E.; Verhaar, H.; Van Der Schouw, Y.; Emmelot-Vonk, M.; Van Der Schouw, Y.T. The association between vitamin D and cognition: A systematic review. *Ageing Res. Rev.* **2013**, *12*, 1013–1023. [CrossRef]
20. Zhao, Y.; Sun, Y.; Ji, H.F.; Shen, L. Vitamin D levels in Alzheimer's and Parkinson's diseases: A meta-analysis. *Nutrition* **2013**, *29*, 828–832. [CrossRef]
21. Annweiler, C.; Montero-Odasso, M.; Llewellyn, D.J.; Richard-Devantoy, S.; Duque, G.; Beauchet, O. Meta-Analysis of Memory and Executive Dysfunctions in Relation to Vitamin D. *J. Alzheimer Dis.* **2013**, *37*, 147–171. [CrossRef]
22. Timpini, A.; Pini, L.; Tantucci, C.; Cossi, S.; Grassi, V. Vitamin D and health status in elderly. *Intern. Emerg. Med.* **2010**, *6*, 11–21. [CrossRef] [PubMed]
23. Rossom, R.C.; Espeland, M.A.; Manson, J.E.; Dysken, M.W.; Johnson, K.C.; Lane, R.S.; Leblanc, E.S.; Lederle, F.A.; Masaki, K.H.; Margolis, K.L. Calcium and vitamin D supplementation and cognitive impairment in the women's health initiative. *J. Am. Geriatr. Soc.* **2012**, *60*, 2197–2205. [CrossRef] [PubMed]
24. Shaffer, J.A.; Edmondson, D.; Wasson, L.T.; Falzon, L.; Homma, K.; Ezeokoli, N.; Li, P.; Davidson, K.W. Vitamin D Supplementation for Depressive Symptoms: A Systematic Review and Meta-Analysis of Randomized Controlled Trials. *Psychosom. Med.* **2014**, *76*, 190–196. [CrossRef] [PubMed]
25. Zajac, I.; Cavuoto, P.; Danthiir, V.; Wittert, G.A.; Krause, D.; Lawson, L.; Noakes, M.; Weaver, J.; Bennett, L.E. A randomised, double blinded, placebo-controlled clinical trial testing the effects of a vitamin D-enriched mushroom supplement on cognitive performance and mood in healthy elderly adults: Study protocol. *Healthy Aging Res.* **2016**, *5*, 1–14. [CrossRef]
26. Chai-Coetzer, C.L.; Antic, N.A.; Rowland, L.S.; Catcheside, P.G.; Esterman, A.; Reed, R.L.; Williams, H.; Dunn, S.V.; McEvoy, R.D. A simplified model of screening questionnaire and home monitoring for obstructive sleep apnoea in primary care. *Thorax* **2011**, *66*, 213–219. [CrossRef]
27. Folstein, M.F.; Folstein, S.E.; McHugh, P.R. "Mini-mental state". A practical method for grading the cognitive state of patients for the clinician. *J. Psychiatr. Res.* **1975**, *12*, 189–198. [CrossRef]
28. Bennett, L.; Kersaitis, C.; Macaulay, S.L.; Münch, G.; Niedermayer, G.; Nigro, J.; Payne, M.; Sheean, P.; Vallotton, P.; Zabaras, D.; et al. Vitamin D2-Enriched Button Mushroom (Agaricus bisporus) Improves Memory in Both Wild Type and APPswe/PS1dE9 Transgenic Mice. *PLoS ONE* **2013**, *8*, e76362. [CrossRef]
29. Wesnes, K.A. Assessing cognitive function in clinical trials: Latest developments and future directions. *Drug Discov. Today* **2002**, *7*, 29–35. [CrossRef]
30. Pipingas, A.; Harris, E.; Tournier, E.; King, R.; Kras, M.; Stough, C.K. Assessing the Efficacy of Nutraceutical Interventions on Cognitive Functioning in the Elderly. *Curr. Top. Nutraceutical Res.* **2010**, *8*, 79–87.
31. Barnes, M.B.; Danthiir, V.; Noakes, M.; Macaulay, S.L.; Zajac, I.; Bennett, L.E. Cross-sectional relationships of serum 25-OH-D metabolite of vitamin D with cognition and mood in a cognitively-healthy older cohort. *Curr. Psychopharmacol.* **2016**, *5*, 47–60. [CrossRef]
32. Danthiir, V.; Burns, N.; Nettelbeck, T.; Wilson, C.; Wittert, G. The older people, omega-3, and cognitive health (EPOCH) trial design and methodology: A randomised, double-blind, controlled trial investigating the effect of long-chain omega-3 fatty acids on cognitive ageing and wellbeing in cognitively healthy older adults. *Nutr. J.* **2011**, *10*, 117. [CrossRef] [PubMed]
33. Crawford, J.R.; Henry, J.D. The Positive and Negative Affect Schedule (PANAS): Construct validity, measurement properties and normative data in a large non-clinical sample. *Br. J. Clin. Psychol.* **2004**, *43*, 245–265. [CrossRef] [PubMed]

34. Antony, M.M.; Bieling, P.J.; Cox, B.J.; Enns, M.W.; Swinson, R.P. Psychometric properties of the 42-item and 21-item versions of the Depression Anxiety Stress Scales in clinical groups and a community sample. *Psychol. Assess.* **1998**, *10*, 176–181. [CrossRef]
35. Lyubomirsky, S.; Lepper, H.S. A measure of subjective happiness: Preliminary reliability and construct validation. *Soc. Indic. Res.* **1999**, *46*, 137–155. [CrossRef]
36. Fudge, A.N.; Galettis, P.; O'Loughlin, P.D. Measurement of 25-hydroxyvitamin D by high throughput liquid chromatography tandem mass spectroscopy. *Clin. Biochem. Rev.* **2012**, *33*, S34.
37. Hanwell, H.; Vieth, R.; Cole, D.; Scillitani, A.; Modoni, S.; Frusciante, V.; Ritrovato, G.; Chiodini, I.; Minisola, S.; Carnevale, V. Sun exposure questionnaire predicts circulating 25-hydroxyvitamin D concentrations in Caucasian hospital workers in southern Italy. *J. Steroid Biochem. Mol. Biol.* **2010**, *121*, 334–337. [CrossRef]
38. Battault, S.; Whiting, S.J.; Peltier, S.L.; Sadrin, S.; Gerber, G.; Maixent, J.M. Vitamin D metabolism, functions and needs: From science to health claims. *Eur. J. Nutr.* **2013**, *52*, 429–441. [CrossRef]
39. Stephensen, C.B.; Zerofsky, M.; Burnett, D.J.; Lin, Y.-P.; Hammock, B.D.; Hall, L.M.; McHugh, T. Ergocalciferol from Mushrooms or Supplements Consumed with a Standard Meal Increases 25-Hydroxyergocalciferol but Decreases 25-Hydroxycholecalciferol in the Serum of Healthy Adults. *J. Nutr.* **2012**, *142*, 1246–1252. [CrossRef]
40. Itkonen, S.T.; Skaffari, E.; Saaristo, P.; Saarnio, E.M.; Erkkola, M.; Jakobsen, J.; Cashman, K.D.; Lamberg-Allardt, C. Effects of vitamin D2-fortified bread v. supplementation with D2 or D3 on serum 25-hydroxyvitamin D metabolites: An 8-week randomised-controlled trial in young Finnish women. *Br. J. Nutr.* **2016**, *115*, 1232–1239. [CrossRef]
41. Goldberg, T.E.; Harvey, P.D.; Wesnes, K.A.; Snyder, P.J.; Schneider, L.S. Practice effects due to serial cognitive assessment: Implications for preclinical Alzheimer's disease randomized controlled trials. *Alzheimer Dement. Diagn. Assess. Dis. Monit.* **2015**, *1*, 103–111. [CrossRef]
42. Jorde, R.; Sneve, M.; Figenschau, Y.; Svartberg, J.; Waterloo, K. Effects of vitamin D supplementation on symptoms of depression in overweight and obese subjects: Randomized double blind trial. *J. Intern. Med.* **2008**, *264*, 599–609. [CrossRef] [PubMed]
43. Khoraminya, N.; Tehrani-Doost, M.; Jazayeri, S.; Hosseini, A.; Djazayery, A. Therapeutic effects of vitamin D as adjunctive therapy to fluoxetine in patients with major depressive disorder. *Aust. N. Z. J. Psychiatry* **2013**, *47*, 271–275. [CrossRef] [PubMed]
44. Ferry, M.; Coley, N.; Andrieu, S.; Bonhomme, C.; Caubère, J.P.; Cesari, M.; Gautry, J.; Sánchez, I.G.; Hugonot, L.; Mansuy, L.; et al. How to design nutritional intervention trials to slow cognitive decline in apparently healthy populations and apply for efficacy claims: A statement from the International Academy on Nutrition and Aging Task Force. *J. Nutr. Health Aging* **2013**, *17*, 619–623. [CrossRef]
45. Lee, G.; Elashoff, D.; Di, L.; Teng, E.; Melchor, S.; Kim, J.; Lu, P.H. P3-238: Age-associated memory impairment increases risk of conversion to MCI and dementia. *Alzheimer Dement.* **2012**, *8*, P544. [CrossRef]

4

Low Serum 25-Hydroxyvitamin D Levels are Related to Frailty and Sarcopenia in Patients with Chronic Liver Disease

Chisato Saeki [1,2,*], Tomoya Kanai [1,2], Masanori Nakano [1,2], Tsunekazu Oikawa [1], Yuichi Torisu [1,2], Masayuki Saruta [1] and Akihito Tsubota [3,*]

1 Division of Gastroenterology and Hepatology, Department of Internal Medicine, The Jikei University School of Medicine, 3-25-8 Nishi-shimbashi, Minato-ku, Tokyo 105-8461, Japan; tomoyaaust@hotmail.com (T.K.); masanori-nakano@jikei.ac.jp (M.N.); oitsune@jikei.ac.jp (T.O.); torisu@jikei.ac.jp (Y.T.); m.saruta@jikei.ac.jp (M.S.)

2 Division of Gastroenterology, Department of Internal Medicine, Fuji City General Hospital, 50 Takashima-cho, Fuji-shi 417-8567, Shizuoka, Japan

3 Core Research Facilities, Research Center for Medical Science, The Jikei University School of Medicine, 3-25-8 Nishi-shimbashi, Minato-ku, Tokyo 105-8461, Japan

* Correspondence: chisato@jikei.ac.jp (C.S.); atsubo@jikei.ac.jp (A.T.)

Abstract: Low vitamin D status is related to frailty and/or sarcopenia in elderly individuals. However, these relationships are unclear in patients with chronic liver disease (CLD). This study aimed at exploring the relationship between serum 25-hydroxyvitamin D [25(OH)D] levels and frailty or sarcopenia in 231 patients with CLD. Frailty was determined based on five factors (weight loss, low physical activity, weakness, slowness, and exhaustion). Sarcopenia was diagnosed by applying the Japan Society of Hepatology criteria. The patients were classified into three groups according to baseline 25(OH)D levels: low (L), intermediate (I), and high (H) vitamin D (VD) groups. Of the 231 patients, 70 (30.3%) and 66 (28.6%) had frailty and sarcopenia, respectively. The prevalence rate of frailty and sarcopenia significantly increased stepwise with a decline in the vitamin D status. The L-VD group showed the highest prevalence rates of frailty and sarcopenia (49.1% (28/57), $p < 0.001$ for both), whereas the H-VD group showed the lowest prevalence rates of frailty (15.3% (9/59)) and sarcopenia (18.6% (11/59)) ($p < 0.001$ for both). Multivariate analysis identified serum 25(OH)D levels as a significant independent factor related to frailty and sarcopenia. Serum 25(OH)D levels significantly correlated with handgrip strength, skeletal muscle mass index, and gait speed. In conclusion, low serum vitamin D level, especially severe vitamin D deficient status, is closely related to frailty and sarcopenia in patients with CLD.

Keywords: chronic liver disease; sarcopenia; frailty; vitamin D

1. Introduction

Sarcopenia, characterized by a generalized decline of skeletal muscle mass and strength, is a serious complication in patients with chronic liver disease (CLD) [1,2]. Frailty is defined as increased vulnerability to stressors due to multisystem physiological impairment and is associated with, but not equivalent to, sarcopenia [3–5]. Sarcopenia and frailty negatively impact the quality of life, resulting in disability, and increase the risk of institutionalization and mortality [5–9]. In general, poor nutritional status, including low levels of branched-chain amino acids (BCAAs), vitamin D, zinc, and long-chain omega-3 fatty acids, is considered one of the causes of sarcopenia and frailty [10,11]. Therefore, nutritional evaluations and early therapeutic interventions for these disorders are imperative in patients with CLD.

The liver plays a crucial role in the metabolism of vitamin D, which is included in a group of fat-soluble secosteroids. Vitamin D_3 (cholecalciferol) and D_2 (ergocalciferol) are synthesized in the skin under ultraviolet exposure and ingested from the diet and/or supplements. These two vitamin D forms are inactive until they are hydroxylated in the liver to form 25-hydroxyvitamin D [25(OH)D]. 25(OH)D is the main circulating form of vitamin D and is used as a representative biomarker of a person's vitamin D status. Subsequently, 25(OH)D undergoes further hydroxylation in the kidneys to form active 1,25-dihydroxyvitamin D [1,25(OH)D] [12]. Therefore, a reduction in circulating vitamin D levels reflect an impaired liver function or malnutrition. In addition, bile production is impeded in patients with CLD, leading to decreased fat absorption, and consequently, impaired uptake of vitamin D [13]. Accordingly, patients with CLD are frequently accompanied by low vitamin D status; vitamin D deficiency (≤20 ng/mL) occurs more frequently among patients with CLD (47–78%) than in the general population (34–59%) [12,14–21]. Importantly, vitamin D deficiency causes high mortality in patients with liver cirrhosis (LC), irrespective of the impact of hepatocellular carcinoma [16,22].

Recently, several investigators have focused on the association between 25(OH)D levels and skeletal muscle function [23,24]. Previous studies have demonstrated that low vitamin D levels were related to sarcopenia, frailty, impaired physical performance, and an increased risk of mortality in elderly individuals [25–32]. In addition, a recent study affirmed that low vitamin D levels were associated with sarcopenia in patients with CLD [15]. However, the relationship between 25(OH)D levels, sarcopenia, and frailty in patients with CLD has not yet been reported and thus, remains unknown. Therefore, in the present study, we aimed at exploring the relationship between serum 25(OH)D levels and the prevalence of sarcopenia and frailty in patients with CLD.

2. Patients and Methods

2.1. *Study Design and Patients*

The present cross-sectional study included 231 consecutive patients in whom CLD was diagnosed at Fuji City General Hospital (Shizuoka, Japan) between 2017 and 2020. The inclusion criteria were as follows: (1) the presence of CLD; (2) the availability of data on skeletal muscle mass index (SMI) measured using bioimpedance analysis (InBody S10; InBody, Seoul, Korea), and grip strength using a dynamometer (T.K.K5401 GRIP-D; Takei Scientific Instruments, Niigata, Japan); and (4) the availability of frailty data evaluated based on the diagnostic criteria proposed by Fried et al. [33]. The exclusion criteria were as follows: (1) patients with refractory ascites or implants or undergoing hemodialysis, as previously described [2]; (2) patients with alcoholic liver disease because heavy alcohol consumption frequently leads to malnutrition, including vitamin D deficiency; and (3) patients who had been receiving vitamin D supplementation within 12 months before the date of entry. This study was conducted according to the criteria set by the 2013 revision of the Declaration of Helsinki. The Ethics Committee of Fuji City General Hospital approved this study (approval no. 156).

2.2. *Diagnosis of Sarcopenia and Frailty*

A diagnosis of sarcopenia was made based on the criteria published by the Japan Society of Hepatology [1]. Briefly, sarcopenia was defined as a physical condition with reduced handgrip strength (<18 kg for women and <26 kg for men) and muscle mass (SMI <5.7 kg/m^2 for women and <7.0 kg/m^2 for men). The SMI was computed from the total muscle mass of the four limbs divided by the square of height (kg/m^2). Gait speed was measured using the 6-m walk test (low gait speed was defined as <1.0 m/s). A diagnosis of frailty was made using a validated screening tool based on the following five components [33,34]: (1) weight loss (≥2 kg during the last six months); (2) weakness (handgrip strength <18 kg for women and <26 kg for men); (3) exhaustion, which was determined based on an agreement to the question: "In the last two weeks, have you felt tired without a reason?"; (4) slowness (gait speed of <1.0 m/s); and (5) low physical activity, which was established based on negative answers to the following two questions: "Do you engage in moderate levels of physical exercise or sports aimed at health?" or "Do you engage in low levels of physical exercise aimed at health?". Frailty was determined by three or more agreements [34].

2.3. Clinical and Laboratory Assessments

Serum was collected from each patient in an early morning fasting state. The following blood tests were measured using routine, conventional methods: prothrombin time-international normalized ratio (PT-INR), albumin, total bilirubin, and BCAA. The level of serum 25(OH)D, a biomarker of a person's vitamin D status, was measured using a chemiluminescent immunoassay (Hitachi Chemical Diagnostics Systems, Tokyo, Japan). Vitamin D deficiency, insufficiency, and sufficiency were defined as serum 25(OH)D levels of ≤20.0 ng/mL, 20.1–29.9 ng/mL, and ≥30.0 ng/mL, respectively, based on the conventional classification of vitamin D status [35].

2.4. Provisional Reclassification Based on the Serum 25-Hydroxyvitamin D Levels

The median serum 25(OH)D level for all patients was 14.0 (interquartile range, 10.5–18.1) ng/mL. The patients were reclassified into three groups according to the first and third quartiles (Figure S1): (1) low 25(OH)D (L-VD) group with levels ≤10.5 ng/mL (first quartile); (2) intermediate 25(OH)D (I-VD) group with levels between 10.5 and 18.1 ng/mL (third quartile); and (3) high 25(OH)D (H-VD) group with levels ≥18.1 ng/mL.

2.5. Statistics

Categorical and continuous data are expressed as number (percentage) and median (interquartile range), respectively. The chi-squared test was performed to compare frequencies in categorical data between two groups. The Mann–Whitney U test was performed to compare differences in continuous data between two groups. The Kruskal–Wallis test followed by the Steel–Dwass post hoc test was performed for multiple continuous data comparisons among three groups. Univariate and multiple logistic regression analyses were done to determine significant and independent factors associated with sarcopenia and frailty. The Cochran–Armitage trend test was performed to evaluate whether a trend was present between one variable with two categories and one variable with multiple categories. The Spearman's rank correlation test was used to analyze correlations between two continuous variables. These analyses were done using the SPSS software (ver. 26, IBM, Japan, Tokyo, Japan). A value of $p < 0.05$ was considered statistically significant.

3. Results

3.1. Baseline Characteristics of Patients

The baseline characteristics of the 231 CLD patients in the present study are shown in Table 1. The patients consisted of 95 men (41.1%) and 136 women (58.9%), with a median age of 70.0 (60.0–76.0) years for all patients. Ninety-eight (42.4%) patients were diagnosed with LC. The median 25(OH)D level was 14.0 (10.5–18.1) ng/mL. The median values of handgrip strength, SMI, and gait speed were 22.1 (17.4–29.4) kg, 6.30 (5.54–7.12) kg/m^2, and 1.10 (0.91–1.25) m/s, respectively. Eighty-one (35.1%) patients had slow gait speed.

Table 1. Baseline clinical characteristics among patients with and without sarcopenia.

Variable	All Patients	Sarcopenia Group	Non-Sarcopenia Group	p Value
Patients, n (%)	231	66 (28.6)	165 (71.4)	
Man, n (%)	95 (41.1)	23 (34.8)	72 (43.6)	0.220
Age (years)	70.0 (60.0–76.0)	76.0 (72.8–80.3)	68.0 (58.0–73.0)	<0.001
BMI (kg/m^2)	23.1 (20.7–26.0)	20.5 (19.2–22.6)	24.2 (21.8–26.6)	<0.001
Liver cirrhosis, n (%)	98 (42.4)	40 (60.6)	58 (35.2)	<0.001
Etiology				
HBV/HCV/PBC/other, n	42/90/60/39)	5/36/19/6	37/54/41/33)	0.002
Total bilirubin (mg/dL)	0.7 (0.5–0.9)	0.6 (0.5–0.9)	0.7 (0.5–0.9)	0.610
Albumin (g/dL)	4.1 (3.9–4.4)	3.9 (3.6–4.3)	4.2 (3.9–4.4)	0.003
Prothrombin time INR	1.02 (0.96–1.11)	1.05 (0.96–1.13)	1.02 (0.96–1.10)	0.130
BCAA (μmol/L)	408 (357–475)	364 (302–425)	432 (381–488)	<0.001
25(OH)D (ng/mL)	14.0 (10.5–18.1)	12.2 (8.8–15.7)	14.7 (11.4–18.4)	0.001
Vitamin D insufficiency, n (%)	26 (11.3)	4 (6.1)	22 (13.3)	0.114
Vitamin D deficiency, n (%)	201 (87.0)	62 (93.9)	139 (84.2)	0.048
SMI (kg/m^2)				
All patients	6.30 (5.54–7.12)	5.20 (4.82–5.71)	6.75 (5.98–7.44)	<0.001
Man	7.13 (6.48–7.87)	6.18 (5.49–6.84)	7.49 (7.05–8.15)	<0.001
Woman	5.86 (5.20–6.44)	5.09 (4.67–5.30)	6.05 (5.83–6.59)	<0.001
Handgrip strength (kg)				
All patients	22.1 (17.4–29.4)	16.8 (13.8–18.4)	24.5 (19.9–32.6)	<0.001
Man	30.5 (24.1–37.5)	22.8 (18.3–24.2)	33.4 (28.5–38.9)	<0.001
Woman	18.8 (15.1–22.5)	15.0 (12.8–17.2)	21.3 (18.5–24.0)	<0.001
Gait speed (m/s)	1.10 (0.91–1.25)	0.90 (0.68–1.07)	1.15 (1.02–1.28)	<0.001
Slow gait speed, n (%)	81 (35.1)	49 (74.2)	32 (19.4)	<0.001
Frailty, n (%)	70 (30.3)	51 (77.3)	19 (11.5)	<0.001

Values are presented as median (interquartile range) or number (percentage). Statistical analysis was carried out using the chi-squared test or the Mann–Whitney U test, as appropriate. 25(OH)D, 25-hydroxyvitamin D; BCAA, branched-chain amino acid; BMI, body mass index; HBV, hepatitis B virus; HCV, hepatitis C virus; INR, international normalized ratio; PBC, primary biliary cholangitis; SMI, skeletal muscle mass index.

3.2. *Comparison of Clinical Characteristics among Patients with and without Sarcopenia*

Sixty-six (28.6%) were diagnosed with sarcopenia among the 231 patients (Table 1). The patients in the sarcopenia group were significantly older and had a lower body mass index (BMI) than those in the non-sarcopenia group ($p < 0.001$ for both). The sarcopenia group had a higher prevalence of LC than the non-sarcopenia group (60.6% vs. 35.2%; $p < 0.001$). As for the biochemical findings, the levels of albumin ($p = 0.003$), BCAA ($p < 0.001$), and 25(OH)D ($p = 0.001$) in the sarcopenia group were significantly lower than those in the non-sarcopenia group. Vitamin D deficiency was significantly more frequent in the sarcopenia group than in the non-sarcopenia group ($p = 0.048$). The sarcopenia group showed significantly higher rates of frailty (77.3% vs. 11.5%; $p < 0.001$) and slow gait speed (74.2% vs. 19.4%; $p < 0.001$) than the non-sarcopenia group.

3.3. *Significant Factors Related to Sarcopenia among Patients with Chronic Liver Disease*

The univariate analysis showed that the following eight variables were significantly associated with sarcopenia: age, BMI, LC, serum levels of albumin, BCAA, and 25(OH)D, PT-INR deficiency vitamin D (Table S1). Finally, the following four variables remained significant and independent on the multivariate analysis (Table 2): advanced age (odds ratio (OR), 1.087; 95% confidence interval (CI), 1.044–1.130; $p < 0.001$); the presence of LC (OR, 2.493; 95% CI, 1.180–5.266; $p = 0.017$); lower BMI (OR, 0.720; 95% CI, 0.635–0.817; $p < 0.001$); and lower 25 (OH)D levels (OR, 0.863; 95% CI, 0.794–0.937; $p < 0.001$).

Table 2. Significant factors related to sarcopenia in patients with chronic liver disease.

Variable	Univariate		Multivariate	
	OR (95% CI)	*p*-Value	OR (95% CI)	*p* Value
Age (years)	1.083 (1.047–1.121)	<0.001	1.087 (1.044–1.130)	<0.001
BMI (kg/m^2)	0.726 (0.649–0.813)	<0.001	0.720 (0.635–0.817)	<0.001
Liver cirrhosis	2.838 (1.576–5.111)	0.001	2.493 (1.180–5.266)	0.017
Albumin (g/dL)	0.334 (0.184–0.605)	<0.001		
Prothrombin time INR	11.004 (1.104–109.651)	0.041		
BCAA (μmol/L)	0.992 (0.988–0.995)	<0.001		
25(OH)D (ng/mL)	0.896 (0.841–0.953)	0.001	0.863 (0.794–0.937)	<0.001
Vitamin D deficiency	2.899 (0.971–8.661)	0.057		

25(OH)D, 25-hydroxyvitamin D; BCAA, branched-chain amino acid; BMI, body mass index; CI, confidence interval; INR, international normalized ratio; OR, odds ratio.

3.4. Comparison of Clinical Characteristics among Patients with and without Frailty

The prevalence rate of frailty was 30.3% (70/231) (Table S2). The patients with frailty were significantly older and had a higher prevalence of LC (68.6% vs. 31.1%) and lower BMI than those without frailty ($p < 0.001$ for all). The patients in the frail group had significantly lower levels of 25(OH)D ($p < 0.001$), albumin ($p < 0.001$), BCAA ($p < 0.001$), and longer PT-INR ($p = 0.014$) than those in the non-frail group. The frail group had significantly higher rates of sarcopenia (72.9% vs. 9.3%; $p < 0.001$) and slow gait speed (92.9% vs. 9.9%; $p < 0.001$) than the non-frail group.

3.5. Significant Factors Related to Frailty among Patients with Chronic Liver Disease

On the univariate analysis, the following eight variables were significantly related to frailty: age, BMI, LC, serum levels of albumin, BCAA, and 25(OH)D, PT-INR, and vitamin D deficiency (Table S3). The following four variables remained significant and independent on the multivariate analysis (Table 3): advanced age (OR, 1.094; 95% CI, 1.052–1.138; $p < 0.001$); the presence of LC (OR, 3.749; 95% CI, 1.843–7.626; $p < 0.001$); lower BCAA levels (OR, 0.994; 95% CI, 0.990–0.998; $p = 0.008$); and lower 25(OH)D levels (OR, 0.887; 95% CI, 0.822–0.957; $p = 0.002$).

Table 3. Significant factors related to frailty in patients with chronic liver disease.

Variable	Univariate		Multivariate	
	OR (95% CI)	*p*-Value	OR (95% CI)	*p* Value
Age (years)	1.091 (1.054–1.129)	<0.001	1.094 (1.052–1.138)	<0.001
BMI (kg/m^2)	0.869 (0.801–0.943)	0.001		
Liver cirrhosis	4.844 (2.645–8.870)	<0.001	3.749 (1.843–7.626)	<0.001
Albumin (g/dL)	0.292 (0.159–0.534)	<0.001		
Prothrombin time INR	18.162 (1.821–181.168)	0.013		
BCAA (μmol/L)	0.991 (0.988–0.995)	<0.001	0.994 (0.990–0.998)	0.008
25(OH)D (ng/mL)	0.893 (0.840–0.950)	0.001	0.887 (0.822–0.957)	0.002
Vitamin D deficiency	2.390 (0.875–6.526)	0.089		

25(OH)D, 25-hydroxyvitamin D; BCAA, branched-chain amino acid; BMI, body mass index; CI, confidence interval; INR, international normalized ratio; OR, odds ratio.

3.6. Prevalence of Sarcopenia and Frailty Defined according to the Conventional Classification of Vitamin D Status

Vitamin D deficiency, insufficiency, and sufficiency were present in 87.0% (201/231), 11.3% (26/231), and 1.7% (4/231) of the patients, respectively (Table 1, Figure 1A). The vitamin D deficient group had the highest prevalence of sarcopenia (30.8% (62/201), Figure 1B) and frailty (32.3% (65/201), Figure 1C) among the three groups, although the difference was not statistically significant.

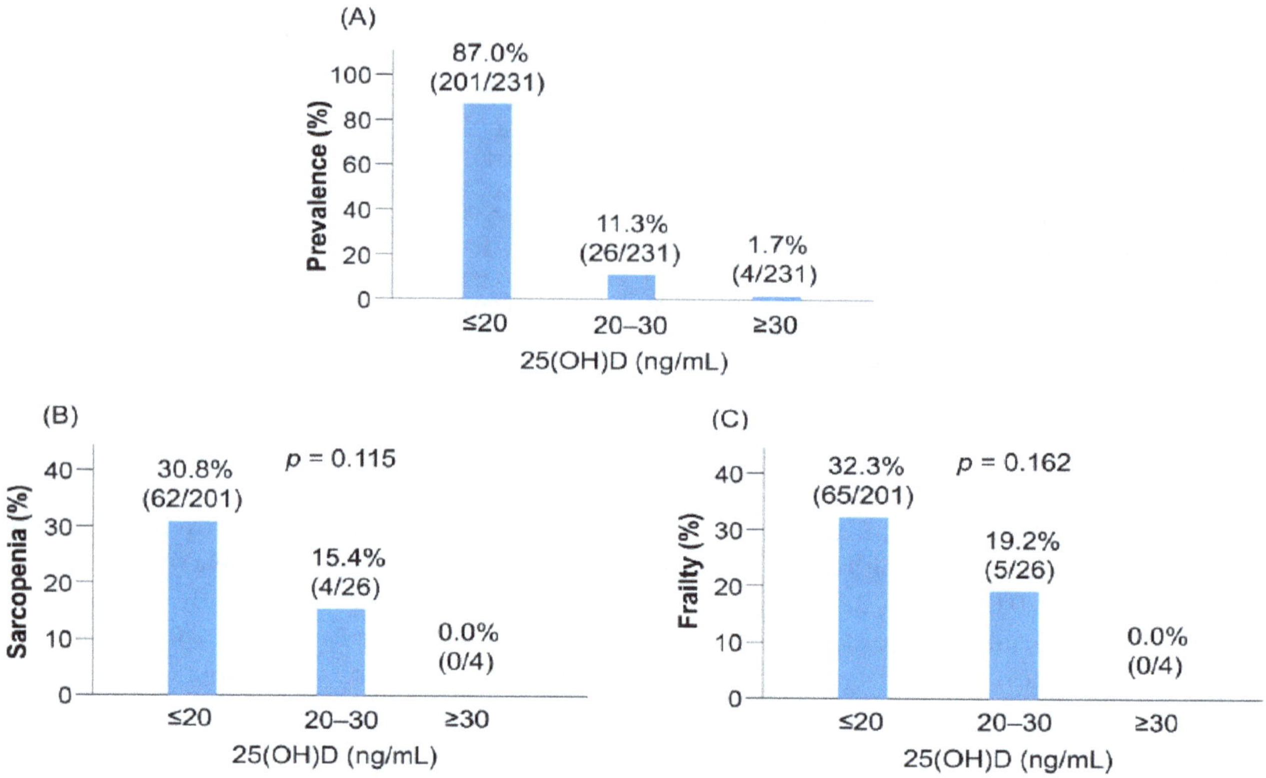

Figure 1. (**A**) Distribution of the serum 25-hydroxyvitamin D [25(OH)D] levels in patients with chronic liver disease. (**B**,**C**) The prevalence rates of sarcopenia and frailty based on the serum 25(OH)D levels.

3.7. Clinical Characteristics Based on the Provisional Reclassification of Vitamin D Status

As described previously, most patients (87.0%) had vitamin D deficiency (as defined by the conventional classification). Therefore, we could not confirm the statistical correlation between vitamin D deficiency/insufficiency and sarcopenia or frailty. To resolve this issue and explore the association between vitamin D status and disease conditions in more detail, we reclassified the patients into three groups provisionally according to the baseline serum 25(OH)D levels (as described in the Methods section). The distribution of the L-VD, I-VD, and H-VD groups was 24.7% (57/231), 49.8% (115/231), and 25.5% (59/231), respectively (Table 4). Gender ($p = 0.012$), BCAA ($p < 0.001$), SMI ($p = 0.002$), and handgrip strength ($p < 0.001$) were significantly different among these groups. Notably, the L-VD group had the highest prevalence rate of sarcopenia (49.1% (28/57); $p < 0.001$; adjusted residual = |4.0|) and frailty (49.1% (28/57); $p < 0.001$; adjusted residual = |3.6|) among these groups, while the H-VD group had the lowest prevalence rate of sarcopenia (18.6% (11/59); $p < 0.001$; adjusted residual = |2.0|) and frailty (15.3% (9/59); $p < 0.001$; adjusted residual = |2.9|) (Table 4, Figure 2A,B). The prevalence rates of sarcopenia and frailty significantly increased in a stepwise manner with a decline in the 25(OH)D levels ($p < 0.001$ for both).

Table 4. Characteristics of the three groups classified based on the serum 25-hydroxyvitamin D levels.

Variable	L-VD	M-VD	H-VD	*p* Value
Patients, n (%)	57 (24.7)	115 (49.8)	59 (25.5)	
Man, n (%)	20 (35.1)	41 (35.7)	34 (57.6)	0.012
Age (years)	68.0 (55.0–77.0)	70.0 (61.0–76.0)	72.0 (64.0–77.0)	0.317
BMI (kg/m^2)	22.2 (20.2–26.0)	22.8 (20.4–26.1)	23.6 (22.3–25.8)	0.489
Liver cirrhosis, n (%)	30 (52.6)	48 (41.7)	20 (33.9)	0.122
Etiology				
HBV/HCV/PBC/other, n	8/21/15/13	20/50/27/18	14/19/18/8	0.499
Total bilirubin (mg/dL)	0.7 (0.5–1.3)	0.6 (0.5–0.8)	0.7 (0.5–0.9)	0.238
Albumin (g/dL)	4.1 (3.7–4.5)	4.1 (3.8–4.3)	4.2 (4.0–4.4)	0.209
Prothrombin time INR	1.06 (0.96–1.16)	1.01 (0.95–1.11)	1.00 (0.97–1.07)	0.139
BCAA (μmol/L)	382 (312–432)	420 (364–478)	438 (379–501)	<0.001
25(OH)D (ng/mL)	8.4 (6.9–9.7)	14.0 (12.4–15.9)	20.1 (18.7–23.5)	<0.001
SMI (kg/m^2)				
ALL patients	5.87 (5.08–6.96)	6.16 (5.66–6.95)	7.04 (5.97–7.43)	0.002
Man	7.07 (6.44–8.27)	6.98 (6.17–7.76)	7.23 (7.01–8.11)	0.152
Woman	5.39 (4.87–5.94)	5.97 (5.44–6.49)	5.90 (5.16–6.70)	0.014
Handgrip strength (kg)				
ALL patients	18.6 (14.8–25.1)	22.1 (17.8–27.1)	26.9 (20.6–33.2)	<0.001
Man	26.3 (18.3–33.5)	30.2 (23.9–37.0)	32.5 (27.0–38.9)	0.036
Woman	17.4 (14.1–19.9)	19.1 (16.5–22.5)	19.4 (16.7–24.0)	0.082
Sarcopenia, n (%)	28 (49.1)	27 (23.5)	11 (18.6)	<0.001
Gait speed (m/s)	1.00 (0.69–1.16)	1.11 (0.92–1.25)	1.17 (1.00–1.38)	0.003
Slow gait speed, n (%)	29 (50.9)	38 (33.0)	14 (23.7)	0.007
Frailty, n (%)	28 (49.1)	33 (28.7)	9 (15.3)	<0.001

Values are presented as median (interquartile range) or number (percentage). Statistical analysis was carried out using the chi-squared test or the Kruskal–Wallis test, as appropriate. 25(OH)D, 25-hydroxyvitamin D; BCAA, branched-chain amino acid; BMI, body mass index; HBV, hepatitis B virus; HCV, hepatitis C virus; INR, international normalized ratio; PBC, primary biliary cholangitis; SMI, skeletal muscle mass index.

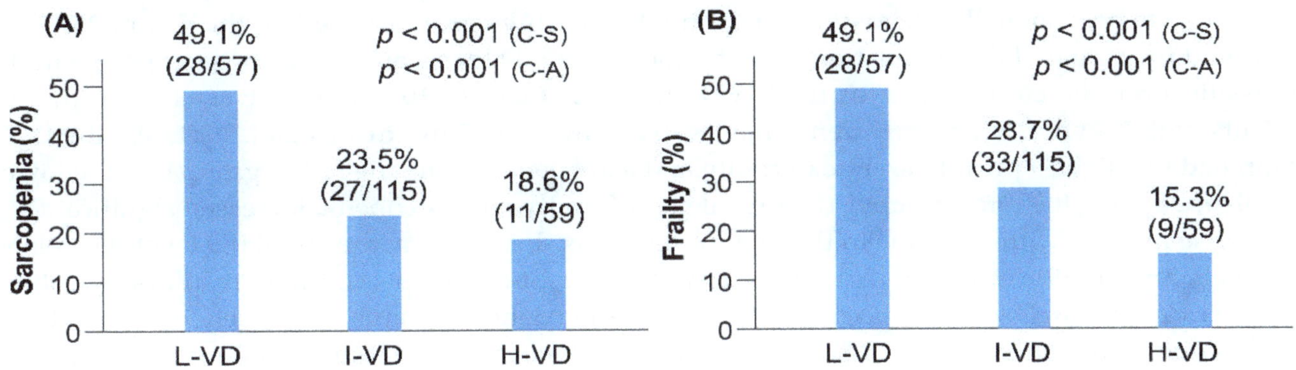

Figure 2. Comparison of clinical characteristics among the low vitamin D (L-VD), intermediate vitamin D (I-VD), and high vitamin D (H-VD) groups. (**A**) The L-VD group had the highest prevalence rate of sarcopenia (chi-squared test: $p < 0.001$), while the H-VD group had the lowest prevalence rate of sarcopenia (chi-squared test: $p < 0.001$) among the three groups. The prevalence of sarcopenia significantly increased in a stepwise manner with a decline in the serum 25-hydroxyvitamin D [25(OH)D] level (Cochran–Armitage trend test: $p < 0.001$). (**B**) The L-VD group had the highest prevalence rate of frailty (chi-squared test: $p < 0.001$), while the H-VD group had the lowest prevalence rate of frailty (chi-squared test: $p < 0.001$) among the three groups. The prevalence of frailty significantly increased in a stepwise manner with a decline in the 25(OH)D level (Cochran–Armitage trend test: $p < 0.001$). C-A, Cochran–Armitage trend test; C-S, chi-squared test.

3.8. Correlation between Serum 25(OH)D Levels and Baseline Clinical Characteristics

The serum 25(OH)D levels correlated significantly with the following baseline factors: BCAA, handgrip strength, SMI, and gait speed. The correlation coefficients for handgrip strength, SMI, and gait speed were 0.304 ($p < 0.001$), 0.220 ($p = 0.001$), and 0.251 ($p < 0.001$), respectively (Figure 3, Table S4).

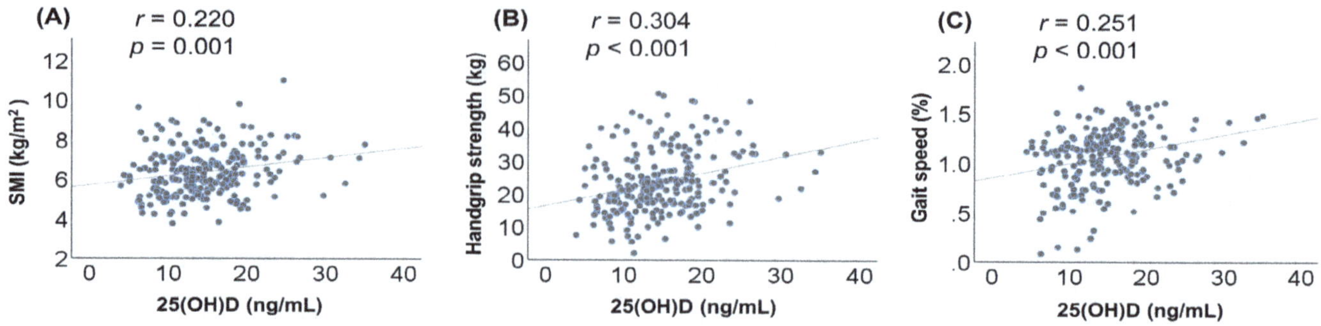

Figure 3. Correlations between the serum 25-hydroxyvitamin D [25(OH)D] levels and skeletal muscle mass index (SMI), handgrip strength, and gait speed in patients with chronic liver disease. The serum 25(OH)D levels were significantly correlated with the (**A**) SMI ($r = 0.220$, $p = 0.001$), (**B**) handgrip strength ($r = 0.304$, $p < 0.001$), and (**C**) gait speed ($r = 0.251$, $p < 0.001$).

4. Discussion

Some studies on elderly adults reported that vitamin D deficiency was associated with sarcopenia and impaired physical performance [25–28], while others reported that low vitamin D levels were related to frailty and mortality [29–32]. These results suggest that lower serum vitamin D levels are closely related to frailty and sarcopenia in elderly individuals. However, these relationships have not yet been reported and remain unclear in CLD. In this study, we focused on the relationships between serum vitamin D levels and frailty or sarcopenia in patients with CLD and showed that lower serum 25(OH)D levels were significantly and independently related to frailty and sarcopenia in such patients.

However, we failed to confirm a statistically significant relationship between the conventional classification of vitamin D status and frailty or sarcopenia, as most patients were vitamin D deficient. Therefore, we provisionally reclassified the patients into three groups based on the serum 25(OH)D levels and investigated the association between the vitamin D levels and frailty or sarcopenia. In this reclassification, the cutoff value for the L-VD group [25(OH)D ≤10.5 ng/mL] was close to that for patients with "severe" vitamin D deficiency (≤10 ng/mL or ≤12 ng/mL) [16,36]. Notably, the L-VD group had the highest prevalence rate of frailty and sarcopenia, while the H-VD group had the lowest prevalence among the three groups. The prevalence of frailty and sarcopenia increased significantly in a stepwise manner with a decline in the vitamin D status. In addition, the 25(OH)D levels correlated positively and significantly with handgrip strength, SMI, and gait speed. These results suggest that lower serum vitamin D levels, especially severe vitamin D deficient status, are closely related to frailty and sarcopenia in patients with CLD. In addition, the provisional reclassification used in the present study may be useful in clinically treating patients with CLD and frailty and/or sarcopenia.

The vitamin D molecule and vitamin D receptor (VDR) play crucial roles in regulating the musculoskeletal system [24,27,37]. The VDR is expressed in murine and human skeletal muscles, which suggests that vitamin D has direct effects on muscle tissue [27,38,39]. However, the expression level of VDR declines with increasing age [27]. Mice with vitamin D deficiency and global VDR knockout mice showed reduced muscle mass and strength, and muscle decline progressed with age and an increase in the duration of vitamin D deficiency [40]. In addition, both the mouse models showed significant increases in the expression level of myostatin, a member of the transforming growth factor-β family and a negative regulator of muscle protein synthesis [40]. An in vitro study has shown that vitamin D stimulates myogenic cell differentiation by modulating the expression of pro- and anti-myogenic factors [41].

Skeletal muscle fibers are classified into type I (slow-twitch) and type II (fast-twitch) fibers [27,42]. Type I muscle fibers are characterized by low-power production and high endurance capacity, while type II fibers are characterized by high speed and high strength contractions and are important for sprinting exercises [27]. Sarcopenia is characterized by a reduction in the size and proportion of type II fibers [42]. Histological assessment of muscle biopsy specimens from patients with vitamin D deficiency demonstrated a predominance of type II fiber atrophy accompanied by fat cell and glycogen granule infiltration and increased fibrosis [43]. These clinical and basic research findings indicate that both vitamin D deficiency and decreased VDR levels in muscle tissues are associated with sarcopenia and impaired physical performance. Indeed, in the present study, vitamin D deficiency was present in 87.0% (201/231) of the patients. Notably, approximately half of the patients in the L-VD group had both frailty and sarcopenia. These findings suggest that we must pay more careful attention to patients with severe vitamin D deficiency, especially those with CLD. However, this study did not investigate the expression of VDR in muscle tissues and the association between VDR expression levels and frailty/sarcopenia. Future studies should assess whether the levels of circulating vitamin D and VDR expression in muscle tissues are involved with these complications in patients with CLD.

As described previously, a long period of vitamin D deficiency exacerbates muscle weakness. Therefore, maintaining sufficient vitamin D levels is important to prevent the loss of muscle function [40]. A randomized controlled study of stroke survivors demonstrated that supplementation of vitamin D increased the number and size of type II muscle fibers and improved muscle strength, and consequently, reduced the frequency of falls and hip fractures [44]. Furthermore, vitamin D supplementation for four months increased the expression level of intramyonuclear VDR and the size of muscle fibers in older women with vitamin D insufficiency [45]. A systematic review with meta-analysis reported that daily supplementation of vitamin D improved muscle strength and balance in elderly adults, although its effect on gait was not observed [46]. Another meta-analysis of vitamin D supplementation trials showed positive effects on muscle strength; however, the effect was confined to the lower limbs, and vitamin D supplementation had no impact on muscle mass [47]. Hence, the effects of vitamin D supplementation on skeletal muscle mass and strength are controversial. Considering that sarcopenia has a multifactorial etiology, including nutrition, hormonal status, physical activity, and lifestyle, a comprehensive management strategy, including vitamin D supplementation, physical exercise, and awareness of complications, is required to treat and prevent sarcopenia.

This study has some limitations. First, we did not investigate the nutritional intakes and daily activities, including their exposure to sunlight, which might influence the serum 25(OH)D levels. Second, we did not investigate the mental state (including a depressed mood) and the use of antidepressants, which are associated with impaired physical activity and sarcopenia [48,49]. The severity of depression inversely correlates with serum vitamin D levels in patients with CLD [50].

5. Conclusions

In this study, we showed that lower serum 25(OH)D levels were significantly and independently related to frailty and sarcopenia in patients with CLD. The prevalence rates of frailty and sarcopenia significantly increased in a stepwise manner with a decline in the vitamin D status (the status was reclassified provisionally). The optimal classification of vitamin D status for patients with CLD may need to be reconsidered to treat those with frailty and/or sarcopenia. Comprehensive assessment (including serum 25(OH)D levels) and early therapeutic interventions (including vitamin D supplementation) are imperative, especially for patients with CLD and severe vitamin D deficiency.

Author Contributions: C.S. participated in the conception and design of the study. C.S., T.K., M.N., and Y.T. acquired, analyzed, and interpreted the data. C.S. and A.T. drafted the manuscript. T.O., M.S., and A.T. interpreted the data and revised the manuscript. A.T. substantively revised and completed the manuscript. All authors read and approved the final version of the manuscript.

Acknowledgments: We thank the medical staff at Fuji City General Hospital who were involved in the collection of the data.

References

1. Nishikawa, H.; Shiraki, M.; Hiramatsu, A.; Moriya, K.; Hino, K.; Nishiguchi, S. Japan Society of Hepatology guidelines for sarcopenia in liver disease (1st edition): Recommendation from the working group for creation of sarcopenia assessment criteria. *Hepatol. Res.* **2016**, *46*, 951–963. [CrossRef] [PubMed]
2. Saeki, C.; Takano, K.; Oikawa, T.; Aoki, Y.; Kanai, T.; Takakura, K.; Nakano, M.; Torisu, Y.; Sasaki, N.; Abo, M.; et al. Comparative assessment of sarcopenia using the JSH, AWGS, and EWGSOP2 criteria and the relationship between sarcopenia, osteoporosis, and osteosarcopenia in patients with liver cirrhosis. *BMC Musculoskelet. Disord.* **2019**, *20*, 615. [CrossRef] [PubMed]
3. Clegg, A.; Young, J.; Iliffe, S.; Rikkert, M.O.; Rockwood, K. Frailty in elderly people. *Lancet* **2013**, *38*, 752–762. [CrossRef]
4. Saeki, C.; Kanai, T.; Nakano, M.; Oikawa, T.; Torisu, Y.; Abo, M.; Saruta, M.; Tsubota, A. Relationship between Osteosarcopenia and Frailty in Patients with Chronic Liver Disease. *J. Clin. Med.* **2020**, *26*, 2381. [CrossRef] [PubMed]
5. Bhanji, R.A.; Narayanan, P.; Moynagh, M.R.; Takahashi, N.; Angirekula, M.; Kennedy, C.C.; Mara, K.C.; Dierkhising, R.A.; Watt, K.D. Differing Impact of Sarcopenia and Frailty in Nonalcoholic Steatohepatitis and Alcoholic Liver Disease. *Liver Transpl.* **2019**, *25*, 14–24. [CrossRef]
6. Tsekoura, M.; Kastrinis, A.; Katsoulaki, M.; Billis, E.; Gliatis, J. Sarcopenia and Its Impact on Quality of Life. *Adv. Exp. Med. Biol.* **2017**, *987*, 213–218.
7. Hanai, T.; Shiraki, M.; Nishimura, K.; Ohnishi, S.; Imai, K.; Suetsugu, A.; Takai, K.; Shimizu, M.; Moriwaki, H. Sarcopenia impairs prognosis of patients with liver cirrhosis. *Nutrition* **2015**, *31*, 193–199. [CrossRef]
8. Lai, J.C.; Covinsky, K.E.; Dodge, J.L.; Boscardin, W.J.; Segev, D.L.; Roberts, J.P.; Feng, S. Development of a novel frailty index to predict mortality in patients with end-stage liver disease. *Hepatology* **2017**, *66*, 564–574. [CrossRef]
9. Lai, J.C.; Rahimi, R.S.; Verna, E.C.; Kappus, M.R.; Dunn, M.A.; McAdams DeMarco, M.; Haugen, C.E.; Volk, M.L.; Duarte-Rojo, A.; Ganger, D.R.; et al. Frailty Associated With Waitlist Mortality Independent of Ascites and Hepatic Encephalopathy in a Multicenter Study. *Gastroenterology* **2019**, *156*, 1675–1682. [CrossRef]
10. Cruz-Jentoft, A.J.; Kiesswetter, E.; Drey, M.; Sieber, C.C. Nutrition, frailty, and sarcopenia. *Aging Clin. Exp. Res.* **2017**, *29*, 43–48. [CrossRef]
11. Bloom, I.; Shand, C.; Cooper, C.; Robinson, S.; Baird, J. Diet Quality and Sarcopenia in Older Adults: A Systematic Review. *Nutrients* **2018**, *10*, 308. [CrossRef] [PubMed]
12. Arteh, J.; Narra, S.; Nair, S. Prevalence of vitamin D deficiency in chronic liver disease. *Dig. Dis. Sci.* **2010**, *55*, 2624–2628. [CrossRef] [PubMed]
13. Nakchbandi, I.A. Osteoporosis and fractures in liver disease: Relevance, pathogenesis and therapeutic implications. *World J. Gastroenterol.* **2014**, *20*, 9427–9438. [PubMed]
14. Konstantakis, C.; Tselekouni, P.; Kalafateli, M.; Triantos, C. Vitamin D deficiency in patients with liver cirrhosis. *Ann. Gastroenterol.* **2016**, *29*, 297–306. [CrossRef]
15. Okubo, T.; Atsukawa, M.; Tsubota, A.; Yoshida, Y.; Arai, T.; Iwashita, A.N.; Itokawa, N.; Kondo, C.; Iwakiri, K. Relationship between serum vitamin D level and sarcopenia in chronic liver disease. *Hepatol. Res.* **2020**, *50*, 588–597. [CrossRef]
16. Buonomo, A.R.; Scotto, R.; Zappulo, E.; Nerilli, M.; Pinchera, B.; Perruolo, G.; Formisano, P.; Nappa, S.; Gentile, I. Severe Vitamin D Deficiency Increases Mortality Among Patients With Liver Cirrhosis Regardless of the Presence of HCC. *In Vivo* **2019**, *33*, 177–182. [CrossRef]
17. Atsukawa, M.; Tsubota, A.; Shimada, N.; Yoshizawa, K.; Abe, H.; Asano, T.; Ohkubo, Y.; Araki, M.; Ikegami, T.; Kondo, C.; et al. Influencing factors on serum 25-hydroxyvitamin D3 levels in Japanese chronic hepatitis C patients. *BMC Infect. Dis.* **2015**, *15*, 344. [CrossRef]

18. Aspell, N.; Laird, E.; Healy, M.; Shannon, T.; Lawlor, B.; O'Sullivan, M. The Prevalence and Determinants of Vitamin D Status in Community-Dwelling Older Adults: Results from the English Longitudinal Study of Ageing (ELSA). *Nutrients.* **2019**, *11*, 1253. [CrossRef]
19. Nakamura, K.; Tsugawa, N.; Saito, T.; Ishikawa, M.; Tsuchiya, Y.; Hyodo, K.; Maruyama, K.; Oshiki, R.; Kobayashi, R.; Nashimoto, M.; et al. Vitamin D status, bone mass, and bone metabolism in home-dwelling postmenopausal Japanese women: Yokogoshi Study. *Bone* **2008**, *42*, 271–277. [CrossRef]
20. Cashman, K.D.; Dowling, K.G.; Škrabáková, Z.; Gonzalez-Gross, M.; Valtueña, J.; De Henauw, S.; Moreno, L.; Damsgaard, C.T.; Michaelsen, K.F.; Mølgaard, C.; et al. Vitamin D deficiency in Europe: Pandemic? *Am. J. Clin. Nutr.* **2016**, *103*, 1033–1044. [CrossRef]
21. Liu, X.; Baylin, A.; Levy, P.D. Vitamin D deficiency and insufficiency among US adults: Prevalence, predictors and clinical implications. *Br. J. Nutr.* **2018**, *119*, 928–936. [CrossRef] [PubMed]
22. Paternostro, R.; Wagner, D.; Reiberger, T.; Mandorfer, M.; Schwarzer, R.; Ferlitsch, M.; Trauner, M.; Peck-Radosavljevic, M.; Ferlitsch, A. Low 25-OH-vitamin D levels reflect hepatic dysfunction and are associated with mortality in patients with liver cirrhosis. *Wien. Klin. Wochenschr.* **2017**, *29*, 8–15. [CrossRef] [PubMed]
23. Granic, A.; Hill, T.R.; Davies, K.; Jagger, C.; Adamson, A.; Siervo, M.; Kirkwood, T.B.; Mathers, J.C.; Sayer, A.A. Vitamin D Status, Muscle Strength and Physical Performance Decline in Very Old Adults: A Prospective Study. *Nutrients* **2017**, *9*, 379. [CrossRef] [PubMed]
24. Wintermeyer, E.; Ihle, C.; Ehnert, S.; Stöckle, U.; Ochs, G.; de Zwart, P.; Flesch, I.; Bahrs, C.; Nussler, A.K. Crucial Role of Vitamin D in the Musculoskeletal System. *Nutrients* **2016**, *8*, 319. [CrossRef]
25. Kim, M.K.; Baek, K.H.; Song, K.H.; Il Kang, M.; Park, C.Y.; Lee, W.Y.; Oh, K.W. Vitamin D deficiency is associated with sarcopenia in older Koreans, regardless of obesity: The Fourth Korea National Health and Nutrition Examination Surveys (KNHANES IV) 2009. *J. Clin. Endocrinol. Metab.* **2011**, *96*, 3250–3256. [CrossRef]
26. Houston, D.K.; Tooze, J.A.; Davis, C.C.; Chaves, P.H.; Hirsch, C.H.; Robbins, J.A.; Arnold, A.M.; Newman, A.B.; Kritchevsky, S.B. Serum 25-hydroxyvitamin D and physical function in older adults: The Cardiovascular Health Study All Stars. *J. Am. Geriatr Soc.* **2011**, *59*, 1793–1801. [CrossRef]
27. Remelli, F.; Vitali, A.; Zurlo, A.; Volpato, S. Vitamin D Deficiency and Sarcopenia in Older Persons. *Nutrients* **2019**, *11*, 2861. [CrossRef]
28. Tieland, M.; Brouwer-Brolsma, E.M.; Nienaber-Rousseau, C.; van Loon, L.J.; De Groot, L.C. Low vitamin D status is associated with reduced muscle mass and impaired physical performance in frail elderly people. *Eur. J. Clin. Nutr.* **2013**, *67*, 1050–1055. [CrossRef]
29. Wilhelm-Leen, E.R.; Hall, Y.N.; Deboer, I.H.; Chertow, G.M. Vitamin D deficiency and frailty in older Americans. *J. Intern. Med.* **2010**, *268*, 171–180. [CrossRef]
30. Vaes, A.M.M.; Brouwer-Brolsma, E.M.; Toussaint, N.; de Regt, M.; Tieland, M.; van Loon, L.J.C.; de Groot, L.C. The association between 25-hydroxyvitamin D concentration, physical performance and frailty status in older adults. *Eur. J. Nutr.* **2019**, *58*, 1173–1181. [CrossRef]
31. Wong, Y.Y.; McCaul, K.A.; Yeap, B.B.; Hankey, G.J.; Flicker, L. Low vitamin D status is an independent predictor of increased frailty and all-cause mortality in older men: The Health in Men Study. *J. Clin. Endocrinol. Metab.* **2013**, *98*, 3821–3828. [CrossRef] [PubMed]
32. Smit, E.; Crespo, C.J.; Michael, Y.; Ramirez-Marrero, F.A.; Brodowicz, G.R.; Bartlett, S.; Andersen, R.E. The effect of vitamin D and frailty on mortality among non-institutionalized US older adults. *Eur. J. Clin. Nutr.* **2012**, *66*, 1024–1028. [CrossRef] [PubMed]
33. Fried, L.P.; Tangen, C.M.; Walston, J.; Newman, A.B.; Hirsch, C.; Gottdiener, J.; Seeman, T.; Tracy, R.; Kop, W.J.; Burke, G.; et al. Cardiovascular Health Study Collaborative Research Group. Frailty in older adults: Evidence for a phenotype. *J. Gerontol. A Biol. Sci. Med. Sci.* 2001; 5, M146–M156.
34. Tsutsumimoto, K.; Doi, T.; Makizako, H.; Hotta, R.; Nakakubo, S.; Makino, K.; Suzuki, T.; Shimada, H. Aging-related anorexia and its association with disability and frailty. *J. Cachexia Sarcopenia Muscle* **2018**, *9*, 834–843. [CrossRef] [PubMed]
35. Holick, M.F.; Binkley, N.C.; Bischoff-Ferrari, H.A.; Gordon, C.M.; Hanley, D.A.; Heaney, R.P.; Murad, M.H.; Weaver, C.M. Evaluation, treatment, and prevention of vitamin D deficiency: An Endocrine Society clinical practice guideline. *J. Clin. Endocrinol. Metab.* **2011** *96*, 1911–1930. [CrossRef]

36. Amrein, K.; Scherkl, M.; Hoffmann, M.; Neuwersch-Sommeregger, S.; Köstenberger, M.; Berisha, A.T.; Martucci, G.; Pilz, S.; Malle, O. Vitamin D deficiency 2.0: An update on the current status worldwide. *Eur. J. Clin. Nutr.* **2020**, *20*, 1–16. [CrossRef]
37. Pojednic, R.M.; Ceglia, L. The emerging biomolecular role of vitamin D in skeletal muscle. *Exerc. Sport Sci. Rev.* **2014**, *42*, 76–81. [CrossRef]
38. Girgis, C.M.; Mokbel, N.; Cha, K.M.; Houweling, P.J.; Abboud, M.; Fraser, D.R.; Mason, R.S.; Clifton-Bligh, R.J.; Gunton, J.E. The vitamin D receptor (VDR) is expressed in skeletal muscle of male mice and modulates 25-hydroxyvitamin D (25OHD) uptake in myofibers. *Endocrinology* **2014**, *155*, 3227–3237. [CrossRef]
39. Pojednic, R.M.; Ceglia, L.; Olsson, K.; Gustafsson, T.; Lichtenstein, A.H.; Dawson-Hughes, B.; Fielding, R.A. Effects of 1,25-dihydroxyvitamin D3 and vitamin D3 on the expression of the vitamin d receptor in human skeletal muscle cells. *Calcif. Tissue Int.* **2015**, *96*, 256–263. [CrossRef]
40. Girgis, C.M.; Cha, K.M.; Houweling, P.J.; Rao, R.; Mokbel, N.; Lin, M.; Clifton-Bligh, R.J.; Gunton, J.E. Vitamin D Receptor Ablation and Vitamin D Deficiency Result in Reduced Grip Strength, Altered Muscle Fibers, and Increased Myostatin in Mice. *Calcif. Tissue Int.* **2015**, *97*, 602–610. [CrossRef]
41. Garcia, L.A.; King, K.K.; Ferrini, M.G.; Norris, K.C.; Artaza, J.N. 1,25(OH)2vitamin D3 stimulates myogenic differentiation by inhibiting cell proliferation and modulating the expression of promyogenic growth factors and myostatin in C2C12 skeletal muscle cells. *Endocrinology* **2011**, *152*, 2976–2986. [CrossRef]
42. Talbot, J.; Maves, L. Skeletal muscle fiber type: Using insights from muscle developmental biology to dissect targets for susceptibility and resistance to muscle disease. *Wiley Interdiscip. Rev. Dev. Biol.* **2016**, *5*, 518–534. [CrossRef] [PubMed]
43. Ceglia, L.; Harris, S.S. Vitamin D and its role in skeletal muscle. *Calcif. Tissue Int.* **2013**, *92*, 151–162. [CrossRef] [PubMed]
44. Sato, Y.; Iwamoto, J.; Kanoko, T.; Satoh, K. Low-dose vitamin D prevents muscular atrophy and reduced falls and hip fractures in women after stroke: A randomized controlled trial. *Cerebrovasc. Dis.* **2005**, *20*, 187–192, Retracted in *Cerebrovasc. Dis.* **2017**, *44*, 240. [CrossRef] [PubMed]
45. Ceglia, L.; Niramitmahapanya, S.; da Silva Morais, M.; Rivas, D.A.; Harris, S.S.; Bischoff-Ferrari, H.; Fielding, R.A.; Dawson-Hughes, B. A randomized study on the effect of vitamin D_3 supplementation on skeletal muscle morphology and vitamin D receptor concentration in older women. *J. Clin. Endocrinol. Metab.* **2013**, *98*, E1927–E1935. [CrossRef] [PubMed]
46. Muir, S.W.; Montero-Odasso, M. Effect of vitamin D supplementation on muscle strength, gait and balance in older adults: A systematic review and meta-analysis. *J. Am. Geriatr. Soc.* **2011**, *59*, 2291–2300. [CrossRef]
47. Beaudart, C.; Buckinx, F.; Rabenda, V.; Gillain, S.; Cavalier, E.; Slomian, J.; Petermans, J.; Reginster, J.Y.; Bruyère, O. The effects of vitamin D on skeletal muscle strength, muscle mass, and muscle power: A systematic review and meta-analysis of randomized controlled trials. *J. Clin. Endocrinol. Metab.* **2014**, *99*, 4336–4345. [CrossRef]
48. Nishikawa, H.; Enomoto, H.; Yoh, K.; Iwata, Y.; Sakai, Y.; Kishino, K.; Ikeda, N.; Takashima, T.; Aizawa, N.; Takata, R.; et al. Association between Sarcopenia and Depression in Patients with Chronic Liver Diseases. *J. Clin. Med.* **2019**, *8*, 634. [CrossRef]
49. An, R.; Lu, L. Antidepressant use and functional limitations in U.S. older adults. *J. Psychosom. Res.* **2016**, *80*, 31–36. [CrossRef]
50. Stokes, C.S.; Grünhage, F.; Baus, C.; Volmer, D.A.; Wagenpfeil, S.; Riemenschneider, M.; Lammert, F. Vitamin D supplementation reduces depressive symptoms in patients with chronic liver disease. *Clin. Nutr.* **2016**, *35*, 950–957. [CrossRef]

5

Vitamin D and Sarcopenia: Potential of Vitamin D Supplementation in Sarcopenia Prevention and Treatment

Ran Uchitomi †, Mamoru Oyabu † and Yasutomi Kamei *

Graduate School of Life and Environmental Sciences, Kyoto Prefectural University, Kyoto 606-8522, Japan; s820731001@kpu.ac.jp (R.U.); s820631011@kpu.ac.jp (M.O.)

* Correspondence: kamei@kpu.ac.jp

† These authors contributed equally to this work.

Abstract: Skeletal muscle, the largest organ in the human body, accounting for approximately 40% of body weight, plays important roles in exercise and energy expenditure. In the elderly, there is often a progressive decline in skeletal muscle mass and function, a condition known as sarcopenia, which can lead to bedridden conditions, wheelchair confinement as well as reducing the quality of life (QOL). In developed countries with aging populations, the prevention and management of sarcopenia are important for the improvement of health and life expectancy in these populations. Recently, vitamin D, a fat-soluble vitamin, has been attracting attention due to its importance in sarcopenia. This review will focus on the effects of vitamin D deficiency and supplementation on sarcopenia.

Keywords: vitamin D; sarcopenia; atrophy; skeletal muscle; gene regulation; nuclear receptor

---

1. Sarcopenia

The term "sarcopenia" was first proposed by Rosenberg in 1989 and is derived from the Greek "sarx", meaning flesh and "penia", meaning loss [1,2]. Originally, sarcopenia referred only to the loss of skeletal muscle mass with aging. In 2010, the European Working Group on Sarcopenia in Older People (EWGSOP) defined sarcopenia as a syndrome characterized by the progressive and generalized loss of skeletal muscle mass and strength with a risk of adverse outcomes such as physical disability, poor quality of life (QOL), and death [3]. Another definition by the International Working Group on Sarcopenia described sarcopenia as an age-associated loss of skeletal muscle mass and function [4].

Sarcopenia has been associated with the propensity of elderly people to fall. It has been reported that sarcopenic individuals aged 80 years or older were over three times more likely to fall during a two-year observation period compared with non-sarcopenic individuals [5]. Furthermore, evidence from nine prospective cohort studies has shown that people with a high skeletal muscle mass and a fast walking speed have greater longevity as they are less likely to suffer from sarcopenia [6].

1.1. *Etiology of Sarcopenia*

Sarcopenia is classified as either primary or secondary based on etiological factors (Table 1). Sarcopenia is considered "primary" when no other specific cause other than aging is evident, while it is considered "secondary" when causal factors besides aging are apparent. Sarcopenia can occur secondary to a systemic disease, especially inflammatory diseases, e.g., malignancy or organ failure, and endocrine diseases such as diabetes mellitus. Physical inactivity also contributes to the development of sarcopenia. Moreover, sarcopenia can develop as a result of undernutrition or malabsorption.

Table 1. Etiology of primary and secondary sarcopenia.

Categories	Causes
Primary sarcopenia	
Aging	Age-related muscle loss
Secondary sarcopenia	
Disease	Inflammatory conditions (e.g., malignancy or organ failure) Endocrine disease (e.g., diabetes mellitus)
Inactivity	Sedentary lifestyle (e.g., bedridden, dependent on a wheelchair or disease-related limited mobility)
Malnutrition	Undernutrition or malabsorption Medication-related anorexia

1.2. *Diagnosis of Sarcopenia*

The most widely accepted method of diagnosing sarcopenia is from the EWGSOP, which considers the reduction in muscle mass and function (muscle strength or physical ability) as the standard criteria [3]. This has been further developed by a second convening of EWGSOP (EWGSOP2) to emphasize low muscle strength as the primary indicator of sarcopenia [7]. When low muscle strength is detected, it is increasingly likely that sarcopenia is present. The diagnosis is confirmed when low muscle strength is accompanied by low muscle quantity or quality. If physical performance is also poor, then the sarcopenia is considered severe.

Appendicular muscle mass is most commonly assessed using dual-energy X-ray absorptiometry (DXA) and bioelectrical impedance analysis (BIA). Walking speed (<0.8 m/s) and the 400 m walking test (>6 min) are recommended for the evaluation of physical performance [7]. The Asian Working Group for Sarcopenia (AWGS) has revised cutoff values for some diagnostic criteria: low muscle strength is defined as handgrip strength of <28 kg and <18 kg for men and women, respectively, reduced physical performance in the 6 m walking test is a speed of <1.0 m/s, and a time of ≥12 s in the chair stand test for five rises [8].

1.3. *Prevalence of Sarcopenia*

The prevalence of sarcopenia in 1882 elderly Japanese individuals, aged 65 to 89 years, was observed to be 21.8% and 22.1% for men and women, respectively, with diagnosis based on the EWGSOP criteria [9]. Other research with 243 elderly Thai participants indicated a sarcopenia prevalence of 30.5% (33.9% for men and 29.3% for women) [10]. Few studies have reported the prevalence of sarcopenia based on the EWGSOP2 criteria. EWGSOP2-defined sarcopenia prevalence was lower than that defined using EWGSOP-1 criteria due to the difference in diagnostic factors to detect sarcopenia. Reiss et al. reported a sarcopenia prevalence of 18.1% using the EWGSOP2 criteria versus a 27.7% prevalence with the EWGSOP criteria in 144 geriatric patients [11]. Similarly, in a study with 501 subjects, Locquet et al. observed a prevalence of sarcopenia of 7.4% and 13.6% for EWGSOP2 and EWGSOP, respectively [12].

On the other hand, the revisions made to the AWGS criteria appear to have the opposite effect on prevalence. In a study with 2123 elderly participants, aged 70–84 years, the prevalence of sarcopenia in men and women was 21.3% and 13.8%, respectively, with the revised AWGS criteria. The older AWGS criteria yielded a prevalence of 10.3% for men and 8.1% for women. In this case, revising the AWGS criteria seems to have relaxed the conditions under which sarcopenia is diagnosed [13]. The prevalence of sarcopenia is heavily dependent on the criteria that are used to diagnose it and since no criteria are used universally, the prevalence may vary widely.

2. Vitamin D

Vitamin D is a fat-soluble vitamin that can act as a hormone through a nuclear receptor. Vitamin D was discovered in cod liver oil as the anti-rickets factor in the 1930s. Since then, research on the metabolism of vitamin D has been conducted in a variety of species, and the metabolic pathways have been elucidated [14]. The most important function of vitamin D is in the regulation of Ca^{2+}

concentration in the circulating blood, whose deficiency leads to diseases such as rickets in children and osteomalacia in adults [14]. It has recently been proven that deficiency or insufficiency in vitamin D is positively correlated with the risk of several diseases including sarcopenia, cardiovascular diseases, obesity, and cancer. Indeed, Remelli et al. reviewed the biological, clinical and epidemiological evidence supporting the association between vitamin D and an increased risk of sarcopenia in older people [15]. Consequently, attention has been drawn to the other aspects of vitamin D metabolism other than Ca^{2+} homeostasis. Vitamin D has significant effects on several other tissues [16], and the following sections will review its effects on skeletal muscle, including recent progress, and consequences on sarcopenia.

2.1. *Synthesis and Metabolism of Vitamin D*

Vitamin D is primarily produced in the skin when it has been exposed to ultraviolet (UV) rays. A product of cholesterol synthesis, 7-dehydrocholesterol, is converted into previtamin D by irradiation with ultraviolet light B (UVB) of wavelengths from 290 to 320 nm. The previtamin D is in turn non-enzymatically converted to vitamin D via double bond transfer which occurs at body temperature. However, it is required to ingest some dietary vitamin D to compensate for the shortage caused by insufficient de novo synthesis of vitamin D in the skin. Dietary vitamin D is divided into two groups: vitamin D_3 (cholecalciferol), present in fish and egg yolk, and vitamin D_2 (ergocalciferol) which is found in mushrooms. Approximately 80% of vitamin D is synthesized in the skin upon UVB exposure and the remainder is derived from the diet. These values may differ depending on factors such as ethnicity, duration of exposure to sunlight, and season [17,18]. Vitamin D is absorbed in the small intestine, then incorporated into chylomicrons that are transported via lymphatic vessels into the veins for distribution throughout the body. Serum vitamin D is conjugated to a vitamin D binding protein and transported to the liver where vitamin D is metabolized. Metabolism of vitamin D is mediated by cytochrome P450 oxidases (CYPs) [19] (Figure 1). Vitamin D is hydroxylated at the C25 site by CYP2R1 or CYP27A1 in the liver leading to the production of 25-hydroxyvitamin D [25(OH)D]. Serum 25(OH)D levels are used to determine vitamin D sufficiency. The 25(OH)D is hydroxylated at the C1α site by CYP27B1 in the kidney, producing 1α,25-dihydroxyvitamin D [1,25$(OH)_2$D]. The 1,25$(OH)_2$D then binds to a vitamin D receptor (VDR), a nuclear, ligand-dependent transcription factor, eliciting several physiological responses through the regulation of multiple VDR target gene expressions. Both 25(OH)D and 1,25$(OH)_2$D are metabolized by CYP24A1, inactivated and in part excreted into the feces as bile or in urine [20] (Figure 1).

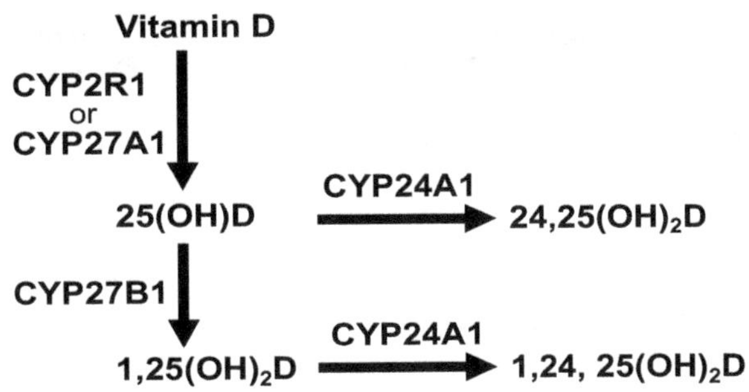

Figure 1. Vitamin D metabolic pathway by cytochrome P450 oxidases (CYPs). Vitamin D is hydroxylated at the C25 site by CYP2R1 or CYP27A1 in the liver leading to the production of 25-hydroxyvitamin D [25(OH)D]. The 25(OH)D is hydroxylated at the C1α site by CYP27B1 in the kidney, producing 1α,25-dihydroxyvitamin D [1,25$(OH)_2$D]. Both 25(OH)D and 1,25$(OH)_2$D are metabolized by CYP24A1, inactivated and in part excreted into the feces as bile or in urine.

2.2. *Vitamin D Deficiency and Hypervitaminosis D*

Vitamin D deficiency reduces calcium and phosphorus absorption from the intestinal tract. This results in hypocalcemia and hypophosphatemia which can cause rickets in children and osteomalacia in adults [20]. The primary cause of vitamin D deficiency is reduced vitamin D synthesis in the skin which can be caused by: inadequate UV exposure, excessive use of sunscreen, and limited outdoor activity. Deficiency is also associated with decreased ingestion of dietary vitamin D, aging, and hepatic or renal disorders. The nutritional status of vitamin D is evaluated by measuring the serum 25(OH)D concentration. A concentration of 30 ng/mL is indicative of vitamin D insufficiency and that of 20 ng/mL and less reflects deficiency [21].

Hypervitaminosis D, excess vitamin D, is responsible for hypercalcemia, renal dysfunction, and nephrocalcinosis. However, vitamin D is relatively safe as hypervitaminosis D is caused by the substantial consumption of vitamin D over an extended period (a few months). Furthermore, elevated 1,25$(OH)_2$D levels due to increased intake of vitamin D inhibit the activity of the renal enzyme CYP27B1 and stimulate CYP24A1 activity, leading to reduced serum 1,25$(OH)_2$D levels [22].

2.3. Regulation of Gene Expression by the Vitamin D/VDR

The VDR is a nuclear receptor, ligand-dependent transcription factor [23], which forms complexes with co-factor proteins [24,25]; these complexes regulate gene expression in numerous physiological processes. Once the 1,25$(OH)_2$D binds to the VDR as a ligand, VDR interacts with its heterodimer partner, retinoid X receptor, and subsequently binds to the vitamin D response element (VDRE) located on the target genes [26,27]. Activated VDR induces the gene expression of CYP24A1 (Figure 2), which inactivates 1,25$(OH)_2$D by hydroxylation at C24, as a negative feedback machinery [28]. Transient receptor potential vanilloid—subfamily V, member 6 (TRPV6), a calcium channel in the small intestinal mucous membrane—is also a target gene of VDR [29]. In addition, there are more VDR-target genes, such as fibroblast growth factor-23 (FGF23) and receptor activator of NF-kappaB ligand (RANKL), involved in calcium and phosphate homeostasis [30,31]. Recently, dystrobrevin alpha (DTNA), a member of the dystrophin-associated protein complex (DPAC), was also identified as the VDR-target gene in skeletal muscle cells [32]. Moreover, 1,25$(OH)_2$D increases the expression of the VDR gene itself [33] (Figure 2). Meanwhile, the activation of VDR has been reported to be caused by bile acids, as an endogenous ligand [34,35] (Figure 2). Vitamin D is also known to act independently of VDR. Recently, Asano et al. demonstrated that 25(OH)D induces the degradation of sterol regulatory element-binding protein (SREBP) cleavage-activating protein (SCAP) without VDR, consequently suppressing SREBP-2, a transcription factor that induces cholesterol synthesis [36].

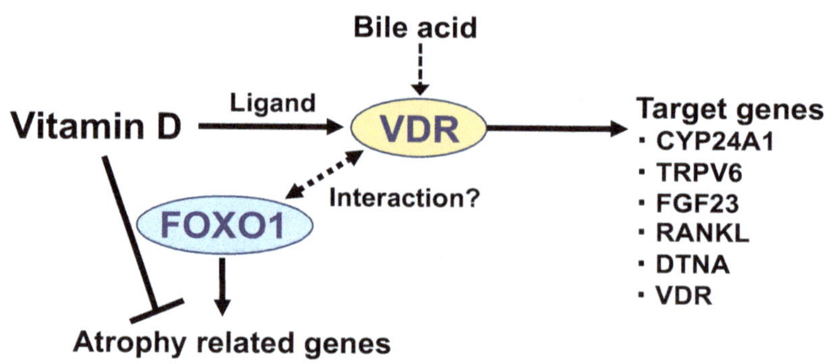

Figure 2. Vitamin D regulates the expression of the target genes by binding to the vitamin D receptor (VDR). The primary target genes for VDR [28–33] are shown in Figure 2. CYP24A1, cytochrome P450 family 24 subfamily A member 1; TRPV6, transient receptor potential cation channel subfamily V member 6; FGF23, fibroblast growth factor 23; RANKL, receptor activator of nuclear factor-kappaB-ligand; DTNA, dystrobrevin alpha; and VDR. In skeletal muscle, vitamin D has been shown to suppress the expression of muscle atrophy-related genes (atrogin-1 and cathepsin L). Possibly, this is achieved by the ability of vitamin D to repress the transcriptional activity of the forkhead box protein O1 (FOXO1), which activates the genes involved in protein degradation (discussed in later section). FOXO1 has been reported to physically interact with multiple nuclear receptors (possibly with VDR) [37,38], which may be responsible for the suppression of atrophy-related gene expression. However, further investigations are required to shed light on the relationship between vitamin D and FOXO1.

3. Vitamin D and Sarcopenia

3.1. Vitamin D Deficiency and Sarcopenia

A positive correlation has been shown to exist between serum 25(OH)D concentration and muscle function. Serum 25(OH)D concentrations <30 ng/mL (75 nM) and <20 ng/mL (50 nM) are indicative of vitamin D insufficiency and deficiency, respectively [21]. In a study by Okuno et al., vitamin D insufficiency was reported in 89% and deficiency in 28% of a sample of 80 elderly Japanese women over the age of 65 years [39]. Of those whose vitamin D levels were insufficient or deficient, 56.3% experienced falls during a three-month observation period. In another report, a meta-analysis of five randomized controlled trials investigating the effects of vitamin D supplementation (20 μg/day, 800 IU/day) on falls and bone fractures in the elderly revealed that vitamin D supplementation lowered the risk of falling by 22% compared with calcium alone or a placebo. Furthermore, vitamin D supplementation at 20 μg/day resulted in a significantly lower incidence of bone fracturing compared with a supplementation rate of 10 μg/day (400 IU/day) [40]. It has been concluded that elderly individuals with low serum 25(OH)D concentrations are susceptible to sarcopenia [41]. A decline in serum 25(OH)D concentration with advanced age results in reduced bone density, leading to a higher risk of falling and bone fractures. It has been observed that the expression of CYP24A1, an enzyme that inactivates $1,25(OH)_2D$, increases with age in the rat kidney [28]. MacLaughlin and Holick concluded that reduced outdoor activity with aging results in a decline in the ability to synthesize vitamin D and a two-fold decrease in previtamin D production by the skin [42]. These factors culminate in low serum 25(OH)D concentrations in elderly individuals. Another consequence of aging is the reduced ability to synthesize $1,25(OH)_2D$ in the kidneys [43].

Sarcopenic patients often become obese (sarcopenic obesity) as a result of the negative correlation that exists between serum 25(OH)D concentration and body fat mass. Vitamin D deficiency is frequently observed in obese people [44]. It has been shown that vitamin D inhibits the differentiation of 3T3-L1 preadipocytes to mature adipocytes [33,45]. It follows that low serum concentrations of 25(OH)D would mean that there is a reduced inhibitory effect on the differentiation of preadipocytes, hence obesity becomes probable.

3.2. Vitamin D and Muscle Strength

Studies on vitamin D supplementation have shown an increase in muscle strength due to supplementation. A systematic review of twenty-nine studies investigating the implications of vitamin D supplementation on muscle strength revealed that vitamin D supplementation significantly increased muscle strength—more so in individuals with serum 25(OH)D concentrations <30 ng/mL versus those with >30 ng/mL. This implies that vitamin D supplementation is more effective in cases were serum 25(OH)D concentrations are low, as is the case with elderly individuals [46]. A separate study also showed that muscle nuclear VDR was increased by 30% and augmented muscle fiber size by 10% in elderly females (mean age of 78 years) taking vitamin D orally at a rate of 100 μg/day (4000 IU/day) for 4 months [47]. On the contrary, a meta-analysis of seven controlled trials with vitamin D supplementation showed an improvement in upper and lower limb muscle strength in healthy 18–40-year-old participants. This shows that the benefits of vitamin D supplementation are not limited to the elderly and frail [48]. The administration of vitamin D may improve muscle strength and muscle mass and may be useful for the prevention and therapeutic intervention of sarcopenia. However, vitamin D supplementation does not always improve muscle function as seen in the meta-analysis of 16 randomized, controlled trials investigating the effects of vitamin D supplementation on muscle function in postmenopausal women. Vitamin D supplementation did not improve grip strength and back muscle strength, which are indicators of general muscle strength [49]. These differences in the effects of vitamin D supplementation may be due to several reasons such as the amount and type of vitamin D used, the duration of the intervention, and the state of vitamin D sufficiency in the subjects. Further research is needed in this area.

4. Mechanism of Action of Vitamin D on Skeletal Muscle

4.1. Expression of VDR in Skeletal Muscle

Vitamin D is metabolically converted into active 1,25$(OH)_2$D by the metabolic enzyme CYP27B1 in the kidney, and subsequently binds to the nuclear receptor VDR to regulate the target gene expression. The expression of VDR and CYP27B1 was observed in neonatal and damaged skeletal muscle, and to a lesser extent in mature skeletal muscle tissue [50,51]. Systemic VDR knockout (KO) mice have been observed to have reduced muscle mass, muscle fiber size, and muscle strength (grip strength) compared with wild-type mice [52]. Another phenotypic study with VDR-KO mice showed muscle fiber size atrophy at three weeks of age and pronounced muscle atrophy at eight weeks. There was also delayed skeletal muscle maturation characterized by persistent immature neonatal-type myosin heavy chain expression up to 3 weeks of age in skeletal muscle of the VDR-KO mice [53]. Similarly, in skeletal muscle-specific VDR-KO mice, decreased voluntary activity in rotating cages, declined muscle function (examined as lower grip strength), and reduced muscle mass were all recorded. Additionally, the expression of sarcoendoplasmic reticulum calcium transport ATPase (SERCA) and Calbindin, genes involved in the regulation of intracellular calcium concentration, decreased in skeletal muscle of skeletal muscle-specific VDR-KO mice [54]. These reports suggest that vitamin D improves muscle function and muscle mass through the mediation of VDR, although the detailed mechanisms are still unclear.

4.2. Vitamin D Effects on the Expression of Atrophy-Related Genes

Vitamin D can suppress the activity of atrophy-related transcription factors. We have been investigating the mechanisms underlying the regulation of skeletal muscle metabolism by FOXO1. Based on the fact that energy deprivation increases FOXO1 gene expression in skeletal muscle, genetically modified mice with an overexpression of FOXO1 specifically in skeletal muscle have been generated and used to show that FOXO1 causes muscle atrophy [55]. The increased expression of FOXO1 is commonly observed during muscle atrophy under multiple pathophysiological conditions such as malnutrition, inactivity, and cancer [56,57]. FOXO1 and its analog FOXO3a are known to induce muscle atrophy by mechanisms that include enhanced protein degradation through the ubiquitin-proteasome system and autophagy induction [55,58]. A reporter assay system was prepared with the intention of measuring the transcriptional activity of FOXO1. After screening several compounds derived from various foods and plants, it was found that 1,25$(OH)_2$D suppressed the transcriptional activity of FOXO1 [59]. Moreover, 1,25$(OH)_2$D suppressed the increased expression of atrogin-1 and cathepsin L, target genes for FOXO1, which induces muscle atrophy in C2C12 myoblasts [59] (Figure 2). Interestingly, Yang et al. recently reported that physical inactivity and low serum vitamin D can synergistically promote sarcopenia in the elderly [60]. Under inactive conditions, vitamin D deficiency accelerated the loss of muscle mass, muscle cross-sectional area, and grip strength, and conversely increased protein expression of FOXO3a and its target genes (Atrogin-1 and MuRF1). In older adults, serum 25 (OH) D_3 and physical activity showed interactive effects on physical performance (timed up and go test) and muscle strength (grip strength) [60].

4.3. Vitamin D Effects on Protein Synthesis and Skeletal Muscle Hypertrophy

Recent evidence indicated that vitamin D can also stimulate protein synthesis via mammalian target of rapamycin complex 1 (mTORC1) signaling and induce skeletal muscle hypertrophy. Bass et al. demonstrated that overexpression of VDR in rats induced muscle hypertrophy, which was characterized by the increased muscle cross-sectional area, and that it enhanced anabolic signaling and translational efficacy, resulting in increased phosphorylated mTOR (p-mTOR) and downstream targets (p-4E-BP and p-p70S6K) [61]. Conversely, vitamin D deficiency in rats inhibited mTORC1 signaling and contributed to decreased protein synthesis in skeletal muscle [62]. These reports suggest that VDR in skeletal muscle plays important roles in muscle hypertrophy.

4.4. *Effects of Vitamin D on Skeletal Muscle Mitochondria*

Mitochondrial dysfunction results in mild but chronic inflammation due to increased production of reactive oxygen species, leading to qualitative/quantitative deterioration of skeletal muscle, which is thought to be one of the major causes of sarcopenia onset [63]. Reports suggest that 1,25$(OH)_2D$ supplementation improves the function of mitochondrial oxidative phosphorylation in the skeletal muscle in vitamin D deficient humans [64]. Furthermore, the introduction of 1,25$(OH)_2D$ to human skeletal muscle cells enhances the oxygen consumption rate of mitochondria and activates pyruvate dehydrogenase [65]. The regulation of mitochondrial respiration via 1,25$(OH)_2D$ is dependent on the VDR because silencing of the VDR in skeletal muscle cells reduces mitochondrial oxygen consumption rate and adenosine triphosphate (ATP) production derived from oxidative phosphorylation [66]. In addition, 1,25$(OH)_2D$ also ameliorates the palmitic acid (PA)-induced mitochondrial dysfunction and triglyceride (TG) accumulation in skeletal muscle cells [67]. In elderly individuals aged 60 to 80, vitamin D has been reported to reduce intramyocellular lipid accumulation in combination with treadmill aerobic training [68]. Hence, 1,25$(OH)_2D$ may have beneficial effects on skeletal muscle by regulating mitochondrial function.

5. Guidelines of Vitamin D Intake and Actual Intake

The Dietary Reference Intake (2020) in Japan determines the Adequate Intake (AI) for vitamin D which was recently reviewed upwards from 5.5 μg/day (220 IU) to 8.5 μg/day (340 IU) (Table 2) [69]. However, this value is still much lower than in other countries. Previously, the Dietary Reference Intake of the United States and Canada specified the AI for vitamin D, but changed to the Estimated Average Requirement and Recommended Dietary Allowance in 2011 [70]. The recommended quantities are: 15 μg/day (600 IU) for people under 70 years old; 20 μg/day (800 IU) for those 71 years and older. According to the International Osteoporosis Foundation, dietary vitamin D intake from 20 to 25 μg/day (800 to 1000 IU/day) is required to prevent both falls and bone fractures in elderly women (Table 2) [71].

Table 2. Comparison of vitamin D requirements.

Dietary Reference Intake for Japanese	
2005	5.0 μg/day (200 IU)
2015	5.5 μg/day (220 IU)
2020	8.5 μg/day (340 IU)
Dietary Reference Intake for the U.S. and Canada (2011)	
9–70 years	15 μg/day (600 IU)
>70 years	20 μg/day (800 IU)
International Osteoporosis Foundation (IOF) Position Statement	
Fracture prevention	20 μg/day (800 IU)
Fall prevention	25 μg/day (1000 IU)

6. Vitamin D Fortified Foods

Dairy products make up the bulk of the foods that are fortified with vitamin D. Programs to develop vitamin D fortified foods such as milk, margarine, and yogurt have been introduced in several countries, including the United States, Canada, and Finland [18]. A recent study reported that garden pea protein-based, small vitamin D nanoemulsion (233 nm) increased the efficiency of vitamin D transport into Caco-2 cells by up to 5.3 times that of a free vitamin D suspension [72]. Similarly, Almajwal et al. found that Wistar rats fed a vitamin D deficient diet (vitamin D < 50 IU/kg (25 μg/kg)) for 6 weeks were soon restored to normal serum 25(OH)D levels by oral administration of garden pea protein-based vitamin D fortified nanoemulsion (containing 81 μg of vitamin D) given every other day for one week (three times in total). In contrast, there was no improvement in serum 25(OH)D in the group given canola oil supplemented with the same amount of vitamin D [73]. In the future, studies on the development of foods fortified with vitamin D by way of nanoemulsion technology, as well as functional foods containing vitamin D, may significantly increase the bioavailability of vitamin D in the elderly, ultimately contributing to improved vitamin D deficiency interventions.

7. Closing Remarks

In developed countries with large proportions of elderly citizens, the prevention of sarcopenia and the management of its progression are important issues in terms of reducing health care costs and improvement of QOL. Evidence is given from several studies on the efficacy of vitamin D as an intervention in cases of sarcopenia in the elderly. However, whether supplementation with vitamin D in sarcopenia patients has beneficial effects such as suppression of muscle atrophy and increased muscle strength is controversial, in part because of the complicated mechanisms underlying the action of vitamin D on muscle tissue. Further studies on vitamin D and sarcopenia will be useful in shedding more light on the matter.

Author Contributions: R.U., M.O. and Y.K. wrote the paper, evaluated the data and participated in preparing the manuscript. All authors have read and agreed to the published version of the manuscript.

References

1. Rosenberg, I.H. Sarcopenia: Origins and clinical relevance. *J. Nutr.* **1997**, *127* (Suppl. 5), 990S–991S. [CrossRef] [PubMed]
2. Rosenberg, I.H. Sarcopenia: Origins and clinical relevance. *Clin. Geriatr. Med.* **2011**, *27*, 337–339. [CrossRef] [PubMed]
3. Cruz-Jentoft, A.J.; Baeyens, J.P.; Bauer, J.M.; Boirie, Y.; Cederholm, T.; Landi, F.; Martin, F.C.; Michel, J.P.; Rolland, Y.; Schneider, S.M.; et al. Sarcopenia: European consensus on definition and diagnosis: Report of the European Working Group on Sarcopenia in Older People. *Age Ageing* **2010**, *39*, 412–423. [CrossRef] [PubMed]
4. Fielding, R.A.; Vellas, B.; Evans, W.J.; Bhasin, S.; Morley, E.; Newman, A.B.; Abellan van Kan, G.; Andrieu, S.; Bauer, J.; Breuille, D.; et al. Sarcopenia: An undiagnosed condition in older adults. Current consensus definition: Prevalence, etiology, and consequences. International working group on sarcopenia. *J. Am. Med. Dir. Assoc.* **2011**, *12*, 249–256. [CrossRef] [PubMed]
5. Landi, F.; Liperoti, R.; Russo, A.; Giovannini, S.; Tosato, M.; Capoluongo, E.; Bernabei, R.; Onder, G. Sarcopenia as a risk factor for falls in elderly individuals: Results from the ilSIRENTE study. *Clin. Nutr.* **2012**, *31*, 652–658. [CrossRef]
6. Studenski, S.; Perera, S.; Patel, K.; Rosano, C.; Faulkner, K.; Inzitari, M.; Brach, J.; Chandler, J.; Cawthon, P.; Connor, E.B.; et al. Gait speed and survival in older adults. *JAMA* **2011**, *305*, 50–58. [CrossRef]
7. Cruz-Jentoft, A.J.; Bahat, G.; Bauer, J.; Boirie, Y.; Bruyere, O.; Cederholm, T.; Cooper, C.; Landi, F.; Rolland, Y.; Sayer, A.A.; et al. Sarcopenia: Revised European consensus on definition and diagnosis. *Age Ageing* **2019**, *48*, 601. [CrossRef]
8. Chen, L.K.; Woo, J.; Assantachai, P.; Auyeung, T.W.; Chou, M.Y.; Iijima, K.; Jang, H.C.; Kang, L.; Kim, M.; Kim, S.; et al. Asian Working Group for Sarcopenia: 2019 Consensus Update on Sarcopenia Diagnosis and Treatment. *J. Am. Med. Dir. Assoc.* **2020**, *21*, 300–307.e2. [CrossRef]
9. Yamada, M.; Nishiguchi, S.; Fukutani, N.; Tanigawa, T.; Yukutake, T.; Kayama, H.; Aoyama, T.; Arai, H. Prevalence of sarcopenia in community-dwelling Japanese older adults. *J. Am. Med. Dir. Assoc.* **2013**, *14*, 911–915. [CrossRef]

10. Khongsri, N.; Tongsuntud, S.; Limampai, P.; Kuptniratsaikul, V. The prevalence of sarcopenia and related factors in a community-dwelling elders Thai population. *Osteoporos. Sarcopenia* **2016**, *2*, 110–115. [CrossRef]
11. Reiss, J.; Iglseder, B.; Alzner, R.; Mayr-Pirker, B.; Pirich, C.; Kässmann, H.; Kreutzer, M.; Dovjak, P.; Reiter, R. Consequences of applying the new EWGSOP2 guideline instead of the former EWGSOP guideline for sarcopenia case finding in older patients. *Age Ageing* **2019**, *48*, 719–724. [CrossRef] [PubMed]
12. Locquet, M.; Beaudart, C.; Petermans, J.; Reginster, J.Y.; Bruyère, O. EWGSOP2 Versus EWGSOP1: Impact on the Prevalence of Sarcopenia and Its Major Health Consequences. *J. Am. Med. Dir. Assoc.* **2019**, *20*, 384–385. [CrossRef]
13. Kim, M.; Won, C.W. Sarcopenia in Korean Community-Dwelling Adults Aged 70 Years and Older: Application of Screening and Diagnostic Tools From the Asian Working Group for Sarcopenia 2019 Update. *J. Am. Med Dir. Assoc.* **2020**, *21*, 752–758. [CrossRef]
14. Deluca, H.F. History of the discovery of vitamin D and its active metabolites. *Bonekey Rep.* **2014**, *3*, 479. [CrossRef] [PubMed]
15. Remelli, F.; Vitali, A.; Zurlo, A.; Volpato, S. Vitamin D Deficiency and Sarcopenia in Older Persons. *Nutrients* **2019**, *11*, 2861. [CrossRef]
16. Ceglia, L.; Harris, S.S. Vitamin D and its role in skeletal muscle. *Calcif. Tissue Int.* **2013**, *92*, 151–162. [CrossRef] [PubMed]
17. Macdonald, H.M.; Mavroeidi, A.; Fraser, W.D.; Darling, A.L.; Black, A.J.; Aucott, L.; O'Neill, F.; Hart, K.; Berry, J.L.; Lanham-New, S.A.; et al. Sunlight and dietary contributions to the seasonal vitamin D status of cohorts of healthy postmenopausal women living at northerly latitudes: A major cause for concern? *Osteoporos Int.* **2011**, *22*, 2461–2472. [CrossRef] [PubMed]
18. Pilz, S.; Marz, W.; Cashman, K.D.; Kiely, M.E.; Whiting, S.J.; Holick, M.F.; Grant, W.B.; Pludowski, P.; Hiligsmann, M.; Trummer, C.; et al. Rationale and Plan for Vitamin D Food Fortification: A Review and Guidance Paper. *Front. Endocrinol.* **2018**, *9*, 373. [CrossRef] [PubMed]
19. Christakos, S.; Dhawan, P.; Verstuyf, A.; Verlinden, L.; Carmeliet, G. Vitamin D: Metabolism, Molecular Mechanism of Action, and Pleiotropic Effects. *Physiol. Rev.* **2016**, *96*, 365–408. [CrossRef] [PubMed]
20. Matyjaszek-Matuszek, B.; Lenart-Lipinska, M.; Wozniakowska, E. Clinical implications of vitamin D deficiency. *Przeglad Menopauzalny* **2015**, *14*, 75–81. [CrossRef]
21. Okazaki, R.; Ozono, K.; Fukumoto, S.; Inoue, D.; Yamauchi, M.; Minagawa, M.; Michigami, T.; Takeuchi, Y.; Matsumoto, T.; Sugimoto, T. Assessment criteria for vitamin D deficiency/insufficiency in Japan: Proposal by an expert panel supported by the Research Program of Intractable Diseases, Ministry of Health, Labour and Welfare, Japan, the Japanese Society for Bone and Mineral Research and the Japan Endocrine Society [Opinion]. *J. Bone Miner. Metab.* **2017**, *35*, 1–5. [CrossRef] [PubMed]
22. Tebben, P.J.; Singh, R.J.; Kumar, R. Vitamin D-Mediated Hypercalcemia: Mechanisms, Diagnosis, and Treatment. *Endocr. Rev.* **2016**, *37*, 521–547. [CrossRef] [PubMed]
23. Kamei, Y.; Kawada, T.; Fukuwatari, T.; Ono, T.; Kato, S.; Sugimoto, E. Cloning and sequencing of the gene encoding the mouse vitamin D receptor. *Gene* **1995**, *152*, 281–282. [CrossRef]
24. Kamei, Y.; Xu, L.; Heinzel, T.; Torchia, J.; Kurokawa, R.; Gloss, B.; Lin, S.C.; Heyman, R.A.; Rose, D.W.; Glass, C.K.; et al. A CBP integrator complex mediates transcriptional activation and AP-1 inhibition by nuclear receptors. *Cell* **1996**, *85*, 403–414. [CrossRef]
25. Kamei, Y.; Ohizumi, H.; Fujitani, Y.; Nemoto, T.; Tanaka, T.; Takahashi, N.; Kawada, T.; Miyoshi, M.; Ezaki, O.; Kakizuka, A. PPARgamma coactivator 1beta/ERR ligand 1 is an ERR protein ligand, whose expression induces a high-energy expenditure and antagonizes obesity. *Proc. Natl. Acad. Sci. USA* **2003**, *100*, 12378–12383. [CrossRef] [PubMed]
26. Umesono, K.; Murakami, K.K.; Thompson, C.C.; Evans, R.M. Direct repeats as selective response elements for the thyroid hormone, retinoic acid, and vitamin D3 receptors. *Cell* **1991**, *65*, 1255–1266. [CrossRef]
27. Carlberg, C.; Bendik, I.; Wyss, A.; Meier, E.; Sturzenbecker, L.J.; Grippo, J.F.; Hunziker, W. Two nuclear signalling pathways for vitamin D. *Nature* **1993**, *361*, 657–660. [CrossRef] [PubMed]
28. Matkovits, T.; Christakos, S. Variable in vivo regulation of rat vitamin D-dependent genes (osteopontin, Ca,Mg-adenosine triphosphatase, and 25-hydroxyvitamin D3 24-hydroxylase): Implications for differing mechanisms of regulation and involvement of multiple factors. *Endocrinology* **1995**, *136*, 3971–3982. [CrossRef]

29. Meyer, M.B.; Watanuki, M.; Kim, S.; Shevde, N.K.; Pike, J.W. The human transient receptor potential vanilloid type 6 distal promoter contains multiple vitamin D receptor binding sites that mediate activation by 1,25-dihydroxyvitamin D3 in intestinal cells. *Mol. Endocrinol.* **2006**, *20*, 1447–1461. [CrossRef]
30. Kim, S.; Yamazaki, M.; Zella, L.A.; Shevde, N.K.; Pike, J.W. Activation of receptor activator of NF-kappaB ligand gene expression by 1,25-dihydroxyvitamin D3 is mediated through multiple long-range enhancers. *Mol. Cell. Biol.* **2006**, *26*, 6469–6486. [CrossRef]
31. Saini, R.K.; Kaneko, I.; Jurutka, P.W.; Forster, R.; Hsieh, A.; Hsieh, J.C.; Haussler, M.R.; Whitfield, G.K. 1,25-dihydroxyvitamin D(3) regulation of fibroblast growth factor-23 expression in bone cells: Evidence for primary and secondary mechanisms modulated by leptin and interleukin-6. *Calcif. Tissue Int.* **2013**, *92*, 339–353. [CrossRef]
32. Tsoumpra, M.K.; Sawatsubashi, S.; Imamura, M.; Fukumoto, S.; Takeda, S.; Matsumoto, T.; Aoki, Y. Dystrobrevin alpha gene is a direct target of the vitamin D receptor in muscle. *J. Mol. Endocrinol.* **2020**, *64*, 195–208. [CrossRef]
33. Kamei, Y.; Kawada, T.; Kazuki, R.; Ono, T.; Kato, S.; Sugimoto, E. Vitamin D receptor gene expression is up-regulated by 1, 25-dihydroxyvitamin D3 in 3T3-L1 preadipocytes. *Biochem. Biophys. Res. Commun.* **1993**, *193*, 948–955. [CrossRef]
34. Makishima, M.; Lu, T.T.; Xie, W.; Whitfield, G.K.; Domoto, H.; Evans, R.M.; Haussler, M.R.; Mangelsdorf, D.J. Vitamin D receptor as an intestinal bile acid sensor. *Science* **2002**, *296*, 1313–1316. [CrossRef] [PubMed]
35. Ishizawa, M.; Akagi, D.; Makishima, M. Lithocholic Acid Is a Vitamin D Receptor Ligand That Acts Preferentially in the Ileum. *Int. J. Mol. Sci.* **2018**, *19*, 1975. [CrossRef] [PubMed]
36. Asano, L.; Watanabe, M.; Ryoden, Y.; Usuda, K.; Yamaguchi, T.; Khambu, B.; Takashima, M.; Sato, S.I.; Sakai, J.; Nagasawa, K.; et al. Vitamin D Metabolite, 25-Hydroxyvitamin D, Regulates Lipid Metabolism by Inducing Degradation of SREBP/SCAP. *Cell Chem. Biol.* **2017**, *24*, 207–217. [CrossRef]
37. Schuur, E.R.; Loktev, A.V.; Sharma, M.; Sun, Z.; Roth, R.A.; Weigel, R.J. Ligand-dependent interaction of estrogen receptor-alpha with members of the forkhead transcription factor family. *J. Biol. Chem.* **2001**, *276*, 33554–33560. [CrossRef]
38. Zhao, H.H.; Herrera, R.E.; Coronado-Heinsohn, E.; Yang, M.C.; Ludes-Meyers, J.H.; Seybold-Tilson, K.J.; Nawaz, Z.; Yee, D.; Barr, F.G.; Diab, S.G.; et al. Forkhead homologue in rhabdomyosarcoma functions as a bifunctional nuclear receptor-interacting protein with both coactivator and corepressor functions. *J. Biol. Chem.* **2001**, *276*, 27907–27912. [CrossRef]
39. Okuno, J.; Tomura, S.; Yabushita, N.; Kim, M.J.; Okura, T.; Tanaka, K.; Yanagi, H. Effects of serum 25-hydroxyvitamin D(3) levels on physical fitness in community-dwelling frail women. *Arch. Gerontol. Geriatr.* **2010**, *50*, 121–126. [CrossRef]
40. Bischoff-Ferrari, H.A.; Dawson-Hughes, B.; Staehelin, H.B.; Orav, J.E.; Stuck, A.E.; Theiler, R.; Wong, J.B.; Egli, A.; Kiel, D.P.; Henschkowski, J. Fall prevention with supplemental and active forms of vitamin D: A meta-analysis of randomised controlled trials. *BMJ* **2009**, *339*, b3692. [CrossRef] [PubMed]
41. Visser, M.; Deeg, D.J.; Lips, P. Low vitamin D and high parathyroid hormone levels as determinants of loss of muscle strength and muscle mass (sarcopenia): The Longitudinal Aging Study Amsterdam. *J. Clin. Endocrinol. Metab.* **2003**, *88*, 5766–5772. [CrossRef] [PubMed]
42. MacLaughlin, J.; Holick, M.F. Aging decreases the capacity of human skin to produce vitamin D3. *J. Clin. Investig.* **1985**, *76*, 1536–1538. [CrossRef] [PubMed]
43. Tsai, K.S.; Heath, H., 3rd; Kumar, R.; Riggs, B.L. Impaired vitamin D metabolism with aging in women. Possible role in pathogenesis of senile osteoporosis. *J. Clin. Investig.* **1984**, *73*, 1668–1672. [CrossRef] [PubMed]
44. Gallagher, J.C.; Yalamanchili, V.; Smith, L.M. The effect of vitamin D supplementation on serum 25(OH)D in thin and obese women. *J. Steroid Biochem. Mol. Biol.* **2013**, *136*, 195–200. [CrossRef]
45. Kawada, T.; Kamei, Y.; Sugimoto, E. The possibility of active form of vitamins A and D as suppressors on adipocyte development via ligand-dependent transcriptional regulators. *Int. J. Obes. Relat. Metab. Disord.* **1996**, *20* (Suppl. 3), S52–S57.
46. Beaudart, C.; Buckinx, F.; Rabenda, V.; Gillain, S.; Cavalier, E.; Slomian, J.; Petermans, J.; Reginster, J.Y.; Bruyere, O. The effects of vitamin D on skeletal muscle strength, muscle mass, and muscle power: A systematic review and meta-analysis of randomized controlled trials. *J. Clin. Endocrinol. Metab.* **2014**, *99*, 4336–4345. [CrossRef]

47. Ceglia, L.; Niramitmahapanya, S.; da Silva Morais, M.; Rivas, D.A.; Harris, S.S.; Bischoff-Ferrari, H.; Fielding, R.A.; Dawson-Hughes, B. A randomized study on the effect of vitamin D(3) supplementation on skeletal muscle morphology and vitamin D receptor concentration in older women. *J. Clin. Endocrinol. Metab.* **2013**, *98*, E1927–E1935. [CrossRef]
48. Tomlinson, P.B.; Joseph, C.; Angioi, M. Effects of vitamin D supplementation on upper and lower body muscle strength levels in healthy individuals. A systematic review with meta-analysis. *J. Sci. Med. Sport* **2015**, *18*, 575–580. [CrossRef]
49. Tabrizi, R.; Hallajzadeh, J.; Mirhosseini, N.; Lankarani, K.B.; Maharlouei, N.; Akbari, M.; Asemi, Z. The effects of vitamin D supplementation on muscle function among postmenopausal women: A systematic review and meta-analysis of randomized controlled trials. *EXCLI J.* **2019**, *18*, 591–603. [CrossRef]
50. Srikuea, R.; Zhang, X.; Park-Sarge, O.K.; Esser, K.A. VDR and CYP27B1 are expressed in C2C12 cells and regenerating skeletal muscle: Potential role in suppression of myoblast proliferation. *Am. J. Physiol. Cell Physiol.* **2012**, *303*, C396–C405. [CrossRef]
51. Girgis, C.M.; Mokbel, N.; Cha, K.M.; Houweling, P.J.; Abboud, M.; Fraser, D.R.; Mason, R.S.; Clifton-Bligh, R.J.; Gunton, J.E. The vitamin D receptor (VDR) is expressed in skeletal muscle of male mice and modulates 25-hydroxyvitamin D (25OHD) uptake in myofibers. *Endocrinology* **2014**, *155*, 3227–3237. [CrossRef] [PubMed]
52. Girgis, C.M.; Cha, K.M.; Houweling, P.J.; Rao, R.; Mokbel, N.; Lin, M.; Clifton-Bligh, R.J.; Gunton, J.E. Vitamin D Receptor Ablation and Vitamin D Deficiency Result in Reduced Grip Strength, Altered Muscle Fibers, and Increased Myostatin in Mice. *Calcif. Tissue Int.* **2015**, *97*, 602–610. [CrossRef] [PubMed]
53. Endo, I.; Inoue, D.; Mitsui, T.; Umaki, Y.; Akaike, M.; Yoshizawa, T.; Kato, S.; Matsumoto, T. Deletion of vitamin D receptor gene in mice results in abnormal skeletal muscle development with deregulated expression of myoregulatory transcription factors. *Endocrinology* **2003**, *144*, 5138–5144. [CrossRef]
54. Girgis, C.M.; Cha, K.M.; So, B.; Tsang, M.; Chen, J.; Houweling, P.J.; Schindeler, A.; Stokes, R.; Swarbrick, M.M.; Evesson, F.J.; et al. Mice with myocyte deletion of vitamin D receptor have sarcopenia and impaired muscle function. *J. Cachex- Sarcopenia Muscle* **2019**, *10*, 1228–1240. [CrossRef]
55. Kamei, Y.; Miura, S.; Suzuki, M.; Kai, Y.; Mizukami, J.; Taniguchi, T.; Mochida, K.; Hata, T.; Matsuda, J.; Aburatani, H.; et al. Skeletal muscle FOXO1 (FKHR) transgenic mice have less skeletal muscle mass, down-regulated Type I (slow twitch/red muscle) fiber genes, and impaired glycemic control. *J. Biol. Chem.* **2004**, *279*, 41114–41123. [CrossRef] [PubMed]
56. Kamei, Y.; Mizukami, J.; Miura, S.; Suzuki, M.; Takahashi, N.; Kawada, T.; Taniguchi, T.; Ezaki, O. A forkhead transcription factor FKHR up-regulates lipoprotein lipase expression in skeletal muscle. *FEBS Lett.* **2003**, *536*, 232–236. [CrossRef]
57. Lecker, S.H.; Jagoe, R.T.; Gilbert, A.; Gomes, M.; Baracos, V.; Bailey, J.; Price, S.R.; Mitch, W.E.; Goldberg, A.L. Multiple types of skeletal muscle atrophy involve a common program of changes in gene expression. *FASEB J.* **2004**, *18*, 39–51. [CrossRef]
58. Reed, S.A.; Sandesara, P.B.; Senf, S.M.; Judge, A.R. Inhibition of FoxO transcriptional activity prevents muscle fiber atrophy during cachexia and induces hypertrophy. *FASEB J. Off. Publ. Fed. Am. Soc. Exp. Biol.* **2012**, *26*, 987–1000. [CrossRef]
59. Hirose, Y.; Onishi, T.; Miura, S.; Hatazawa, Y.; Kamei, Y. Vitamin D Attenuates FOXO1-Target Atrophy Gene Expression in C2C12 Muscle Cells. *J. Nutr. Sci. Vitaminol.* **2018**, *64*, 229–232. [CrossRef]
60. Yang, A.; Lv, Q.; Chen, F.; Wang, Y.; Liu, Y.; Shi, W.; Liu, Y.; Wang, D. The effect of vitamin D on sarcopenia depends on the level of physical activity in older adults. *J. Cachex- Sarcopenia Muscle* **2020**, *11*, 678–689. [CrossRef]
61. Bass, J.J.; Nakhuda, A.; Deane, C.S.; Brook, M.S.; Wilkinson, D.J.; Phillips, B.E.; Philp, A.; Tarum, J.; Kadi, F.; Andersen, D.; et al. Overexpression of the vitamin D receptor (VDR) induces skeletal muscle hypertrophy. *Mol. Metab.* **2020**, *42*, 101059. [CrossRef] [PubMed]
62. Gogulothu, R.; Nagar, D.; Gopalakrishnan, S.; Garlapati, V.R.; Kallamadi, P.R.; Ismail, A. Disrupted expression of genes essential for skeletal muscle fibre integrity and energy metabolism in Vitamin D deficient rats. *J. Steroid Biochem. Mol. Biol.* **2020**, *197*, 105525. [CrossRef] [PubMed]
63. Coen, P.M.; Musci, R.V.; Hinkley, J.M.; Miller, B.F. Mitochondria as a Target for Mitigating Sarcopenia. *Front. Physiol.* **2018**, *9*, 1883. [CrossRef]

64. Sinha, A.; Hollingsworth, K.G.; Ball, S.; Cheetham, T. Improving the vitamin D status of vitamin D deficient adults is associated with improved mitochondrial oxidative function in skeletal muscle. *J. Clin. Endocrinol. Metab.* **2013**, *98*, E509–E513. [CrossRef] [PubMed]
65. Ryan, Z.C.; Craig, T.A.; Folmes, C.D.; Wang, X.; Lanza, I.R.; Schaible, N.S.; Salisbury, J.L.; Nair, K.S.; Terzic, A.; Sieck, G.C.; et al. 1alpha,25-Dihydroxyvitamin D3 Regulates Mitochondrial Oxygen Consumption and Dynamics in Human Skeletal Muscle Cells. *J. Biol. Chem.* **2016**, *291*, 1514–1528. [CrossRef]
66. Ashcroft, S.P.; Bass, J.J.; Kazi, A.A.; Atherton, P.J.; Philp, A. The vitamin D receptor regulates mitochondrial function in C2C12 myoblasts. *Am. J. Physiol. Cell Physiol.* **2020**, *318*, C536–C541. [CrossRef]
67. Chang, E.; Kim, Y. Vitamin D Ameliorates Fat Accumulation with AMPK/SIRT1 Activity in C2C12 Skeletal Muscle Cells. *Nutrients* **2019**, *11*, 2806. [CrossRef]
68. Thomas, D.T.; Schnell, D.M.; Redzic, M.; Zhao, M.; Abraha, H.; Jones, D.; Brim, H.; Yu, G. Local In Vivo Measures of Muscle Lipid and Oxygen Consumption Change in Response to Combined Vitamin D Repletion and Aerobic Training in Older Adults. *Nutrients* **2019**, *11*, 930. [CrossRef]
69. Asakura, K.; Etoh, N.; Imamura, H.; Michikawa, T.; Nakamura, T.; Takeda, Y.; Mori, S.; Nishiwaki, Y. Vitamin D Status in Japanese Adults: Relationship of Serum 25-Hydroxyvitamin D with Simultaneously Measured Dietary Vitamin D Intake and Ultraviolet Ray Exposure. *Nutrients* **2020**, *12*, 743. [CrossRef]
70. Institute of Medicine Committee to Review Dietary Reference Intakes for Vitamin, D. Calcium. The National Academies Collection: Reports funded by National Institutes of Health. In *Dietary Reference Intakes for Calcium and Vitamin D*; Ross, A.C., Taylor, C.L., Yaktine, A.L., Del Valle, H.B., Eds.; National Academy of Sciences: Washington, DC, USA, 2011. [CrossRef]
71. Institute of Medicine Standing Committee on the Scientific Evaluation of Dietary Reference, I. The National Academies Collection: Reports funded by National Institutes of Health. In *Dietary Reference Intakes for Calcium, Phosphorus, Magnesium, Vitamin D, and Fluoride*; National Academy of Sciences: Washington, DC, USA, 1997. [CrossRef]
72. Walia, N.; Chen, L. Pea protein based vitamin D nanoemulsions: Fabrication, stability and in vitro study using Caco-2 cells. *Food Chem.* **2020**, *305*, 125475. [CrossRef]
73. Almajwal, A.M.; Abulmeaty, M.M.A.; Feng, H.; Alruwaili, N.W.; Dominguez-Uscanga, A.; Andrade, J.E.; Razak, S.; ElSadek, M.F. Stabilization of Vitamin D in Pea Protein Isolate Nanoemulsions Increases Its Bioefficacy in Rats. *Nutrients* **2019**, *11*, 75. [CrossRef] [PubMed]

6

New Insights into the Pros and Cons of the Clinical Use of Vitamin K Antagonists (VKAs) Versus Direct Oral Anticoagulants (DOACs)

Rick H. van Gorp [1,2] **and Leon J. Schurgers** [1,*]

1 Department of Biochemistry, Cardiovascular Research Institute Maastricht, Maastricht University, PO Box 616, 6200 MD Maastricht, The Netherlands; rick.vangorp@maastrichtuniversity

2 Nattopharma ASA, 1363 Høvik, Norway

* Correspondence: l.schurgers@maastrichtuniversity.nl

Abstract: Vitamin K-antagonists (VKA) are the most widely used anticoagulant drugs to treat patients at risk of arterial and venous thrombosis for the past 50 years. Due to unfavorable pharmacokinetics VKA have a small therapeutic window, require frequent monitoring, and are susceptible to drug and nutritional interactions. Additionally, the effect of VKA is not limited to coagulation, but affects all vitamin K-dependent proteins. As a consequence, VKA have detrimental side effects by enhancing medial and intimal calcification. These limitations stimulated the development of alternative anticoagulant drugs, resulting in direct oral anticoagulant (DOAC) drugs, which specifically target coagulation factor Xa and thrombin. DOACs also display non-hemostatic vascular effects via protease-activated receptors (PARs). As atherosclerosis is characterized by a hypercoagulable state indicating the involvement of activated coagulation factors in the genesis of atherosclerosis, anticoagulation could have beneficial effects on atherosclerosis. Additionally, accumulating evidence demonstrates vascular benefit from high vitamin K intake. This review gives an update on oral anticoagulant treatment on the vasculature with a special focus on calcification and vitamin K interaction.

Keywords: oral anticoagulants; vitamin K; vascular calcification; coumarin; DOACs

---

1. Arterial and Venous Thrombosis

In 1856 Rudolf Virchow, often regarded as the founder of modern pathology, delineated three major components that were responsible for the formation of emboli in the venous circulation. These three elements, now known as Virchow's triad, can be briefly summarized as: (1) changes in the composition of blood; (2) alterations in the vessel wall; and (3) disruption of the blood flow. Coagulation is a protective response after vascular injury to prevent bleeding [1] and can be initiated via either the so-called intrinsic or extrinsic pathways, which although simplistic, are still useful schematic models of the coagulation process (Figure 1a). Both pathways are characterized by a series of enzymatic events whereby the activation of members of a hierarchical chain of coagulation enzymes (called coagulation factors) are successively activated by the preceding factor in the chain. Although the initiation steps are different, both pathways converge and lead to activation of pro-thrombin (FII) to produce thrombin (FIIa). An important feature of this coagulation cascade is that it functions as a biochemical amplifier [2] in which the final product, thrombin catalyses the production of fibrin which forms a meshwork clot [3]. The coagulation events leading to the formation of a blood clot (thrombus) that adheres to the wall of a blood vessel and obstructs the flow of blood is termed thrombosis. Thrombosis can take place in both arteries and veins. Atherothrombosis is the term describing the occlusion of a blood vessel by a ruptured atherosclerotic plaque [4,5]. Arterial thrombosis can lead to stroke and myocardial infarction. In contrast to arterial thrombosis, venous thrombosis is associated with dysregulation of coagulation proteins and manifests in deep-vein thrombosis and pulmonary embolism [6]. Obesity and diabetes mellitus are risk factors for both arterial and venous thrombosis whereas other risk factors such as smoking, hypertension and hyperlipidemia increase only the risk for arterial thrombosis [6]. Oral anticoagulant drugs are prescribed to patients to reduce the risk and incidence of both arterial and venous thrombosis, although mainly for the latter.

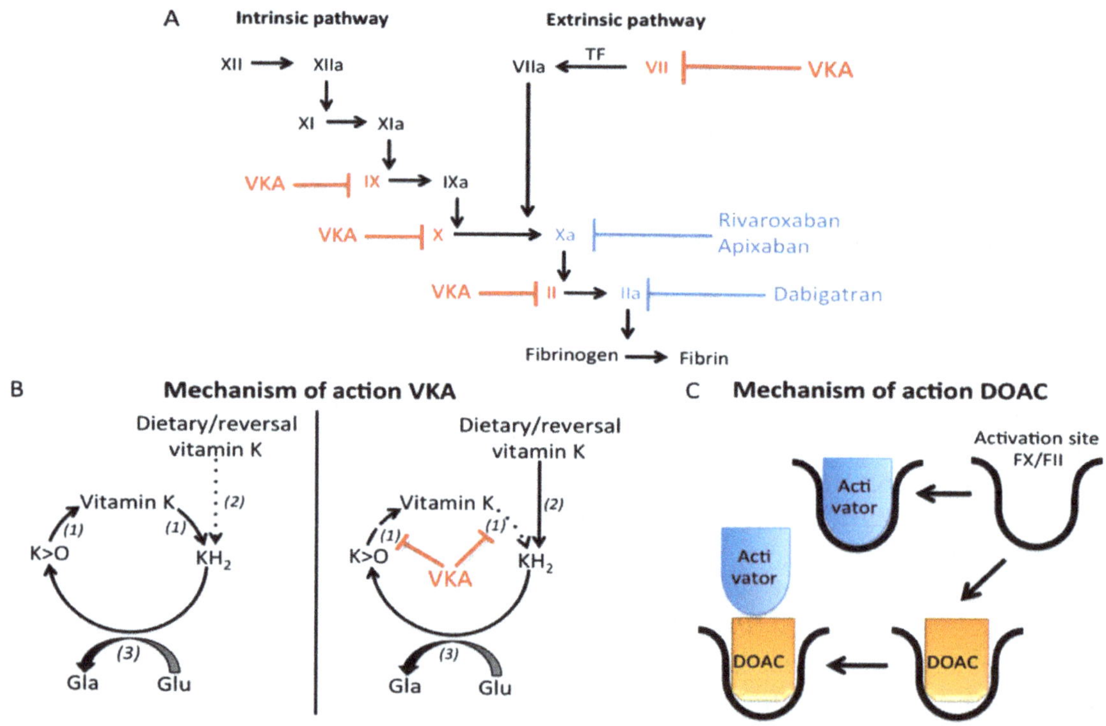

Figure 1. Effects of vitamin K antagonists and direct oral anticoagulants on coagulation. (**A**) The coagulation cascade can be activated by both the intrinsic and extrinsic pathway, which finally results in activation of thrombin and subsequently fibrin formation. Vitamin K antagonists (VKA) induce anticoagulation via inhibiting activation of the coagulation factors depicted in red (factors X, IX, VII, and II). Direct oral anticoagulants (DOACs) induce anticoagulation via blocking the activity of coagulation factors Xa (rivaroxaban and apixaban) and IIa (dabigatran) depicted in blue; (**B**) Vitamin K cycle is required to carboxylate, and thus activate, vitamin K dependent proteins. Vitamin K is converted to vitamin hydroquinone (KH_2), which is oxidized by γ-glutamylcarboxylase (3) to convert glutamate (Glu) residues in γ-carboxyglutamate (Gla) residues. This reaction results in vitamin K epoxide (K > O), which is recycled to vitamin K through vitamin K epoxide reductase (1). VKA disrupts the vitamin K cycle by inhibiting vitamin K epoxide reductase (VKOR) leading to depletion of vitamin K and uncarboxylated vitamin K dependent proteins. In the liver, the inhibition of warfarin can be circumvented via NAD(P)H quinone reductase (2), which can convert vitamin K into KH_2 even in the presence of VKA. In extra-hepatic tissues NAD(P)H quinone reductase activity is *ca.* 100 fold less, resulting in inactive vitamin K dependent proteins in the presence of VKA; (**C**) DOACs induce anticoagulation via inhibiting the activity of FXa and FIIa via binding to the activation site.

2. The Discovery of Oral Anticoagulant Drugs

The story of the discovery of vitamin K antagonists (VKA) began in the 1920s as a result of an often fatal bleeding disorder in cattle that manifested after the animals had been fed on the hay derived from sweet clover [7]. For this reason the haemorrhagic disease became known as "sweet clover disease". A crucial observation was the animals that bled had been fed on sweet clover hay that had become mouldy; those animals fed mould-free hay did not present with bleeding [7]. During the subsequent classical studies by Karl Link's group in Wisconsin it was first shown that bleeding was associated with a low plasma activity of prothrombin as measured by early coagulation assays that were the precursors of the modern day prothrombin time. Link's group then undertook the task of isolating the haemorrhagic component in spoiled sweet clover that was responsible for the prolonged prothrombin time. This proved a long and arduous process but finally resulted in the isolation and identification of the haemorrhagic agent that we now know as the compound dicoumarol and the first VKA [8]. Dicoumarol is a 4-hydroxycoumarin derivative and originated from microbial action on the compound coumarin which is rich in sweet clover.

After animal trials, dicoumarol was rapidly introduced into the clinic with considerable success. At that time, dicoumarol had also been tested in field trials as a potential rodenticide but it was concluded that the anticoagulant activity of dicoumarol in the rat was not high enough to make it practical for rodent control [8]. Therefore, Link's group synthesized a large number of different 4-hydroxycoumarin compounds to try and find a derivative with increased anticoagulant activity over dicoumarol. It turned out that a 4-hydroxycoumarin anticoagulant number 42 (out of 150 synthetic variants) was more potent than dicoumarol and had superior pharmacokinetics [8]. This coumarin derivative is today known as warfarin, the word originating from the combination of the Wisconsin Alumni Research Foundation (WARF) and "arin" from coum"arin". Warfarin revolutionized rodent control but clinicians were reluctant to use a rat poison in humans until an unforeseen event changed their minds. In 1951 an army conscript tried to commit suicide with warfarin. According to Link the slow onset time of warfarin gave him "too much time for thinking" enabling him to reconsider and admit himself to hospital where after receiving vitamin K supplementation he completely recovered. Clinical trials with warfarin in the 1950s confirmed its superiority over dicoumarol, being better absorbed and some 5–10 times more potent, although no head to head comparison was performed. Moreover, it became apparent that an overdose could easily be corrected by vitamin K supplementation [8,9]. Today, warfarin is the most prescribed oral anticoagulant world-wide [10].

2.1. *Vitamin K and Vitamin K Antagonists*

Vitamin K is a fat-soluble vitamin that exists in different forms (Table 1). All forms of vitamin K contain a 2-methyl-1,4-naphthoquinone ring structure, also known as menadione (vitamin K_3). Phylloquinone (vitamins K_1) and menaquinones (vitamin K_2) are classified according to the length and degree of saturation of the aliphatic side chain. Phylloquinone contains a phytyl side chain, and its main dietary sources are green leafy vegetables and certain vegetable oils. Menaquinones have an unsaturated aliphatic side chain comprising a varying number of prenyl units, abbreviated as MK-n (menaquinone with n representing the number of prenyl units). All menaquinones, except MK-4, are produced by bacteria and can be found in fermented foods such as cheese. Additionally, some bacteria in our intestines produce long-chain menaquinones (mainly MK-10 and MK-11) and although they make up the majority of human hepatic reserves their bioavailability for the synthesis of coagulation Gla proteins in the liver is debatable [11]. Both phylloquinone and menaquinones can participate in the γ-glutamylcarboxylation of both hepatic and extra-hepatic vitamin K-dependent proteins, although the longer residence times and better absorption of long chain menaquinones such as MK-7 and MK-9 in the circulation [12,13] makes them more effective for carboxylating both hepatic and extrahepatic vitamin K-dependent proteins [14]. Interestingly, menadione has been shown to act as a endogenous metabolite formed during the *in vivo* conversion of phylloquinone to MK-4 [15]. Furthermore, whereas phylloquinone and menaquinones can reverse VKA induced anticoagulation, menadione per se has no cofactor activity for γ-carboxylation and thus cannot reverse VKA-induced anticoagulation.

Table 1. Structural forms of vitamin K.

Drug	Characterization		Dietary Sources
Phylloquinone (vitamin K_1)	Phytyl side chain		Leafy green vegetables
Menaquinones (vitamin K_2)	Isoprenoid side chain	MK-4	Meat, eggs
		MK-7	Natto, Cheese
		MK-9	Cheese, curd, sauerkraut
Menadione (vitamin K_3)	2-methyl-1,4- naphthoquinone		Non-dietary metabolite. Precursor of MK-4

The molecular function of vitamin K is to serve as an essential cofactor to drive the γ-glutamyl carboxylation reaction (Figure 1b). In this vitamin K-dependent reaction, specific protein bound glutamate residues are modified to γ-glutamate residues, hence the name of the γ-carboxylated protein products as vitamin K-dependent proteins (VKDP). To achieve this protein modification vitamin K is first reduced to the active cofactor vitamin hydroquinone (KH_2) via quinone reductases. Next, the enzyme γ-glutamyl carboxylase (GGCX) oxidizes vitamin KH_2 with vitamin K epoxide (K > O) as the product. This oxidation reaction is intimately linked and essential to the γ-carboxylation modification of VKDP [16]. The metabolite K > O can be recycled by the microsomal enzyme vitamin K epoxide reductase (VKOR), first to vitamin K and then to KH_2. This cyclic pathway is called the "vitamin K-epoxide cycle" or simply the "vitamin K cycle" [17,18]. By this salvage mechanism, one molecule of vitamin K is able to carboxylate some 500 glutamate residues [17].

A deficiency of vitamin K can result from an insufficient dietary intake of vitamin K leading to depletion of local vitamin K tissue stores or via interference with the vitamin K cycle by VKA [18,19]. VKA exert their anticoagulant effect by inhibiting the VKOR enzyme resulting in reduced recycling of K > O, thereby limiting KH_2 production. As the cellular concentrations of KH_2 decline a stage is reached when the cofactor supply to the GGCX becomes insufficient to fully carboxylate the VKDP that are synthesized in a particular tissue. This in turn leads to the secretion of undercarboxylated species of VKDP in the circulation. The anticoagulant balance exerted by VKA can be said to be ultimately determined by the concentrations of γ-carboxylated coagulation proteins II, VII, IX and X that are secreted into the circulation. Changes in nutritional vitamin K intake interfere with VKA treatment by altering the size of the available pool of KH_2 cofactor because dietary vitamin K in its quinone state can be converted to KH_2 by a dehydrogenase enzyme not affected by VKA [18]. Remarkably, despite the long use of VKA the exact mechanism of inhibition of VKOR remains to be elucidated [18].

Owing to their unfavorable pharmacokinetics, VKA have a small therapeutic window, require frequent monitoring, and are susceptible to drug and nutritional interactions. A major disadvantage is that because of their indirect mechanism of action there is a lag phase of 2–3 days before a therapeutic anticoagulant effect is achieved. Therefore, considerable resources have been directed to the discovery of new anticoagulant agents that can directly target specific factors in the coagulation cascade. Several of these so-called direct oral anticoagulants (DOACs) have been approved for clinical use and can be subdivided into agents that either target coagulation factor IIa (FIIa, thrombin) or factor Xa (FXa).

2.2. Direct Thrombin Inhibitors

As with the discovery of VKA, the presence in nature of another anticoagulant (albeit in this case an anticoagulant without a lag phase) proved a catalyst to the future discovery of direct inhibitors of coagulation factors. Here it was the isolation of hirudin, a peptide present in the saliva of leeches as a direct inhibitor of thrombin, and long known to prevent coagulation [20,21]. For a detailed review on hirudin, see [22]. Hirudin binds to both the active and substrate recognition sites of thrombin. In addition, it is slowly reversible and excreted predominantly by the kidneys. In the 1990s, recombinant hirudin was shown to prevent postoperative venous thromboembolism [23]. However, a major concern was the increased bleeding tendency with hirudin treatment [21,24]. As with heparin another major disadvantage of hirudin is that it could only be administered by subcutaneous injection. Despite the specific concerns with hirudin, the theory behind designing a direct thrombin inhibitor as a clinical anticoagulant gained support and in the early 2000s a compound called ximelagatran became the first synthetic direct inhibitor of thrombin to be trialed as an oral anticoagulant. However, although initial human trials were promising, later trials led to concerns of hepatotoxicity, which ultimately prevented ximelagatran from being used in the clinical setting [25,26].

The second direct oral anticoagulant to undergo clinical trials was dabigatran etexilate, and this agent received approval for clinical use in 2008 (Table 2). Dabigatran etexilate is a prodrug that requires hydrolysis by carboxylesterases in the body to the active metabolite dabigatran [27]. Dabigatran binds with high specificity to the active site of thrombin thereby inhibiting both bound and free thrombin activity (Figure 1c). It takes two hours before dabigatran etexilate is metabolically active, which eliminates the need for parental anticoagulation. Dabigatran has a half-life of 12–17 h and is usually taken twice daily. Since 80% of dabigatran is excreted by the kidneys, patients with renal problems are not suited for this drug [25,28,29].

Table 2. Characteristics of VKA and DOACs.

	VKA [10]			Dabigatran Etexilate [24,27,28]	Rivaroxaban [30,31]	Apixaban [32]
	Warfarin	Acenocoumarol	Phenprocoumon			
Target	Vitamin K epoxide reductase	Vitamin K epoxide reductase	Vitamin K epoxide reductase	Thrombin	Factor Xa	Factor Xa
Pro-drug	No	No	No	Yes, active metabolite is dabigatran	No	No
Half-life (hours)	20–60	8–11	120–144	12–17	5–9	9–14
Onset time peak effect (hours)	72–96	36–48	48–72	2	2–3	3
Duration of action	2–5 days	<48 h	7–14 days	24–36 h	24 h	24 h
Metabolism	Via cytochrome P 450	Via cytochrome P 450	Via cytochrome P 450	Via P-Glucoprotein transporter	Via cytochrome P450 (30%), and P-Glucoprotein transporter	Via cytochrome P450 (15%), and P-Glucoprotein transporter
Elimination	Hepatical metabolized	60% Renal 29% Fecal	63% Renal 33% Fecal	85% Renal 6% Fecal	66% Renal 28% Fecal	25% Renal
Bioavailability	79%–100%	60%	>99%	6.5%	80%	66%

2.3. Factor Xa Inhibitors

The idea of using FXa inhibitors as clinical anticoagulants also originates from naturally occurring inhibitors. The first FXa inhibitor to be studied was a compound called antistasin, originally isolated from the Mexican leech *haementeria officinalis* [33]. However, the concept of FXa inhibitors as anticoagulant drugs was not supported until a second FXa inhibitor called the tick anticoagulant peptide (TAP) had been isolated from the soft tick *ornithodors moubata* [34]. *In vitro* and *in vivo* studies demonstrated that FXa inhibitors block the activity of FXa generated via both intrinsic and extrinsic pathways and thus subsequently block the formation of thrombin [35,36].

In 2012 the FXa inhibitor called rivaroxaban was approved for clinical use (Table 2). Rivaroxaban acts via inhibition of the active site of FXa (Figure 1c) [35], and has predictable pharmacokinetic and dynamics [30]. Peak activity of rivaroxaban occurs 2–3 h after intake, with a half-life of 5–9 h [30]. The short half-life suggests that rivaroxaban needs to be taken twice daily, however guidelines for rivaroxaban usage recommend once daily. This recommendation comes from both clinical phase II and III trials, which provided evidence that once daily administration is most beneficial with respect to the balance between safety and efficacy [37]. In addition, the duration of rivaroxaban inhibiting FXa lasts 24 h thereby supporting the once daily policy. Rivaroxaban is mainly excreted by the kidneys (66% with 36% as unchanged drug) with a smaller fraction excreted in the faeces (28% with 7% unchanged) [31].

To date, the most recently approved DOAC is another FXa inhibitor called apixaban (Table 2). Like rivaroxaban, apixaban inhibits both bound and free FXa (Figure 1c). Apixaban activity peaks 3 h after intake and has a half life of 9–14 h [32]. Bioavailability of apixaban is 66%, and apixaban is partly (25%) excreted by the kidneys.

3. Clinical Trials with Oral Anticoagulation Drugs

3.1. *Vitamin K Antagonists (VKA)*

The promise and later importance of VKA as oral anticoagulant drugs for clinical use became apparent in a randomized trial performed in the 1960s [38]. In this trial, patients with pulmonary embolism were divided in two groups receiving either the anticoagulant drug or placebo control. Of the group receiving anticoagulation therapy none of the patients died, whereas 5 patients in the placebo group died of pulmonary embolism [38].

Ever since the clinical introduction of VKA, their clinical efficacy and safety have been monitored through measuring the coagulation activity of the blood, mainly using the prothrombin time (PT) test or a close variant of this test [39]. A central ingredient of the PT test is a biological tissue reagent called thromboplastin. It quickly became apparent that innate variations in the source and batch of thromboplastin led to significant variabilities in PT results which were usually reported as a prothrombin time ratio (PTR) representing the patient's PT divided by normal PT [39]. In principle, when a high or low laboratory PTR is reported, the anticoagulant dosage is adjusted accordingly to reach the target coagulation ratio [39]. In the early 1960s it became apparent that some commercial thromboplastins were insufficiently responsive to the anticoagulant-induced effect leading to an underestimation of the dose of VKA required to achieve the target PTR. The subsequent overdosing with VKA led to an increase in bleeding complications and indicated the importance of using sensitive thromboplastin-based assays to prevent over or under dosing with VKA. Comparison of thromboplastin assays between North America and the UK revealed that increased sensitivity of assays reduced the incidence of hemorrhage [39,40]. These results also addressed the need for increased standardization of PT assays and international guidelines for monitoring anticoagulation therapy. In 1983, the World Health Organization (WHO) adopted a universally standardized system of reporting patient PT data during VKA therapy called the international normalized ratio (INR) which is still used today [41].

3.2. *DOACs*

With the approval of DOACs for clinical use, an alternative to VKA or heparin treatment became available. Recent clinical trials have investigated efficacy and safety profiles of DOACs in comparison to VKA treatment. The outcomes of these comparative trials are briefly described below.

3.2.1. Dabigatran Etexilate

The RE-LY and RE-COVER clinical trials demonstrated non-inferiority of dabigatran etexilate compared to warfarin in atrial fibrillation (AF) patients and patients with acute venous thromboembolism, respectively [25,42]. Additionally, the RE-MODEL clinical trial demonstrated non-inferiority of dabigatran compared to enoxaparin treatment with respect to preventing venous thromboembolism after total knee replacement surgery [43]. Taken together these clinical trials demonstrated the non-inferiority of dabigatran compared to VKA treatment. Thus, dabigatran etexilate seems a suitable alternative for VKA for the treatment of patients with increased thrombosis risk.

3.2.2. Rivaroxaban

The clinical trials ROCKET AF, RECORD, EINSTEIN-DVT and EINSTEIN-Extension demonstrated the non-inferiority of rivaroxaban as compared to VKA and heparin treatment in patients with non-valvular atrial fibrillation, symptomatic venous thromboembolism, deep-vein thrombosis, and recurrent thrombosis in deep-vein thrombosis patients [44–46]. Moreover, rivaroxaban demonstrated no difference in risk for major bleedings in patients undergoing elective hip/knee replacement, though rivaroxaban was more effective in preventing symptomatic venous thromboembolism [47].

3.2.3. Apixaban

The ARISTOTLE and ADVANCE clinical trials showed non-inferiority of apixaban as compared to VKA and heparin in AF patients and for thromboprophylaxis in patients after hip replacement, respectively [48,49]. Similar to dabigatran and rivaroxaban, apixaban showed no difference as compared to VKA treatment with respect to risk for major bleedings.

These clinical trials did not demonstrate superiority of DOACs over VKA, questioning whether DOACs should replace VKA as standard treatment. A meta-analysis comparing DOACs with VKA provided additional insight and showed the superiority over DOACs compared to VKA treatment with respect to major bleedings [50]. However, care is required interpreting these results and more research is needed.

4. Advantages and Disadvantages of VKA and DOACs

The use of VKA treatment over 60 years is one of the major advantages, since this revealed both short and long-term effects in humans. Disadvantages of VKA include the narrow therapeutic window and thus indirectly safety and efficacy. Therefore, VKA therapy requires regular monitoring by measuring the INR [21,51]. Additionally, the pharmacokinetic and pharmacodynamics are unpredictable through drug interactions, cytochrome P450-dependent mechanisms, and the influence of dietary vitamin K intake [10,52]. All the coumarin VKA listed in Table 2 (*i.e.*, warfarin, acenocoumarol, and phenprocoumon) have a slow onset, taking *ca.* two to seven days to be effective in inducing anticoagulation [10,21]. Therefore, VKA therapy requires initial co-administration with other anticoagulants, such as heparin. Moreover, it has been shown recently that patients taking VKA treatment display hitherto unreported non-hemostasis side effects [53]. One of these side effects is VKA-induced vascular calcification. Vascular calcification is associated with an increased risk for cardiovascular disease [53–55]. In addition, VKA treatment is associated with arterial stiffness, which in turn is related to vascular calcification [56,57].

DOACs were developed to circumvent the disadvantages of VKA therapy without negatively influencing safety profiles. Initially, the manufacturers of DOACs promoted the view that a major advantage of DOACs was that they did not require routine coagulation testing (as needed for VKA) or the measurement of circulating drug concentrations. However, data from the dabigatran RE-LY trial suggested that adjusting the dosage of dabigatran based on measurements of plasma dabigatran concentrations may reduce major bleeding events by as much as 30%–40% as compared to well-controlled warfarin [58]. Moreover, monitoring dabigatran plasma concentrations has the potential to improve safety and efficacy profiles as compared to fixed dosage [58,59]. Therapeutic drug monitoring of DOACs is supported by population studies which demonstrated a wide range of plasma dabigatran concentrations in different patient groups and at different time points although drug concentrations remained within the putative therapeutic range [60]. Variations in plasma concentration are ascribed to drug interactions, differences in absorption in the gastrointestinal tract, and clearance by the liver and kidneys [61]. These issues raise the question whether DOAC treatment should be regularly monitored.

A major issue of oral anticoagulation using VKA and DOACs is the need for reversal agents and coagulation assays to monitor the precise degree of anticoagulation. This is of importance in the event of bleeding and to allow surgical procedures or to counteract overdosing. The importance of reversal agents is illustrated by warfarin-related bleeding events, in which 50% of patients die within 90 days, mainly due to intracranial hemorrhage [62]. In the case of VKA, guidelines for the reversal of over-anticoagulation are well established with effective reversal agents (phylloquinone, and prothrombin complex concentrates) and sensitive coagulation assays (e.g., INR) to monitor haemostasis [62]. Vitamin K can counteract the effect of VKA via a

NAD(P)H-dependent quinone reductase, the precise identity of which is uncertain. The enzyme that counteracts VKA is predominantly active in the liver and unlike VKOR is not inhibited by VKA thereby enabling the reduction of vitamin K into KH_2 cofactors needed for γ-glutamyl carboxylation (Figure 1b) [63]. Reversal agents for DOACs were initially lacking, but are currently under development (idarucizumab for dabigatran, and andexanet and PER977 for FXa) [64]. Idarucizumab was developed to inactivate dabigatran, and works by binding to dabigatran with an affinity 350 times higher than thrombin. Recently, the clinical trial RE-VERSE AD investigated the capability and safety of idarucizumab as a reversal agent, and demonstrated a complete reversal of the anticoagulation effect of dabigatran within minutes. Of note, a major limitation in the RE-VERSE AD trial is the lack of a control group [65].

It should be noted that all DOACs are partially excreted by the kidneys (80%, 65%, and 25% for dabigatran, rivaroxaban and apixaban, respectively) [66,67] and are therefore unsuitable for patients with severe renal deficiency. In contrast, VKA are predominantly metabolized through the liver and are thus the best option for anticoagulation with this patient population.

5. Vitamin K Dependent Proteins and Atherosclerosis

5.1. Coagulation and Atherosclerosis

Coagulation factors are effective activators of the vascular system independent of their effects on coagulation and exhibit pleiotropic effects on the vasculature that contribute to cardiovascular disease. More specifically, coagulation factors can affect the vessel wall through regulation of the proliferation, migration and differentiation of vascular smooth muscle cells (VSMCs) as well as by inducing oxidative stress, inflammation and apoptosis [66,67], all processes that contribute to the development of atherosclerosis. In addition, micro plaque ruptures and subclinical thrombosis are pivotal to the progression and increased vulnerability of plaques, thereby increasing the risk for atherothrombosis [67].

5.2. Thrombin and Atherosclerosis

Thrombin is the central player in the coagulation cascade and influences non-hemostasis signaling via the protease-activated receptors (PAR-1, PAR-2, PAR-3, PAR-4) [66]. Thrombin activates these receptors via proteolytic cleavage of the N-terminal domain of PAR-1, PAR-3 and PAR-4 resulting in a tethered ligand activating the receptor [68,69]. In the vasculature, endothelial cells express PAR-1, PAR-2 and PAR-4, whereas VSMCs express PAR-1 and PAR-2 [70]. The effects of thrombin on the different PARs are likely to induce different effects, of which PAR-1 related effects have been most studied [66,71].

Human atherosclerotic plaques express elevated levels of PAR-1 [72], suggesting that PAR-1 plays a role in atherosclerosis development. In line with this hypothesis, thrombin induced PAR-1 activation can lead to VSMC migration and proliferation (Figure 2b). Moreover, thrombin elevates collagen production by VSMCs in a PAR-1 dependent manner [73], indicating a possible role for thrombin in plaque stability. Another feature of atherosclerotic plaque development is apoptosis. VSMCs that undergo apoptosis can generate thrombin via a process that accelerates the assembly of the prothrombinase complex [74]. In addition, thrombin generation is associated with vascular calcification [75].

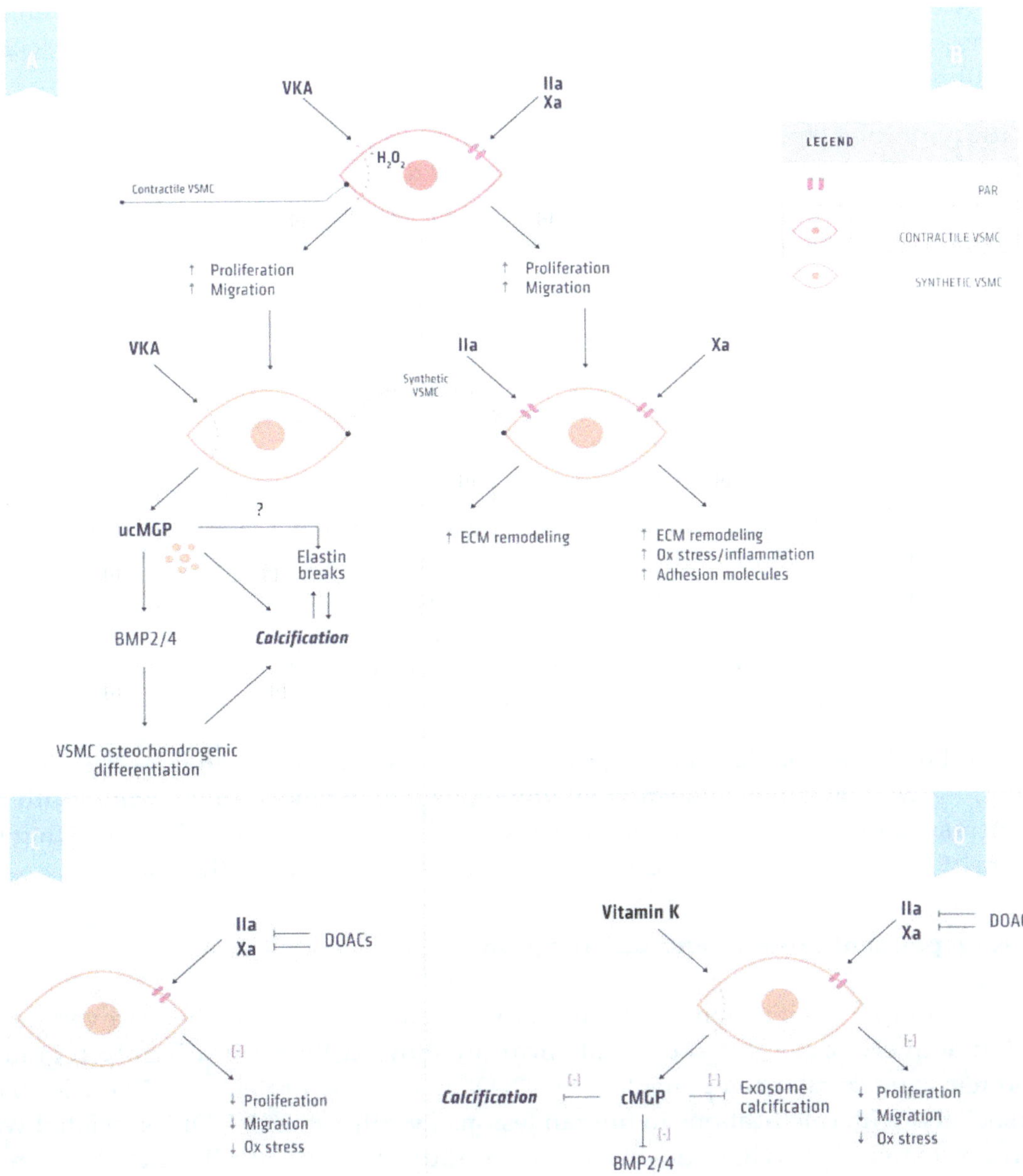

Figure 2. Effects of anticoagulants and vitamin K on vascular calcification. (**A**) Mechanism by which vitamin K antagonist (VKA) induces calcification. VKA induces phenotypic switching of contractile to synthetic vascular smooth muscle cells (VSMCs) by increasing oxidative stress resulting in increased proliferation and migration. Synthetic VSMCs secrete uncarboxylated matrix Gla protein (ucMGP) as a result of vitamin K depletion induced by VKA. ucMGP is unable to inhibit bone morphogenetic protein (BMP) 2 and 4, a marker for osteochondrogenic differentiation. Osteochondrogenic VSMCs are prone to calcification. Additionally, ucMGP is directly associated with increased calcification; (**B**) Thrombin and factor Xa induce non-hemostasis signaling via protease-activated receptors (PARs). Activation of PARs on contractile VSMCs can induce phenotypic switching resulting in increased proliferation and migration. PAR signaling in these synthetic VSMCs increases oxidative stress and adhesion molecules and induces extracellular (ECM) remodeling thereby facilitating calcification; (**C**) DOAC treatment in combination with (**D**) supplemental vitamin K administration has the potential to prevent both hypercoagulability and inhibit vascular calcification.

Of note, rodents lack PAR-1 expression on platelets [71]. Therefore, experiments targeting PAR-1 in rodents can be directly ascribed to PAR-1 expressed by the vessel wall. Indeed, vascular injury is altered in PAR-1 deficient mice possibly via extracellular matrix formation and remodeling [72]. In line with these results, *in vitro* stimulation of VSMCs by thrombin stimulates extracellular matrix production [70].

Dabigatran inhibits thrombin mediated PAR1 function by inhibiting N-terminal cleavage and internalization [76]. The inhibition of thrombin activity by dabigatran may thus inhibit the development of cardiovascular disease by reducing pro-inflammatory signaling [67]. Indeed, dabigatran was shown to attenuate atherosclerosis development [77] and promote plaque stability [78].

5.3. Factor Xa and Atherosclerosis

Like thrombin, FXa induces non-hemostatic signaling via PARs. However, in contrast to thrombin FXa interacts only with PAR-1 and PAR-2 [70,79]. As with PAR-1, the expression of PAR-2 is upregulated in human vascular lesions [70,80]. FXa has been linked to pathophysiological conditions, including inflammation, tissue fibrosis and vascular remodeling [81]. In line with this link, FXa has been shown to induce inflammatory signaling and increase expression of cell adhesion molecules [67]. Moreover, FXa induces proliferation and migration of VSMCs via activation of PAR-2 thereby altering the composition and accumulation of extracellular matrix [82,83]. The *in vivo* importance of PAR-2 in the inflammation process is suggested by findings that PAR-2 deficient mice display lower inflammation in a model of arthritis [84] and from rat studies in which lipopolysaccharide and oxidative stress increased the expression of PAR-2 [85,86].

Taken together, the available data suggests that FXa has a role in atherosclerosis via its interaction with PAR-1 and PAR-2. Recently, treatment of atherosclerosis prone apoE$^{-/-}$ mice with rivaroxaban resulted in increased plaque stability [87]. Since FXa activates prothrombin it is tempting to speculate that inhibition of FXa also prevents thrombin-mediated effects in atherothrombosis.

6. Vitamin K Dependent Proteins and Calcification

Originally, vascular calcification was thought to be a passive process. The discovery of calcification inhibitors that actively prevent vascular calcification showed that it is a highly regulated process involving proteins and cellular components. The VKDP matrix Gla protein (MGP) is a local calcification inhibitor associated with calcifications in human lesions [88,89]. Other VKDP associated with vascular calcification are osteocalcin (OC) and the more recently discovered Gla Rich Protein (GRP) [90]. Moreover, MGP, OC and the downstream regulator bone morphogenetic proteins (BMP) 2 and 4 are associated with microcalcifications in early human atherosclerotic lesions [88]. Microcalcifications in atherosclerosis are associated with increased plaque vulnerability [91–94].

6.1. Osteocalcin

Like all VKDP proteins, OC requires vitamin K for the γ-glutamylcarboxylation of three glutamate-residues, which in turn confers functional protein activity. In tissues and the circulation OC is present in both the carboxylated (cOC) and uncarboxylated (ucOC) conformations. OC is mostly associated with bone metabolism [95] where it promotes bone growth [96–98]. The processes of bone metabolism and soft tissue calcification are closely related, suggesting a possible role of osteocalcin in vascular calcification (Figure 3). As in bone metabolism, OC is thought to both promote [99] and inhibit [100–103] soft tissue calcification in order to regulate remodeling and mineralization [104]. It has been suggested that the inhibitory effect of OC on calcification is via mechanisms that prevent calcium and phosphate precipitation [17].

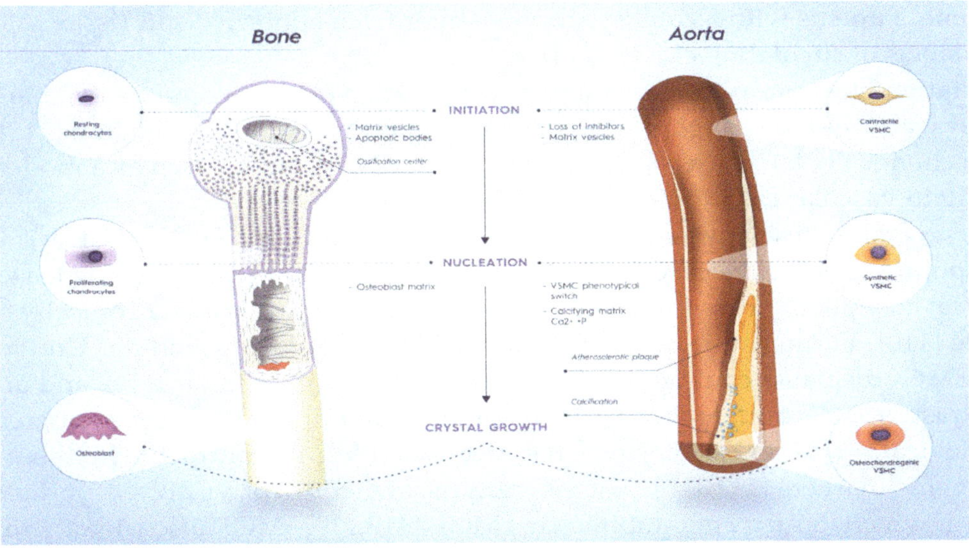

Figure 3. Similarities in bone metabolism and vascular calcification. The calcification process can be divided into three stages: initiation, nucleation and crystal growth. In order to initiate mineralization resting chondrocytes and contractile vascular smooth muscle cells (VSMCs) lose calcification inhibitors. Moreover, vesicles derived from chondrocytes and VSMCs form a nidus for calcification. In both bone metabolism and vascular calcification the matrix plays an important role in the nucleation stage. In bone metabolism, an osteoblast matrix results in proliferation of chondrocytes. Likewise, a calcifying matrix consisting of elastin, collagen and Ca^{2+} and P accompany vascular calcification. Additionally, contractile VSMCs undergo phenotypic switching resulting in synthetic VSMCs, which have increased proliferation and migration in comparison to contractile VSMCs. Finally, osteoblasts and osteochondrogenic VSMCs induce crystal growth in bone metabolism and vascular calcification, respectively.

The role of OC in vascular calcification suggests the possibility that OC measurements can be used as a biomarker of calcification. OC-positive endothelial progenitor cells are elevated in patients with a history of cardiovascular events and were associated with calcification of coronary arteries [105, 106]. During atherosclerosis, VSMCs undergo phenotypic switching resulting in osteoblast-like VSMCs, which are prone to calcification. Calcifying VSMCs express OC [107] and thus increased circulating concentrations of OC may reflect vascular calcification. Indeed, calcification of osteoblast-like VSMCs is associated with OC synthesis [108]. Furthermore, circulating levels of ucOC could provide insights into the relationship between vitamin K status and calcification. Indeed, it has been shown that ucOC concentrations are an independent predictor of carotid artery calcification [109].

6.2. Matrix Gla Protein

MGP is found in a wide range of tissues including heart, lungs, skin and the vasculature. In the vessel wall MGP is secreted by VSMCs [110]. Besides posttranslational carboxylation, MGP can also undergo serine phosphorylation. The precise role of the latter modification is not fully understood, but is thought to play a role in the secretion of MGP [111].

The pivotal role of MGP became clear from MGP-deficient mice, which all died within eight weeks after birth due to rupture of severely calcified arteries [112]. Analyses of the arteries revealed fragmented and calcified elastic fibers and the presence of osteochondrogenic-like cells. Surprisingly, the calcification phenotype of $MGP^{-/-}$ mice was not rescued by restoring circulating levels of MGP via hepatic MGP expression [113]. In contrast, restoring MGP expression in VSMCs rescued the vascular phenotype completely [113]. These data demonstrated that only VSMCs synthesis of carboxylated MGP (cMGP) is able to inhibit vascular calcification. MGP deficiency is also present in humans resulting in

Keutel syndrome. Patients with Keutel syndrome suffer from abnormal soft tissue calcification [104] and have low levels of circulating cMGP [114].

Administration of warfarin results in similar calcification of arteries as observed in MGP$^{-/-}$ mice suggesting that warfarin-induced calcification is via impairment of MGP function [115]. Additionally, since warfarin chemically knocks down γ-carboxylated MGP it can be used as a model to investigate the role of MGP in vascular calcification [115].

There are several routes by which cMGP may inhibit calcification [110]. MGP is present in matrix vesicles and apoptopic bodies released from VSMCs [116]. In the presence of increased extracellular calcium MGP levels initially increase. However, when calcium levels are chronically elevated, MGP levels decrease [110]. Furthermore, MGP blocks VSMC phenotypic switching. Under physiological conditions, VSMCs display a contractile phenotype supporting vascular tone, and are not prone to calcify. In contrast, VSMCs undergoing synthetic or osteochondrogenic differentiation are susceptible to vascular calcification [17]. MGP$^{-/-}$ mice had decreased VSMC contractile markers and increased osteochondrogenic markers [112,117]. The phenotypic switching of VSMCs is under the regulation of BMP 2 and 4, which in turn are inhibited by cMGP [118,119]. MGP also directly inhibits calcium crystal growth by its ability to block nucleation sites through the binding of the negatively charged Gla domain and phosphorylated serine residues of MGP with growing hydroxyapatite crystals [120,121]. Finally, MGP prevents mineralization of elastin fibers by shedding nucleation sites, this process being facilitated by the low molecular weight and small size of MGP allowing it to prevent mineralization within the elastin fibers [122,123].

6.3. Gla Rich Protein

GRP, also termed Upper zone of growth plate and Cartilage Matrix Associated protein (UCMA), is a recently discovered VKDP highly conserved in animals and humans and involved in the inhibition of vascular calcification. Human gene expression and protein accumulation of GRP was shown in the fetal growth plate, vascular system and skin [124]. In human pathological conditions, GRP expression is associated with calcification of skin and arteries [90]. GRP has, like MGP, calcium-binding properties and acts as a calcification inhibitor [125]. The calcification-inhibitory effect of GRP is dose-dependent, requires γ-glutamylcarboxylation, and is thought to act via inhibition of osteochondrogenic switching of VSMCs [125]. GRP knockout mice, however lack phenotypic alterations [126].

7. Role for Vitamin K in Cardiovascular Disease

The first evidence that vitamin K is associated with vascular health came from data from the Rotterdam study [127]. In this observational study the risk for cardiovascular disease was some 50% lower in people in the highest tertile for menaquinone dietary intake (MK4 through MK10) [127]. In epidemiological studies, dietary intakes of menaquinones (MK-4 through MK-10) have been reported to be associated with a reduced risk for cardiovascular mortality [127,128]. Additionally, higher menaquinone intakes (MK-4 through MK-10) or supplementation with MK-7 were associated with reduced calcification, which is presumed to be due to the improved γ-carboxylation and greater functional activity of VKDP [129,130]. Finally, the long chain menaquinone isoprenologue MK-7 has been shown to have a greater impact on restoring coagulation compared to phylloquinone in VKA treated healthy volunteers indicating the overall better efficacy of MK-7 for the γ-carboxylation of the coagulation VKDP synthesized in the liver [14,131]. Explanations for the putative beneficial effect of MK-7 on the vascular system for the γ-carboxylation of MGP and GRP is that long chain menaquinones such as MK7 are mainly transported via low-density lipoproteins and have a slower clearance rate from the circulation [13] as well as a higher co-factor activity for the γ glutamyl-carboxylase [132].

In order to investigate the effect of vitamin K on the vascular system in humans a biomarker that reflects vitamin K status is required. Since vitamin K is essential for carboxylation of VKDP, the carboxylation status of VKDP can be used as a biomarker for vitamin K status. Dialysis patients have significantly increased levels of circulating uncarboxylated MGP (ucMGP) and reduced levels of cMGP indicative of a subclinical vascular vitamin K deficiency [133]. Moreover, circulating levels of ucMGP are positively associated with vascular calcification. Taken together, ucMGP seems a promising biomarker for vascular vitamin K status in relation to vascular calcification [89,133–135]. Therefore, clinical studies investigating the effect of vitamin K on the vascular system and calcification use the carboxylation status of MGP as a biomarker [130]. Currently, clinical trials are ongoing to assess the effect of high intake of vitamin K on vascular calcification progression [136]. In these clinical studies both phylloquinone and menaquinones are under investigation and can therefore provide novel insights into the differential effect of vitamin K forms on vascular calcification.

8. Vitamin K and Direct oral Anticoagulation

Treating patients with hypercoagulability and vascular disease requires personalized medicine. Whereas both VKA and DOACs are equally suitable for treating hypercoagulability, VKA induces vascular calcification thereby affecting the vessel wall in a negative way (Figure 2a). Effects of DOACs on vascular calcification are not known yet, but are unlikely to affect VKDP activity (Figure 2b) [137]. Moreover, high intake of vitamin K has shown to inhibit and even reverse warfarin-induced vascular calcification in experimental animals [56,138] and in adenine treated rats [52]. It is tempting to speculate that co-administration of vitamin K with anticoagulation therapy can target both coagulation and calcification. Since this co-administration is unsuitable with VKA [131], it should be investigated whether combining DOACs and vitamin K can be beneficial for both coagulation and calcification (Figure 2c). Presently, clinical trials assessing these aspects of co-administration are being conducted and the results of these studies should provide novel insights into personalized anticoagulation therapy [136].

9. Conclusions

Currently, VKA are still the most widely prescribed drugs used for anticoagulation therapy. However, owing to the unfavorable pharmacokinetics and actions of VKA, direct thrombin and FXa inhibitors have been introduced as alternatives to VKA. Clinical studies have demonstrated that DOACs are non-inferior to VKA but are likely to lack the calcification-inducing side effect of VKA. Additionally, DOACs exert beneficial effects on atherogenesis via PAR signaling. Presently, ongoing clinical trials are addressing whether vitamin K supplementation can halt or regress vascular calcification. The outcome of these trials will pave the way to test whether co-supplementation of vitamin K with DOACs can benefit both coagulation and calcification.

Acknowledgments: This work was supported in part by research funding from the Trombose Stichting Nederland (grant 2014.02) and by the Norwegian Research Council and NattoPharma ASA.

Author Contributions: Rick van Gorp and Leon Schurgers wrote the manuscript. Leon Schurgers had primary responsibility for the final content.

References

1. Mann, K.G. Biochemistry and physiology of blood coagulation. *Thromb. Haemost.* **1999**, *82*, 165–174. [PubMed]
2. Macfarlane, R.G. An enzyme cascade in the blood clotting mechanism, and its function as a biochemical amplifier. *Nature* **1964**, *202*, 498–499. [CrossRef] [PubMed]
3. Colman, R.W. Are hemostasis and thrombosis two sides of the same coin? *J. Exp. Med.* **2006**, *203*, 493–495. [CrossRef] [PubMed]
4. Badimon, L. Atherosclerosis and thrombosis: Lessons from animal models. *Thromb. Haemost.* **2001**, *86*, 356–365. [PubMed]

5. Fuster, V.; Stein, B.; Ambrose, J.A.; Badimon, L.; Badimon, J.J.; Chesebro, J.H. Atherosclerotic plaque rupture and thrombosis. Evolving concepts. *Circulation* **1990**, *82*, II47–II59. [PubMed]
6. Rosendaal, F.R. Venous thrombosis: A multicausal disease. *Lancet* **1999**, *353*, 1167–1173. [CrossRef]
7. Schofield, F.W. A brief account of a disease in cattle simulating hemorrhagic septicaemia due to feeding sweet clover. *Can. Vet. J. Rev. Vétérinaire Can.* **1984**, *25*, 453–455.
8. Link, K. The discovery of dicumarol and its sequels. *Circulation* **1959**, *19*, 97–107. [CrossRef] [PubMed]
9. Shapiro, S.; Ciferri, F.E. Intramuscular administration of the anticoagulant warfarin (coumadin) sodium. *J. Am. Med. Assoc.* **1957**, *165*, 1377–1380. [CrossRef] [PubMed]
10. Beinema, M.; Brouwers, J.R.B.J.; Schalekamp, T.; Wilffert, B. Pharmacogenetic differences between warfarin, acenocoumarol and phenprocoumon. *Thromb. Haemost.* **2008**, *100*, 1052–1057. [CrossRef] [PubMed]
11. Beulens, J.W.J.; Booth, S.L.; van den Heuvel, E.G.H.M.; Stoecklin, E.; Baka, A.; Vermeer, C. The role of menaquinones (vitamin K2) in human health. *Br. J. Nutr.* **2013**, *110*, 1357–1368. [CrossRef] [PubMed]
12. Schurgers, L.J.; Vermeer, C. Determination of phylloquinone and menaquinones in food. *Eff. Food Matrix Circ. Vitam. K Conc.* **2000**, *30*, 298–307. [CrossRef]
13. Schurgers, L.J.; Vermeer, C. Differential lipoprotein transport pathways of K-vitamins in healthy subjects. *Biochim. Biophys. Acta* **2002**, *1570*, 27–32. [CrossRef]
14. Schurgers, L.J.; Teunissen, K.J.F.; Hamulyak, K.; Knapen, M.H.J.; Vik, H.; Vermeer, C. Vitamin K-containing dietary supplements: Comparison of synthetic vitamin K1 and natto-derived menaquinone-7. *Blood* **2007**, *109*, 3279–3283. [CrossRef] [PubMed]
15. Thijssen, H.H.W.; Vervoort, L.M.T.; Schurgers, L.J.; Shearer, M.J. Menadione is a metabolite of oral vitamin K. *Br. J. Nutr.* **2006**, *95*, 260–266. [CrossRef] [PubMed]
16. Esmon, C.; Sadowski, J.; Suttie, J. A new carboxylation reaction. The vitamin K-dependent incorporation of H-14-CO3- into prothrombin. *J. Biol. Chem.* **1975**, *250*, 4744–4748. [PubMed]
17. Willems, B.A.G.; Vermeer, C.; Reutelingsperger, C.P.M.; Schurgers, L.J. The realm of vitamin K dependent proteins: Shifting from coagulation toward calcification. *Mol. Nutr. Food Res.* **2014**, *58*, 1620–1635. [CrossRef] [PubMed]
18. Van Horn, W.D. Structural and functional insights into human vitamin K epoxide reductase and vitamin K epoxide reductase-like1. *Crit. Rev. Biochem. Mol. Biol.* **2013**, *48*, 357–372. [CrossRef] [PubMed]
19. Stafford, D. The vitamin K cycle. *J. Thromb. Haemost.* **2005**, *3*, 1873–1878. [CrossRef] [PubMed]
20. Weitz, J.I.; Hirsh, J. New antithrombotic agents. *Chest* **1998**, *114*, 715S–727S. [CrossRef] [PubMed]
21. Van Aken, H.; Bode, C.; Darius, H.; Diehm, C.; Encke, A.; Gulba, D.C.; Haas, S.; Hacke, W.; Puhl, W.; Quante, M.; *et al.* State-of-the-art review: Anticoagulation: The present and future. *Clin. Appl. Thromb. Hemost.* **2001**, *7*, 195–204. [CrossRef] [PubMed]
22. Greinacher, A.; Warkentin, T.E. The direct thrombin inhibitor hirudin. *Thromb. Haemost.* **2008**, *99*, 819–829. [CrossRef] [PubMed]
23. Eriksson, B.I.; Wille-Jørgensen, P.; Kälebo, P.; Mouret, P.; Rosencher, N.; Bösch, P.; Baur, M.; Ekman, S.; Bach, D.; Lindbratt, S.; *et al.* A comparison of recombinant hirudin with a low-molecular-weight heparin to prevent thromboembolic complications after total hip replacement. *N. Engl. J. Med.* **1997**, *337*, 1329–1335. [CrossRef] [PubMed]
24. Investigators, G.L. Randomized trial of intravenous heparin *versus* recombinant hirudin for acute coronary syndromes. The Global Use of Strategies to Open Occluded Coronary Arteries (GUSTO) IIa Investigators. *Circulation* **1994**, *90*, 1631–1637.
25. Schulman, S.; Kearon, C.; Kakkar, A.K.; Mismetti, P.; Schellong, S.; Eriksson, H.; Baanstra, D.; Schnee, J.; Goldhaber, S.Z. RE-COVER Study Group Dabigatran *versus* warfarin in the treatment of acute venous thromboembolism. *N. Engl. J. Med.* **2009**, *361*, 2342–2352. [CrossRef] [PubMed]
26. Schulman, S.; Wåhlander, K.; Lundström, T.; Clason, S.B.; Eriksson, H. THRIVE III Investigators Secondary prevention of venous thromboembolism with the oral direct thrombin inhibitor ximelagatran. *N. Engl. J. Med.* **2003**, *349*, 1713–1721. [CrossRef] [PubMed]
27. Laizure, S.C.; Parker, R.B.; Herring, V.L.; Hu, Z.-Y. Identification of carboxylesterase-dependent dabigatran etexilate hydrolysis. *Drug Metab. Dispos. Biol. Fate Chem.* **2014**, *42*, 201–206. [CrossRef] [PubMed]
28. Akwaa, F.; Spyropoulos, A.C. The potential of target-specific oral anticoagulants for the acute and long-term treatment of venous thromboembolism. *Curr. Med. Res. Opin.* **2014**, *30*, 2179–2190. [CrossRef] [PubMed]

29. Yeh, C.H.; Hogg, K.; Weitz, J.I. Overview of the New Oral Anticoagulants: Opportunities and Challenges. *Arterioscler. Thromb. Vasc. Biol.* **2015**, *35*, 1056–1065. [CrossRef] [PubMed]
30. Kubitza, D.; Becka, M.; Wensing, G.; Voith, B.; Zuehlsdorf, M. Safety, pharmacodynamics, and pharmacokinetics of BAY 59–7939—An oral, direct Factor Xa inhibitor—After multiple dosing in healthy male subjects. *Eur. J. Clin. Pharmacol.* **2005**, *61*, 873–880. [CrossRef] [PubMed]
31. Kubitza, D.; Haas, S. Novel factor Xa inhibitors for prevention and treatment of thromboembolic diseases. *Expert Opin. Investig. Drugs* **2006**, *15*, 843–855. [CrossRef] [PubMed]
32. Weitz, J.I. Emerging anticoagulants for the treatment of venous thromboembolism. *Thromb. Haemost.* **2006**, *96*, 274–284. [CrossRef] [PubMed]
33. Nutt, E.M.; Jain, D.; Lenny, A.B.; Schaffer, L.; Siegl, P.K.; Dunwiddie, C.T. Purification and characterization of recombinant antistasin: A leech-derived inhibitor of coagulation factor Xa. *Arch. Biochem. Biophys.* **1991**, *285*, 37–44. [CrossRef]
34. Yeh, C.H.; Fredenburgh, J.C.; Weitz, J.I. Oral direct factor Xa inhibitors. *Circ. Res.* **2012**, *111*, 1069–1078. [CrossRef] [PubMed]
35. Perzborn, E.; Strassburger, J.; Wilmen, A.; Pohlmann, J.; Roehrig, S.; Schlemmer, K.-H.; Straub, A. *In vitro* and *in vivo* studies of the novel antithrombotic agent BAY 59-7939—An oral, direct Factor Xa inhibitor. *J. Thromb. Haemost.* **2005**, *3*, 514–521. [CrossRef] [PubMed]
36. Schurgers, L.J.; Spronk, H.M.H. Differential cellular effects of old and new oral anticoagulants: Consequences to the genesis and progression of atherosclerosis. *Thromb. Haemost.* **2014**, *112*, 909–917. [CrossRef] [PubMed]
37. Kreutz, R. A clinical and pharmacologic assessment of once-daily *versus* twice-daily dosing for rivaroxaban. *J. Thromb. Thrombolysis* **2014**, *38*, 137–149. [CrossRef] [PubMed]
38. Barritt, D.W.; Jordan, S.C. Anticoagulant drugs in the treatment of pulmonary embolism. A controlled trial. *Lancet* **1960**, *1*, 1309–1312. [CrossRef]
39. Duxbury, B.M.; Poller, L. The oral anticoagulant saga: Past, present, and future. *Clin. Appl. Thromb. Hemost.* **2001**, *7*, 269–275. [CrossRef] [PubMed]
40. Hull, R.; Hirsh, J.; Jay, R.; Carter, C.; England, C.; Gent, M.; Turpie, A.G.; McLoughlin, D.; Dodd, P.; Thomas, M.; *et al.* Different intensities of oral anticoagulant therapy in the treatment of proximal-vein thrombosis. *N. Engl. J. Med.* **1982**, *307*, 1676–1681. [CrossRef] [PubMed]
41. Guyatt, G.H.; Akl, E.A.; Crowther, M.; Gutterman, D.D.; Schuünemann, H.J. Executive summary: Antithrombotic therapy and prevention of thrombosis, 9th ed.: American college of chest physicians evidence-based clinical practice guidelines. *Chest* **2012**, *141*, 7S–47S. [CrossRef] [PubMed]
42. Connolly, S.J.; Ezekowitz, M.D.; Yusuf, S.; Eikelboom, J.; Oldgren, J.; Parekh, A.; Pogue, J.; Reilly, P.A.; Themeles, E.; Varrone, J.; *et al.* RE-LY Steering Committee and Investigators Dabigatran *versus* warfarin in patients with atrial fibrillation. *N. Engl. J. Med.* **2009**, *361*, 1139–1151. [CrossRef] [PubMed]
43. Eriksson, B.I.; Dahl, O.E.; Rosencher, N.; Kurth, A.A.; van Dijk, C.N.; Frostick, S.P.; Kälebo, P.; Christiansen, A.V.; Hantel, S.; Hettiarachchi, R.; *et al.* RE-MODEL Study Group Oral dabigatran etexilate *vs.* subcutaneous enoxaparin for the prevention of venous thromboembolism after total knee replacement: The RE-MODEL randomized trial. *J. Thromb. Haemost.* **2007**, *5*, 2178–2185. [CrossRef] [PubMed]
44. Patel, M.R.; Mahaffey, K.W.; Garg, J.; Pan, G.; Singer, D.E.; Hacke, W.; Breithardt, G.; Halperin, J.L.; Hankey, G.J.; Piccini, J.P.; *et al.* ROCKET AF Investigators Rivaroxaban *versus* warfarin in nonvalvular atrial fibrillation. *N. Engl. J. Med.* **2011**, *365*, 883–891. [CrossRef] [PubMed]
45. Eriksson, B.I.; Borris, L.C.; Friedman, R.J.; Haas, S.; Huisman, M.V.; Kakkar, A.K.; Bandel, T.J.; Beckmann, H.; Muehlhofer, E.; Misselwitz, F.; *et al.* RECORD1 Study Group Rivaroxaban *versus* enoxaparin for thromboprophylaxis after hip arthroplasty. *N. Engl. J. Med.* **2008**, *358*, 2765–2775. [CrossRef] [PubMed]
46. EINSTEIN Investigators; Bauersachs, R.; Berkowitz, S.D.; Brenner, B.; Büller, H.R.; Decousus, H.; Gallus, A.S.; Lensing, A.W.; Misselwitz, F.; Prins, M.H.; *et al.* Oral rivaroxaban for symptomatic venous thromboembolism. *N. Engl. J. Med.* **2010**, *363*, 2499–2510.
47. Eriksson, B.I.; Kakkar, A.K.; Turpie, A.G.G.; Gent, M.; Bandel, T.-J.; Homering, M.; Misselwitz, F.; Lassen, M.R. Oral rivaroxaban for the prevention of symptomatic venous thromboembolism after elective hip and knee replacement. *J. Bone Joint Surg. Br.* **2009**, *91*, 636–644. [CrossRef] [PubMed]
48. Granger, C.B.; Alexander, J.H.; McMurray, J.J.V.; Lopes, R.D.; Hylek, E.M.; Hanna, M.; Al-Khalidi, H.R.; Ansell, J.; Atar, D.; Avezum, A.; *et al.* ARISTOTLE Committees and Investigators Apixaban *versus* warfarin in patients with atrial fibrillation. *N. Engl. J. Med.* **2011**, *365*, 981–992. [CrossRef] [PubMed]

49. Lassen, M.R.; Gallus, A.; Raskob, G.E.; Pineo, G.; Chen, D.; Ramirez, L.M. ADVANCE-3 Investigators Apixaban *versus* enoxaparin for thromboprophylaxis after hip replacement. *N. Engl. J. Med.* **2010**, *363*, 2487–2498. [CrossRef] [PubMed]
50. Van Es, N.; Coppens, M.; Schulman, S.; Middeldorp, S.; Büller, H.R. Direct oral anticoagulants compared with vitamin K antagonists for acute venous thromboembolism: Evidence from phase 3 trials. *Blood* **2014**, *124*, 1968–1975. [CrossRef] [PubMed]
51. Haas, S. Medical indications and considerations for future clinical decision making. *Thromb. Res.* **2003**, *109* (Suppl. 1), S31–S37. [CrossRef]
52. McCabe, K.M.; Booth, S.L.; Fu, X.; Shobeiri, N.; Pang, J.J.; Adams, M.A.; Holden, R.M. Dietary vitamin K and therapeutic warfarin alter the susceptibility to vascular calcification in experimental chronic kidney disease. *Kidney Int.* **2013**, *83*, 835–844. [CrossRef] [PubMed]
53. Chatrou, M.L.L.; Winckers, K.; Hackeng, T.M.; Reutelingsperger, C.P.; Schurgers, L.J. Vascular calcification: The price to pay for anticoagulation therapy with vitamin K-antagonists. *Blood Rev.* **2012**, *26*, 155–166. [CrossRef] [PubMed]
54. Rosenhek, R.; Binder, T.; Porenta, G.; Lang, I.; Christ, G.; Schemper, M.; Maurer, G.; Baumgartner, H. Predictors of outcome in severe, asymptomatic aortic stenosis. *N. Engl. J. Med.* **2000**, *343*, 611–617. [CrossRef] [PubMed]
55. Rennenberg, R.J.M.W.; Kessels, A.G.H.; Schurgers, L.J.; van Engelshoven, J.M.A.; de Leeuw, P.W.; Kroon, A.A. Vascular calcifications as a marker of increased cardiovascular risk: A meta-analysis. *Vasc. Health Risk Manag.* **2009**, *5*, 185–197. [CrossRef] [PubMed]
56. Schurgers, L.J.; Spronk, H.M.; Soute, B.A.; Schiffers, P.; DeMey, J.G.R.; Vermeer, C. Regression of warfarin-induced medial elastocalcinosis by high intake of vitamin K in rats. *Blood* **2007**, *109*, 2823–2831. [CrossRef] [PubMed]
57. Mac-Way, F.; Poulin, A.; Utescu, M.S.; De Serres, S.A.; Marquis, K.; Douville, P.; Desmeules, S.; Larivière, R.; Lebel, M.; Agharazii, M. The impact of warfarin on the rate of progression of aortic stiffness in hemodialysis patients: A longitudinal study. *Nephrol. Dial. Transplant.* **2014**, *29*, 2113–2120. [CrossRef] [PubMed]
58. Cohen, D. Dabigatran: How the drug company withheld important analyses. *BMJ (Clin. Res. ed.)* **2014**, *349*. [CrossRef] [PubMed]
59. Moore, T.J.; Cohen, M.R.; Mattison, D.R. Dabigatran, bleeding, and the regulators. *BMJ (Clin. Res. ed.)* **2014**, *349*. [CrossRef] [PubMed]
60. Favaloro, E.J.; Lippi, G. Laboratory testing in the era of direct or non-vitamin K antagonist oral anticoagulants: A practical guide to measuring their activity and avoiding diagnostic errors. *Semin. Thromb. Hemost.* **2015**, *41*, 208–227. [PubMed]
61. Lippi, G.; Favaloro, E.J.; Mattiuzzi, C. Combined administration of antibiotics and direct oral anticoagulants: A renewed indication for laboratory monitoring? *Semin. Thromb. Hemost.* **2014**, *40*, 756–765. [PubMed]
62. Bauer, K.A. Targeted Anti-Anticoagulants. *N. Engl. J. Med.* **2015**, *373*, 569–571. [CrossRef] [PubMed]
63. Shearer, M.J.; Newman, P. Metabolism and cell biology of vitamin K. *Thromb. Haemost.* **2008**, *100*, 530–547. [CrossRef] [PubMed]
64. Crowther, M.; Crowther, M.A. Antidotes for Novel Oral Anticoagulants: Current Status and Future Potential. *Arterioscler. Thromb. Vasc. Biol.* **2015**, *35*, 1736–1745. [CrossRef] [PubMed]
65. Pollack, C.V.; Reilly, P.A.; Eikelboom, J.; Glund, S.; Verhamme, P.; Bernstein, R.A.; Dubiel, R.; Huisman, M.V.; Hylek, E.M.; Kamphuisen, P.W.; *et al.* Idarucizumab for Dabigatran Reversal. *N. Engl. J. Med.* **2015**, *373*, 511–520. [CrossRef] [PubMed]
66. Patterson, C.; Stouffer, G.A.; Madamanchi, N.; Runge, M.S. New tricks for old dogs: Nonthrombotic effects of thrombin in vessel wall biology. *Circ. Res.* **2001**, *88*, 987–997. [CrossRef] [PubMed]
67. Borissoff, J.I.; Spronk, H.M.H.; Ten Cate, H. The hemostatic system as a modulator of atherosclerosis. *N. Engl. J. Med.* **2011**, *364*, 1746–1760. [PubMed]
68. Ma, L.; Dorling, A. The roles of thrombin and protease-activated receptors in inflammation. *Semin. Immunopathol.* **2012**, *34*, 63–72. [CrossRef] [PubMed]
69. Kalz, J.; Ten Cate, H.; Spronk, H.M.H. Thrombin generation and atherosclerosis. *J. Thromb. Thrombolysis* **2014**, *37*, 45–55. [CrossRef] [PubMed]
70. Alberelli, M.A.; De Candia, E. Functional role of protease activated receptors in vascular biology. *Vasc. Pharmacol.* **2014**, *62*, 72–81. [CrossRef] [PubMed]

71. Martorell, L.; Martínez-González, J.; Rodríguez, C.; Gentile, M.; Calvayrac, O.; Badimon, L. Thrombin and protease-activated receptors (PARs) in atherothrombosis. *Thromb. Haemost.* **2008**, *99*, 305–315. [CrossRef] [PubMed]
72. Cheung, W.M.; D'Andrea, M.R.; Andrade-Gordon, P.; Damiano, B.P. Altered vascular injury responses in mice deficient in protease-activated receptor-1. *Arterioscler. Thromb. Vasc. Biol.* **1999**, *19*, 3014–3024. [CrossRef] [PubMed]
73. Dabbagh, K.; Laurent, G.J.; McAnulty, R.J.; Chambers, R.C. Thrombin stimulates smooth muscle cell procollagen synthesis and mRNA levels via a PAR-1 mediated mechanism. *Thromb. Haemost.* **1998**, *79*, 405–409. [PubMed]
74. Flynn, P.; Byrne, C.; Baglin, T.; Weissberg, P.; Bennett, M. Thrombin generation by apoptotic vascular smooth muscle cells. *Blood* **1997**, *89*, 4378–4384. [PubMed]
75. Borissoff, J.I.; Joosen, I.A.; Versteylen, M.O.; Spronk, H.M.; ten Cate, H.; Hofstra, L. Accelerated *In Vivo* Thrombin Formation Independently Predicts the Presence and Severity of CT Angiographic Coronary Atherosclerosis. *JACC Cardiovasc. Imaging* **2012**, *5*, 1201–1210. [CrossRef] [PubMed]
76. Chen, B.; Soto, A.G.; Coronel, L.J.; Goss, A.; van Ryn, J.; Trejo, J. Characterization of Thrombin-Bound Dabigatran Effects on Protease-Activated Receptor-1 Expression and Signaling *In Vitro*. *Mol. Pharmacol.* **2015**, *88*, 95–105. [CrossRef] [PubMed]
77. Pingel, S.; Tiyerili, V.; Mueller, J.; Werner, N.; Nickenig, G.; Mueller, C. Thrombin inhibition by dabigatran attenuates atherosclerosis in ApoE deficient mice. *Arch. Med. Sci.* **2014**, *10*, 154–160. [CrossRef] [PubMed]
78. Kadoglou, N.P.E.; Moustardas, P.; Katsimpoulas, M.; Kapelouzou, A.; Kostomitsopoulos, N.; Schafer, K.; Kostakis, A.; Liapis, C.D. The beneficial effects of a direct thrombin inhibitor, dabigatran etexilate, on the development and stability of atherosclerotic lesions in apolipoprotein E-deficient mice: Dabigatran etexilate and atherosclerosis. *Cardiovasc. Drugs Ther. Spons. Int. Soc. Cardiovasc. Pharmacother.* **2012**, *26*, 367–374. [CrossRef] [PubMed]
79. Borensztajn, K.; Peppelenbosch, M.P.; Spek, C.A. Factor Xa: At the crossroads between coagulation and signaling in physiology and disease. *Trends Mol. Med.* **2008**, *14*, 429–440. [CrossRef] [PubMed]
80. Lee, H.; Hamilton, J.R. Physiology, pharmacology, and therapeutic potential of protease-activated receptors in vascular disease. *Pharmacol. Ther.* **2012**, *134*, 246–259. [CrossRef] [PubMed]
81. Esmon, C.T. Targeting factor Xa and thrombin: Impact on coagulation and beyond. *Thromb. Haemost.* **2014**, *111*, 625–633. [CrossRef] [PubMed]
82. Böhm, A.; Flößer, A.; Ermler, S.; Fender, A.C.; Lüth, A.; Kleuser, B.; Schrör, K.; Rauch, B.H. Factor-Xa-induced mitogenesis and migration require sphingosine kinase activity and S1P formation in human vascular smooth muscle cells. *Cardiovasc. Res.* **2013**, *99*, 505–513. [CrossRef] [PubMed]
83. Borensztajn, K.; Spek, C.A. Blood coagulation factor Xa as an emerging drug target. *Expert Opin. Ther. Targets* **2011**, *15*, 341–349. [CrossRef] [PubMed]
84. Ferrell, W.R.; Lockhart, J.C.; Kelso, E.B.; Dunning, L.; Plevin, R.; Meek, S.E.; Smith, A.J.H.; Hunter, G.D.; McLean, J.S.; McGarry, F.; *et al*. Essential role for proteinase-activated receptor-2 in arthritis. *J. Clin. Investig.* **2003**, *111*, 35–41. [CrossRef] [PubMed]
85. Aman, M.; Hirano, M.; Kanaide, H.; Hirano, K. Upregulation of proteinase-activated receptor-2 and increased response to trypsin in endothelial cells after exposure to oxidative stress in rat aortas. *J. Vasc. Res.* **2010**, *47*, 494–506. [CrossRef] [PubMed]
86. Cicala, C.; Pinto, A.; Bucci, M.; Sorrentino, R.; Walker, B.; Harriot, P.; Cruchley, A.; Kapas, S.; Howells, G.L.; Cirino, G. Protease-activated receptor-2 involvement in hypotension in normal and endotoxemic rats *in vivo*. *Circulation* **1999**, *99*, 2590–2597. [CrossRef] [PubMed]
87. Zhou, Q.; Bea, F.; Preusch, M.; Wang, H.; Isermann, B.; Shahzad, K.; Katus, H.A.; Blessing, E. Evaluation of plaque stability of advanced atherosclerotic lesions in apo E-deficient mice after treatment with the oral factor Xa inhibitor rivaroxaban. *Mediat. Inflamm.* **2011**, *2011*, 1–9. [CrossRef] [PubMed]
88. Roijers, R.B.; Debernardi, N.; Cleutjens, J.P.M.; Schurgers, L.J.; Mutsaers, P.H.A.; van der Vusse, G.J. Microcalcifications in early intimal lesions of atherosclerotic human coronary arteries. *Am. J. Pathol.* **2011**, *178*, 2879–2887. [CrossRef] [PubMed]
89. Schurgers, L.J.; Teunissen, K.J.F.; Knapen, M.H.J.; Kwaijtaal, M.; van Diest, R.; Appels, A.; Reutelingsperger, C.P.; Cleutjens, J.P.M.; Vermeer, C. Novel conformation-specific antibodies against matrix γ-carboxyglutamic acid (Gla) protein: Undercarboxylated matrix Gla protein as marker for vascular

calcification. *Arterioscler. Thromb. Vasc. Biol.* **2005**, *25*, 1629–1633. [CrossRef] [PubMed]
90. Viegas, C.S.B.; Cavaco, S.; Williamson, M.K.; Price, P.A.; Cancela, M.L.; Simes, D.C. Gla-rich protein is a novel vitamin K-dependent protein present in serum that accumulates at sites of pathological calcifications. *Am. J. Pathol.* **2009**, *175*, 2288–2298. [CrossRef] [PubMed]
91. Joshi, N.V.; Vesey, A.T.; Williams, M.C.; Shah, A.S.V.; Calvert, P.A.; Craighead, F.H.M.; Yeoh, S.E.; Wallace, W.; Salter, D.; Fletcher, A.M.; *et al.* 18F-fluoride positron emission tomography for identification of ruptured and high-risk coronary atherosclerotic plaques: A prospective clinical trial. *Lancet* **2014**, *383*, 705–713. [CrossRef]
92. Ehara, S.; Kobayashi, Y.; Yoshiyama, M.; Shimada, K.; Shimada, Y.; Fukuda, D.; Nakamura, Y.; Yamashita, H.; Yamagishi, H.; Takeuchi, K.; *et al.* Spotty calcification typifies the culprit plaque in patients with acute myocardial infarction: An intravascular ultrasound study. *Circulation* **2004**, *110*, 3424–3429. [CrossRef] [PubMed]
93. Bluestein, D.; Alemu, Y.; Avrahami, I.; Gharib, M.; Dumont, K.; Ricotta, J.J.; Einav, S. Influence of microcalcifications on vulnerable plaque mechanics using FSI modeling. *J. Biomech.* **2008**, *41*, 1111–1118. [CrossRef] [PubMed]
94. Vengrenyuk, Y.; Carlier, S.; Xanthos, S.; Cardoso, L.; Ganatos, P.; Virmani, R.; Einav, S.; Gilchrist, L.; Weinbaum, S. A hypothesis for vulnerable plaque rupture due to stress-induced debonding around cellular microcalcifications in thin fibrous caps. *Proc. Natl. Acad. Sci. USA* **2006**, *103*, 14678–14683. [CrossRef] [PubMed]
95. Lombardi, G.; Perego, S.; Luzi, L.; Banfi, G. A four-season molecule: Osteocalcin. Updates in its physiological roles. *Endocrine* **2014**, *48*, 394–404. [CrossRef] [PubMed]
96. Schlieper, G.; Schurgers, L.; Brandenburg, V.; Reutlingsperger, C.; Floege, J. Vascular calcification in chronic kidney disease: An update. *Nephrol. Dial. Transplant.* **2015**. [CrossRef] [PubMed]
97. Yamada, S.; Taniguchi, M.; Tokumoto, M.; Toyonaga, J.; Fujisaki, K.; Suehiro, T.; Noguchi, H.; Iida, M.; Tsuruya, K.; Kitazono, T. The antioxidant tempol ameliorates arterial medial calcification in uremic rats: Important role of oxidative stress in the pathogenesis of vascular calcification in chronic kidney disease. *J. Bone Miner. Res.* **2012**, *27*, 474–485. [CrossRef] [PubMed]
98. Ndip, A.; Wilkinson, F.L.; Jude, E.B.; Boulton, A.J.; Alexander, M.Y. RANKL-OPG and RAGE modulation in vascular calcification and diabetes: Novel targets for therapy. *Diabetologia* **2014**, *57*, 2251–2260. [CrossRef] [PubMed]
99. Lei, Y.; Sinha, A.; Nosoudi, N.; Grover, A.; Vyavahare, N. Hydroxyapatite and calcified elastin induce osteoblast-like differentiation in rat aortic smooth muscle cells. *Exp. Cell Res.* **2014**, *323*, 198–208. [CrossRef] [PubMed]
100. Hunter, G.K.; Hauschka, P.V.; Poole, A.R.; Rosenberg, L.C.; Goldberg, H.A. Nucleation and inhibition of hydroxyapatite formation by mineralized tissue proteins. *Biochem. J.* **1996**, *317*, 59–64. [CrossRef] [PubMed]
101. Ducy, P.; Desbois, C.; Boyce, B.; Pinero, G.; Story, B.; Dunstan, C.; Smith, E.; Bonadio, J.; Goldstein, S.; Gundberg, C.; *et al.* Increased bone formation in osteocalcin-deficient mice. *Nature* **1996**, *382*, 448–452. [CrossRef] [PubMed]
102. Kavukcuoglu, N.B.; Patterson-Buckendahl, P.; Mann, A.B. Effect of osteocalcin deficiency on the nanomechanics and chemistry of mouse bones. *J. Mech. Behav. Biomed. Mater.* **2009**, *2*, 348–354. [CrossRef] [PubMed]
103. Roy, M.E.; Nishimoto, S.K.; Rho, J.Y.; Bhattacharya, S.K.; Lin, J.S.; Pharr, G.M. Correlations between osteocalcin content, degree of mineralization, and mechanical properties of *C. carpio* rib bone. *J. Biomed. Mater. Res.* **2001**, *54*, 547–553. [CrossRef]
104. Evrard, S.; Delanaye, P.; Kamel, S.; Cristol, J.-P.; Cavalier, E. SFBC/SN joined working group on vascular calcifications vascular calcification: From pathophysiology to biomarkers. *Clin. Chim. Acta* **2015**, *438*, 401–414. [CrossRef] [PubMed]
105. Price, P.A.; Otsuka, A.A.; Poser, J.W.; Kristaponis, J.; Raman, N. Characterization of a γ-carboxyglutamic acid-containing protein from bone. *Proc. Natl. Acad. Sci. USA* **1976**, *73*, 1447–1451. [CrossRef] [PubMed]
106. Van de Loo, P.G.F.; Soute, B.; van Haarlem, L.; Vermeer, C. The effect of Gla-containing proteins on the precipitation of insoluble salts. *Biochem. Biophys. Res. Commun.* **1987**, *142*, 113–119. [CrossRef]
107. Kapustin, A.N.; Shanahan, C.M. Osteocalcin: A novel vascular metabolic and osteoinductive factor? *Arterioscler. Thromb. Vasc. Biol.* **2011**, *31*, 2169–2171. [CrossRef] [PubMed]
108. Aikawa, E.; Nahrendorf, M.; Sosnovik, D.; Lok, V.M.; Jaffer, F.A.; Aikawa, M.; Weissleder, R. Multimodality molecular imaging identifies proteolytic and osteogenic activities in early aortic valve disease. *Circulation*

2007, *115*, 377–386. [CrossRef] [PubMed]

109. Okura, T.; Kurata, M.; Enomoto, D.; Jotoku, M.; Nagao, T.; Desilva, V.R.; Higaki, J. Undercarboxylated osteocalcin is a biomarker of carotid calcification in patients with essential hypertension. *Kidney Blood Press. Res.* **2010**, *33*, 66–71. [CrossRef] [PubMed]
110. Schurgers, L.J.; Uitto, J.; Reutelingsperger, C.P. Vitamin K-dependent carboxylation of matrix Gla-protein: A crucial switch to control ectopic mineralization. *Trends Mol. Med.* **2013**, *19*, 217–226. [CrossRef] [PubMed]
111. Wajih, N.; Borras, T.; Xue, W.; Hutson, S.M.; Wallin, R. Processing and transport of matrix γ-carboxyglutamic acid protein and bone morphogenetic protein-2 in cultured human vascular smooth muscle cells: Evidence for an uptake mechanism for serum fetuin. *J. Biochem.* **2004**, *279*, 43052–43060. [CrossRef] [PubMed]
112. Luo, G.; Ducy, P.; McKee, M.; Pinero, G.; Loyer, E.; Behringer, R.; Karsenty, G. Spontaneous calcification of arteries and cartilage in mice lacking matrix GLA protein. *Nature* **1997**, *385*, 78–81. [CrossRef] [PubMed]
113. Murshed, M.; Schinke, T.; McKee, M.D.; Karsenty, G. Extracellular matrix mineralization is regulated locally; different roles of two gla-containing proteins. *J. Cell Biol.* **2004**, *165*, 625–630. [CrossRef] [PubMed]
114. Cranenburg, E.C.M.; van Spaendonck-Zwarts, K.Y.; Bonafe, L.; Mittaz Crettol, L.; Rödiger, L.A.; Dikkers, F.G.; van Essen, A.J.; Superti-Furga, A.; Alexandrakis, E.; Vermeer, C.; *et al.* Circulating matrix γ-carboxyglutamate protein (MGP) species are refractory to vitamin K treatment in a new case of Keutel syndrome. *J. Thromb. Haemost.* **2011**, *9*, 1225–1235. [CrossRef] [PubMed]
115. Price, P.; Faus, S.; Williamson, M. Warfarin causes rapid calcification of the elastic lamellae in rat arteries and heart valves. *Arterioscler. Thromb. Vasc. Biol.* **1998**, *18*, 1400–1407. [CrossRef] [PubMed]
116. Reynolds, J.L.; Joannides, A.J.; Skepper, J.N.; McNair, R.; Schurgers, L.J.; Proudfoot, D.; Jahnen-Dechent, W.; Weissberg, P.L.; Shanahan, C.M. Human vascular smooth muscle cells undergo vesicle-mediated calcification in response to changes in extracellular calcium and phosphate concentrations: A potential mechanism for accelerated vascular calcification in ESRD. *J. Am. Soc. Nephrol.* **2004**, *15*, 2857–2867. [CrossRef] [PubMed]
117. Steitz, S.A.; Speer, M.Y.; Curinga, G.; Yang, H.Y.; Haynes, P.; Aebersold, R.; Schinke, T.; Karsenty, G.; Giachelli, C.M. Smooth muscle cell phenotypic transition associated with calcification: Upregulation of Cbfa1 and downregulation of smooth muscle lineage markers. *Circ. Res.* **2001**, *89*, 1147–1154. [CrossRef] [PubMed]
118. Yao, Y.; Bennett, B.J.; Wang, X.; Rosenfeld, M.E.; Giachelli, C.; Lusis, A.J.; Boström, K.I. Inhibition of bone morphogenetic proteins protects against atherosclerosis and vascular calcification. *Circ. Res.* **2010**, *107*, 485–494. [CrossRef] [PubMed]
119. Boström, K.I.; Rajamannan, N.M.; Towler, D.A. The regulation of valvular and vascular sclerosis by osteogenic morphogens. *Circ. Res.* **2011**, *109*, 564–577. [CrossRef] [PubMed]
120. O'Young, J.; Liao, Y.; Xiao, Y.; Jalkanen, J.; Lajoie, G.; Karttunen, M.; Goldberg, H.A.; Hunter, G.K. Matrix Gla protein inhibits ectopic calcification by a direct interaction with hydroxyapatite crystals. *J. Am. Chem. Soc.* **2011**, *133*, 18406–18412. [CrossRef] [PubMed]
121. Schurgers, L.J.; Spronk, H.M.H.; Skepper, J.N.; Hackeng, T.M.; Shanahan, C.M.; Vermeer, C.; Weissberg, P.L.; Proudfoot, D. Post-translational modifications regulate matrix Gla protein function: Importance for inhibition of vascular smooth muscle cell calcification. *J. Thromb. Haemost.* **2007**, *5*, 2503–2511. [CrossRef] [PubMed]
122. Khavandgar, Z.; Roman, H.; Li, J.; Lee, S.; Vali, H.; Brinckmann, J.; Davis, E.C.; Murshed, M. Elastin haploinsufficiency impedes the progression of arterial calcification in MGP-deficient mice. *J. Bone Miner. Res.* **2014**, *29*, 327–337. [CrossRef] [PubMed]
123. Price, P.A.; Toroian, D.; Lim, J.E. Mineralization by inhibitor exclusion: The calcification of collagen with fetuin. *J. Biol. Chem.* **2009**, *284*, 17092–17101. [CrossRef] [PubMed]
124. Cancela, M.L.; Conceição, N.; Laizé, V. Gla-rich protein, a new player in tissue calcification? *Adv. Nutr.* **2012**, *3*, 174–181. [CrossRef] [PubMed]
125. Viegas, C.S.B.; Rafael, M.S.; Enriquez, J.L.; Teixeira, A.; Vitorino, R.; Luís, I.M.; Costa, R.M.; Santos, S.; Cavaco, S.; Neves, J.; *et al.* Gla-rich protein acts as a calcification inhibitor in the human cardiovascular system. *Arterioscler. Thromb. Vasc. Biol.* **2015**, *35*, 399–408. [CrossRef] [PubMed]
126. Eitzinger, N.; Surmann-Schmitt, C.; Bösl, M.; Schett, G.; Engelke, K.; Hess, A.; von der Mark, K.; Stock, M. Ucma is not necessary for normal development of the mouse skeleton. *Bone* **2012**, *50*, 670–680. [CrossRef] [PubMed]
127. Geleijnse, J.M.; Vermeer, C.; Grobbee, D.E.; Schurgers, L.J.; Knapen, M.H.J.; van der Meer, I.M.; Hofman, A.; Witteman, J.C.M. Dietary intake of menaquinone is associated with a reduced risk of coronary heart disease: The Rotterdam Study. *J. Nutr.* **2004**, *134*, 3100–3105. [PubMed]

128. Juanola-Falgarona, M.; Salas-Salvadó, J.; Martínez-González, M.Á.; Corella, D.; Estruch, R.; Ros, E.; Fitó, M.; Arós, F.; Gómez-Gracia, E.; Fiol, M.; *et al.* Dietary intake of vitamin k is inversely associated with mortality risk. *J. Nutr.* **2014**, *144*, 743–750. [CrossRef] [PubMed]
129. Beulens, J.W.; Bots, M.L.; Atsma, F.; Bartelink, M.L.E.; Prokop, M.; Geleijnse, J.M.; Van Der Schouw, Y.T. High dietary menaquinone intake is associated with reduced coronary calcification. *Atherosclerosis* **2009**, *203*, 489–493. [CrossRef] [PubMed]
130. Westenfeld, R.; Krueger, T.; Schlieper, G.; Cranenburg, E.C.M.; Magdeleyns, E.J.; Heidenreich, S.; Holzmann, S.; Vermeer, C.; Jahnen-Dechent, W.; Ketteler, M.; *et al.* Effect of vitamin K_2 supplementation on functional vitamin K deficiency in hemodialysis patients: A randomized trial. *Am. J. Kidney Dis.* **2012**, *59*, 186–195. [CrossRef] [PubMed]
131. Theuwissen, E.; Teunissen, K.J.; Spronk, H.M.H.; Hamulyak, K.; ten Cate, H.; Shearer, M.J.; Vermeer, C.; Schurgers, L.J. Effect of low-dose supplements of menaquinone-7 (vitamin K_2) on the stability of oral anticoagulant treatment: Dose-response relationship in healthy volunteers. *J. Thromb. Haemost.* **2013**, *11*, 1085–1092. [CrossRef] [PubMed]
132. Buitenhuis, H.C.; Soute, B.A.; Vermeer, C. Comparison of the vitamins K1, K2 and K3 as cofactors for the hepatic vitamin K-dependent carboxylase. *Biochim. Biophys. Acta* **1990**, *1034*, 170–175. [CrossRef]
133. Schlieper, G.; Westenfeld, R.; Krüger, T.; Cranenburg, E.C.; Magdeleyns, E.J.; Brandenburg, V.M.; Djuric, Z.; Damjanovic, T.; Ketteler, M.; Vermeer, C.; *et al.* Circulating nonphosphorylated carboxylated matrix Gla protein predicts survival in ESRD. *J. Am. Soc. Nephrol.* **2011**, *22*, 387–395. [CrossRef] [PubMed]
134. Ueland, T.; Dahl, C.P.; Gullestad, L.; Aakhus, S.; Broch, K.; Skårdal, R.; Vermeer, C.; Aukrust, P.; Schurgers, L.J. Circulating levels of non-phosphorylated undercarboxylated matrix Gla protein are associated with disease severity in patients with chronic heart failure. *Clin. Sci.* **2011**, *121*, 119–127. [CrossRef] [PubMed]
135. Cranenburg, E.C.M.; Vermeer, C.; Koos, R.; Boumans, M.-L.; Hackeng, T.M.; Bouwman, F.G.; Kwaijtaal, M.; Brandenburg, V.M.; Ketteler, M.; Schurgers, L.J. The circulating inactive form of matrix Gla Protein (ucMGP) as a biomarker for cardiovascular calcification. *J. Vasc. Res.* **2008**, *45*, 427–436. [CrossRef] [PubMed]
136. Brandenburg, V.M.; Schurgers, L.J.; Kaesler, N.; Püsche, K.; van Gorp, R.H.; Leftheriotis, G.; Reinartz, S.; Koos, R.; Krüger, T. Prevention of vasculopathy by vitamin K supplementation: Can we turn fiction into fact? *Atherosclerosis* **2015**, *240*, 10–16. [CrossRef] [PubMed]
137. Morishima, Y.; Kamisato, C.; Honda, Y.; Furugohri, T.; Shibano, T. The effects of warfarin and edoxaban, an oral direct factor Xa inhibitor, on γcarboxylated (Gla-osteocalcin) and undercarboxylated osteocalcin (uc-osteocalcin) in rats. *Thromb. Res.* **2013**, *131*, 59–63. [CrossRef] [PubMed]
138. Krüger, T.; Oelenberg, S.; Kaesler, N.; Schurgers, L.J.; van de Sandt, A.M.; Boor, P.; Schlieper, G.; Brandenburg, V.M.; Fekete, B.C.; Veulemans, V.; *et al.* Warfarin induces cardiovascular damage in mice. *Arterioscler. Thromb. Vasc. Biol.* **2013**, *33*, 2618–2624. [CrossRef] [PubMed]

7

Vitamin E Biosynthesis and its Regulation in Plants

Laurent Mène-Saffrané

Department of Biology, University of Fribourg, Chemin du Musée, 10, 1700 Fribourg, Switzerland; laurent.mene-saffrane@unifr.ch

Abstract: Vitamin E is one of the 13 vitamins that are essential to animals that do not produce them. To date, six natural organic compounds belonging to the chemical family of tocochromanols—four tocopherols and two tocotrienols—have been demonstrated as exhibiting vitamin E activity in animals. Edible plant-derived products, notably seed oils, are the main sources of vitamin E in the human diet. Although this vitamin is readily available, independent nutritional surveys have shown that human populations do not consume enough vitamin E, and suffer from mild to severe deficiency. Tocochromanols are mostly produced by plants, algae, and some cyanobacteria. Tocochromanol metabolism has been mainly studied in higher plants that produce tocopherols, tocotrienols, plastochromanol-8, and tocomonoenols. In contrast to the tocochromanol biosynthetic pathways that are well characterized, our understanding of the physiological and molecular mechanisms regulating tocochromanol biosynthesis is in its infancy. Although it is known that tocochromanol biosynthesis is strongly conditioned by the availability in homogentisate and polyprenyl pyrophosphate, its polar and lipophilic biosynthetic precursors, respectively, the mechanisms regulating their biosyntheses are barely known. This review summarizes our current knowledge of tocochromanol biosynthesis in plants, and highlights future challenges regarding the understanding of its regulation.

Keywords: vitamin E; tocochromanol; tocopherol; tocotrienol; plastochromanol-8; tocomonoenol; homogentisate; polyprenyl pyrophosphate; nutrigenomics

---

1. Introduction

Natural compounds exhibiting vitamin E activity in animal cells belong to the chemical family of tocochromanols, a group of organic molecules with a polar chromanol ring and lipophilic polyprenyl side chain that varies according to the type of tocochromanol [1]. The polyprenyl precursor of tocopherols, tocotrienols, plastochromanol-8 (PC-8), and tocomonoenols is phytyl pyrophosphate (PPP), geranylgeranyl pyrophosphate (GGPP), solanesyl pyrophosphate (SPP), and tetrahydrogeranylgeranyl pyrophosphate (THGGPP), respectively (Figure 1). According to the degree of methylation of the chromanol ring, each type of tocochromanol exhibits up to four different forms, named α- (three-methyl groups), β- and γ- (two-methyl groups), and δ-tocochromanol (one-methyl group; Figure 1), respectively. While the four forms of tocopherol, tocotrienol, and tocomonoenol have been identified in wild-type plant extracts, only the γ- form of the solanesyl-derived tocochromanol PC-8 naturally exists.

The first article published on vitamin E relates the finding of an unknown nutritional factor that prevents embryo resorption during rodent gestation [2]. Several years later, this "*factor X*", as it was originally named, was identified as α-tocopherol [3]. In addition to its essential role in animal reproduction, vitamin E has been shown to have beneficial roles in human health [4], notably by inhibiting lung cancer [5], by delaying brain aging and reducing the risk of developing Alzheimer's disease [6], and by suppressing cholesterogenesis [7,8]. Although vitamin E is present in many edible plant-derived products, converging nutritional surveys conducted in both poor and developed countries, respectively, have shown that a significant proportion of human populations exhibit mild to severe vitamin E deficiencies [9–13]. It has been shown, for instance, that 23% of the Seoul metropolitan population exhibited plasma α-tocopherol concentrations below 12 μmol/L, the threshold defining vitamin E deficiency in humans [11]. The consequences of vitamin E deficiency on human health have not yet been fully documented nor investigated. However, it has been clearly established that low plasma vitamin E is strongly associated with miscarriage during the first trimester of woman pregnancy [12]. Moreover, it has been shown that diet supplementation with vitamin E decreased the miscarriage rate of pregnant woman by approximately 50% [12]. Collectively, these results demonstrate the importance of adequate vitamin E intake for proper reproduction.

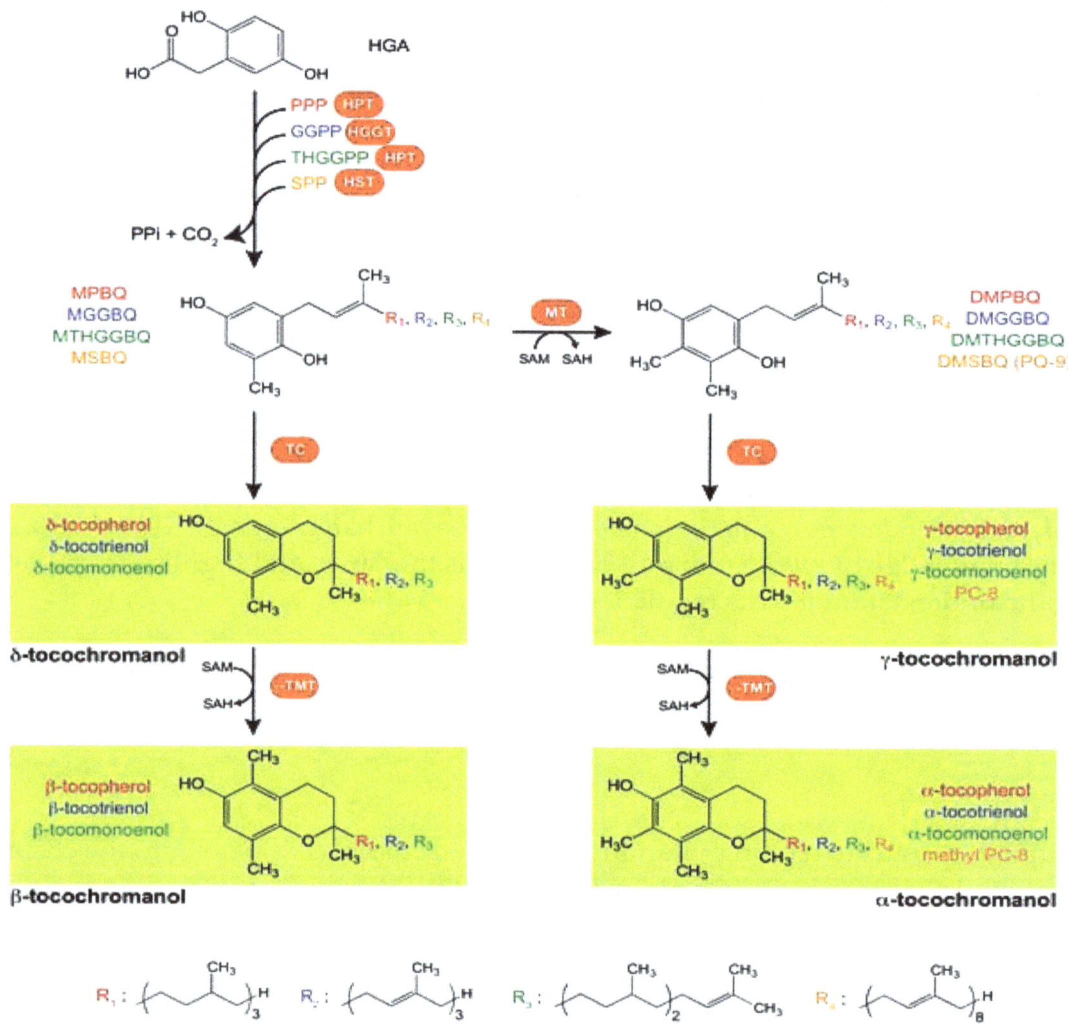

Figure 1. Tocochromanol biosynthetic pathways in plants. Tocochromanol and prenyl benzoquinol chemical structures and biosynthetic enzymes (highlighted in orange). Tocochromanol and prenyl benzoquinol names are color-coded to distinguish each tocochromanol pathway: red for the tocopherol pathway, blue for the tocotrienol pathway, green for the tocomonoenol pathway, and orange for the PC-8 and methyl PC-8 pathway. The α-, β-, γ-, and δ-forms of tocopherols, tocotrienols, and tocomonoenols have been identified in plants. For solanesyl-derived tocochromanols, only PC-8 has been identified in wild-type plants, and only methyl PC-8 has been identified in transgenic Arabidopsis overexpressing the γ-*TMT/VTE4* gene. Abbreviations: HGA, homogentisate; HGGT, homogentisate geranylgeranyltransferase; HPT, homogentisate phytyltransferase; HST, homogentisate solanesyltransferase; GGPP, geranylgeranyl pyrophosphate; γ-TMT, γ-tocopherol methyltransferase; MT, methyltransferase; PC-8, plastochromanol-8; PPi, pyrophosphate; PPP, phytyl pyrophosphate; PQ-9, plastoquinol-9; SAM, *S*-adenosyl-L-methionine; SAH, *S*-adenosyl-L-homocysteine; SPP, solanesyl pyrophosphate; TC, tocopherol cyclase; THGGPP, tetrahydrogeranylgeranyl pyrophosphate. Prenyl benzoquinol acronyms are detailed in the main text.

It has been assumed for a long time that tocochromanol biosynthesis was the exclusive appanage of plants, algae, and some cyanobacteria that are all photosynthetic organisms. However, a recent study showed that *Plasmodium falciparum*, a non-photosynthetic parasite that causes malaria, synthesizes both α- and γ-tocopherols during its intraerythrocytic stages to avoid oxidative stress [14–16]. Besides this exception, tocochromanol metabolism has been primarily studied in angiosperms and in the vitamin E-producing cyanobacteria *Synechocystis*. The present review summarizes our current knowledge on tocochromanol metabolism in plants, including the core tocochromanol biosynthetic pathway that is now well delineated (Section 2); the transcriptional regulation of γ-*TMT* expression, which is the gene encoding the biosynthetic enzyme of the most potent vitamin E form of α-tocopherol in animals (Section 3); the regulation of homogentisate (HGA) biosynthesis, which is the polar precursor of tocochromanols (Section 4); and the regulation of polyprenyl pyrophosphate biosynthesis, which is the lipophilic precursor of tocochromanols (Section 5). Thus, this work complements the very recent review that highlighted the biosynthetic origins and transports of polar and lipophilic tocochromanol biosynthetic precursors in plants [17].

2. Tocochromanol Biosynthetic Pathways

Tocochromanol biosynthesis is initiated by the condensation of the polar aromatic head HGA with various lipophilic polyprenyl pyrophosphates that determine the type of tocochromanol. PPP is the lipophilic biosynthetic precursor of tocopherols, while GGPP is the one for tocotrienols, as is SPP for PC-8, and THGGPP for tocomonoenols (Pellaud and Mène-Saffrané, 2017 [17] and Figure 1). The condensation reaction is catalyzed by three types of HGA prenyltransferases that possess each their substrate specificities. Tocopherol synthesis is initiated by HGA phytyltransferases (HPTs) that condense HGA and PPP. This enzyme has been identified in both Arabidopsis and the cyanobacterium *Synechocystis* [18,19]. While the Arabidopsis HPT (AtHPT), also named VTE2, preferentially utilizes PPP as a prenyl donor, its *Synechocystis* counterpart uses both PPP and GGPP [18]. Although AtHPT poorly utilizes GGPP as a substrate in vitro, and wild-type Arabidopsis accessions do not naturally accumulate tocotrienols, it has been shown that AtHPT catalyzes the synthesis of tocotrienols in transgenic Arabidopsis plants that are overaccumulating HGA [20]. Recently, AtHPT was also shown to be catalyzing the accumulation of γ-tocomonoenol in Arabidopsis seeds, indicating that THGGPP is a substrate for this enzyme [21]. Collectively, these data show that the substrate specificity of HGA phytyl transferases is wider than that originally described, and is notably modulated by HGA availability. In Poaceae, tocotrienol synthesis is initiated by HGA geranylgeranyltransferase (HGGT), which utilizes both GGPP and PPP as prenyl donors in vitro. In addition, overexpression of the barley *HGGT* gene in the Arabidopsis *vte2* mutant induces the quantitative accumulation of both tocotrienols and tocopherols in seeds and leaves, indicating that HGGT utilizes both prenyl donors in vivo as well [22]. The Arabidopsis *vte2-1* mutant lacks tocopherols, but still accumulates PC-8 in both seeds and leaves, confirming in vitro data showing that VTE2 is not involved in the condensation of HGA with the solanesyl derivative SPP [18,23]. This reaction is catalyzed by the HGA solanesyltransferase (HST) that has been identified in both *Chlamydomonas* and Arabidopsis [24,25]. The condensation reaction between HGA and polyprenyl pyrophosphates produces 2-methyl-6-phytyl-1,4-benzoquinol (MPBQ) for tocopherols, 2-methyl-6-geranylgeranyl-1,4-benzoquinol (MGGBQ) for tocotrienols, 2-methyl-6-solanesyl-1,4-benzoquinol (MSBQ) for PC-8, and 2-methyl-6-tetrahydrogeranylgeranyl-1,4-benzoquinol (MTHGGBQ) for tocomonoenols (Figure 1). These compounds are either direct precursors of δ- and β-tocochromanols, or can alternatively be methylated by a methyltransferase (MT/VTE3) that uses *S*-adenosyl-L-methionine (SAM) as a methyl donor [26,27]. The products of the later reaction are prenylated dimethyl-benzoquinols, namely 2,3-dimethyl-6-phytyl-1,4-benzoquinol (DMPBQ) for tocopherols, 2,3-dimethyl-6-geranylgeranyl-1,4-benzoquinol (DMGGBQ) for tocotrienols, 2,3-dimethyl-6-solanesyl-1,4-benzoquinol better known as plastoquinol-9 (PQ-9) for PC-8, and 2,3-dimethyl-6-tetrahydrogeranylgeranyl-1,4-benzoquinol (DMTHGGBQ) for tocomonoenols

(Figure 1). Both methyl- and dimethyl-benzoquinols are then further cyclized by the tocopherol cyclase (TC/VTE1) into δ- and γ-tocochromanols, respectively. Seeds of the Arabidopsis *vte1-1* mutant lack all tocopherols, PC-8, and γ-tocomonoenol, indicating that the cyclase indiscriminately uses mono- and dimethyl-benzoquinols carrying either a phytyl, a solanesyl, or a tetrahydrogeranylgeranyl side chain as substrates [21,23,28,29]. The fourth and final step of tocochromanol biosynthesis consists of the methylation of γ- and δ-tocochromanols into α- and β-tocochromanols, respectively [30,31]. This reaction is catalyzed by the γ-tocopherol methyltransferase (γ-TMT/VTE4) that utilizes SAM as methyl donor (Figure 1). In Arabidopsis leaves and seeds, VTE4 converts γ- and δ-tocopherols into α- and β-tocopherol, respectively, indicating that the methyl transferase efficiently methylates phytyl-derived tocochromanols [30]. In addition, transgenic Arabidopsis lines overexpressing the barley *HGGT* gene notably produce α-tocotrienol [32]. This indicates that the γ-tocopherol methyltransferase VTE4 catalyzes that methylation of geranylgeranyl-derived tocochromanol such as γ-tocotrienol as well.

3. Regulation of the γ-*tocopherol methyltransferase* Expression

The different tocochromanol forms identified in plants do not exhibit the same vitamin E activity in animal cells [1]. Based on the rat fetal resorption assay, α-tocopherol (1.49 IU/mg; 100%) is by far the most potent vitamin E form, followed by β-tocopherol (0.75 IU/mg; 50%), α-tocotrienol (0.45–0.75 IU/mg; 30–50%), γ-tocopherol (0.15 IU/mg; 10%), β-tocotrienol (0.08 IU/mg; 5%), and δ-tocopherol (0.05 IU/mg; 3%). The vitamin E activities of γ- and δ-tocotrienol have been tested and were below the limit of detection, while those of other tocochromanols such as PC-8 and tocomonoenols have not been tested yet. The difference in vitamin E activity among tocochromanol forms results from their differential affinities to the α-tocopherol transfer protein, a cytoplasmic protein that transports tocochromanols from the endosomal fraction of hepatocytes into the bloodstream of animals [33,34]. This implies that at equal molarity, a plant tissue accumulating α-tocopherol instead of γ-tocopherol for instance, exhibits 10 times more vitamin E activity. Based on this, a relevant question regarding the regulation of tocochromanol biosynthesis in plants and the improvement of crops vitamin E activity is: what are the molecular mechanisms regulating γ-*TMT* expression?

The main tocochromanol identified in wild-type leaves analyzed to date is α-tocopherol, indicating that leaf γ-TMT/VTE4 activity is sufficient to quantitatively methylate the γ-tocopherol pool present in this tissue. In contrast, despite the presence of PC-8 (γ-tocochromanol) in wild-type Arabidopsis and maize leaves, methyl PC-8 (α-tocochromanol) has not been detected in any wild-type tissue analyzed to date [23]. In contrast, methyl PC-8 accumulates in transgenic Arabidopsis leaves overexpressing γ-*TMT/VTE4,* demonstrating that PC-8 is a substrate for γ-TMT/VTE4, and that endogenous γ-TMT/VTE4 activity is not sufficient to convert all γ-tocochromanols into α-tocochromanols [35]. This later conclusion is further supported by the tocochromanol composition of transgenic Arabidopsis leaves overexpressing the barley *HGGT* gene. Indeed, while these transgenic lines accumulate tocopherols mostly under the form of α-tocopherol, their tocotrienol pool is mainly under the form of γ-tocotrienol [32]. In contrast to this, another metabolic engineering study in which tocochromanol biosynthesis has been increased by enhancing the production of HPP in chloroplasts suggests that γ-TMT activity might be limiting for α-tocopherol synthesis in leaves. In comparison to controls, these Arabidopsis transgenic lines overaccumulated both γ-tocopherol and γ-tocotrienol, but exhibited control levels for α-tocopherol in leaves [36]. In addition, they did not accumulate any detectable α-tocotrienol, despite the strong accumulation of γ-tocotrienol in leaf tissues. In alfalfa, it has been shown that the overexpression of a Medicago γ-*TMT* modestly but significantly increased α-tocopherol accumulation in leaves [37]. Collectively, these data show that the leaf γ-TMT/VTE4 activity is clearly not sufficient to fully methylate both γ-tocotrienol and PC-8, and is sometimes limiting α-tocopherol biosynthesis. The former conclusion might indicate that γ-TMT/VTE4 has a lower affinity for γ-tocotrienol and PC-8 than for α-tocopherol.

In contrast to leaves, the tocochromanol composition of wild-type seeds is much more variable, and three groups of plant species can be currently distinguished according to this criterion. The seeds of some plant species accumulate mostly γ-tocochromanols and very little or no α-tocochromanols. This is notably the case of wild-type Arabidopsis seeds, which accumulate mostly γ-tocopherol and PC-8, very low levels of α-tocopherol, and no methyl PC-8 [23]. The overexpression of γ-*TMT* genes in Arabidopsis and *Brassica napus* is sufficient to trigger the quantitative accumulation of both α-tocopherol and methyl PC-8 in transgenic seeds, thus demonstrating that the lack of α-tocochromanols in the seeds of these species results from the very low transcriptional activity of the γ-*TMT/VTE4* gene in seeds [30,35,38]. In contrast to Arabidopsis, the seeds of other plant species mostly accumulate α-tocochromanols, and very few γ-tocochromanols. This is notably the case of sunflower and wheat, which accumulate mostly α-tocopherol ± α-tocotrienol, and very low levels of γ-tocochromanols [39,40]. This indicates that the VTE4 activity in seeds of these species is sufficient to quantitatively convert almost all of the γ-tocochromanols into α-tocochromanols. The third type of plants accumulate both α- and γ-tocochromanols in seeds, suggesting that although their VTE4 activity is sufficient to support the synthesis of α-tocochromanols, it is not strong enough to fully methylate the pools of γ-tocochromanols. This group includes species such as rapeseed and maize [41–43]. Our current knowledge of the transcriptional mechanism(s) regulating γ-*TMT/VTE4* expression, notably in seeds, is currently limited to a single study performed in soybean. Tocopherol analysis in seeds of 1109 wild and cultivated soybean varieties showed that while almost all of them produce primarily γ-tocopherol, three varieties accumulate up to seven times more α-tocopherol [44]. Quantitative trait loci (QTL) analysis in high α-tocopherol soybean varieties showed that polymorphism located in the γ-*TMT3* promoter correlated with the higher expression of the methyl transferase, and thus that α-tocopherol level is transcriptionally regulated in soybean seeds as well [45]. Collectively, these data demonstrate that the synthesis of α-tocochromanols, such as α-tocopherol in seeds and leaves, is determined by the mechanism(s) regulating the expression of the γ-*TMT/VTE4* gene. To date, despite many independent research initiatives that led to the identification of numerous α-tocopherol QTLs in Arabidopsis [46], soybean [45,47,48], maize [42,43,49,50], winter oilseed rape [51,52], and barley [53], the transcriptional machinery regulating the expression of γ-*TMT* genes in plants is still unknown.

4. Plastidic Availability in Homogentisate Regulates Tocochromanol Synthesis

Early feeding experiments of safflower, sunflower, and soybean cell cultures with HGA have shown that an exogenous HGA supply significantly increased tocochromanol biosynthesis in plant cells [54–56]. These indicate that the endogenous mechanism(s) regulating HGA biosynthesis and availability in plant cells directly determines the final amount of tocochromanols. The tocochromanol biosynthetic precursor HGA comes from the degradation of the aromatic amino acid L-tyrosine (L-tyr), which is produced by the plastidic shikimate pathway (Figure 2). L-tyr is first converted into 4-hydroxyphenylpyruvate (HPP) by tyrosine aminotransferases (TATs). Among the six to 10 *TAT* genes identified in the genetic model Arabidopsis, the enzymatic activity has been experimentally confirmed only for TAT1 (also named TAT7) and TAT2 [57–60]. Regarding tocochromanol synthesis, it has been shown that TAT1/TAT7 controls 35–50% of α-tocopherol biosynthesis in Arabidopsis leaves [59]. The other TAT(s) involved in the TAT1-independent tocochromanol biosynthesis, as well as the ones involved in seed tocochromanol biosynthesis, have not been identified yet. Following tyrosine transamination, HPP is converted by 4-hydroxyphenylpyruvate dioxygenase (HPPD) into HGA (Figure 2). A corpus of biochemical, genetic, and cell biology data indicate that the cellular compartment hosting HGA biosynthesis is different among plant species. This aspect of tocochromanol biosynthesis has been recently reviewed in detail [17]. In the genetic model Arabidopsis, several studies have provided evidence that HGA biosynthesis is confined to the cytoplasm. The sequence analysis of the Arabidopsis *TAT1/TAT7* and *HPPD* genes have shown that both lack the typical sequence encoding for a chloroplast transit peptide, suggesting that TAT1/AtTAT7 and HPPD are localized in the cytoplasm [60]. This has been confirmed by Western blot for HPPD, and with TAT1:GFP and HPPD:GFP fusion proteins, which were both localized in the cytoplasm of Arabidopsis cells [60,61].

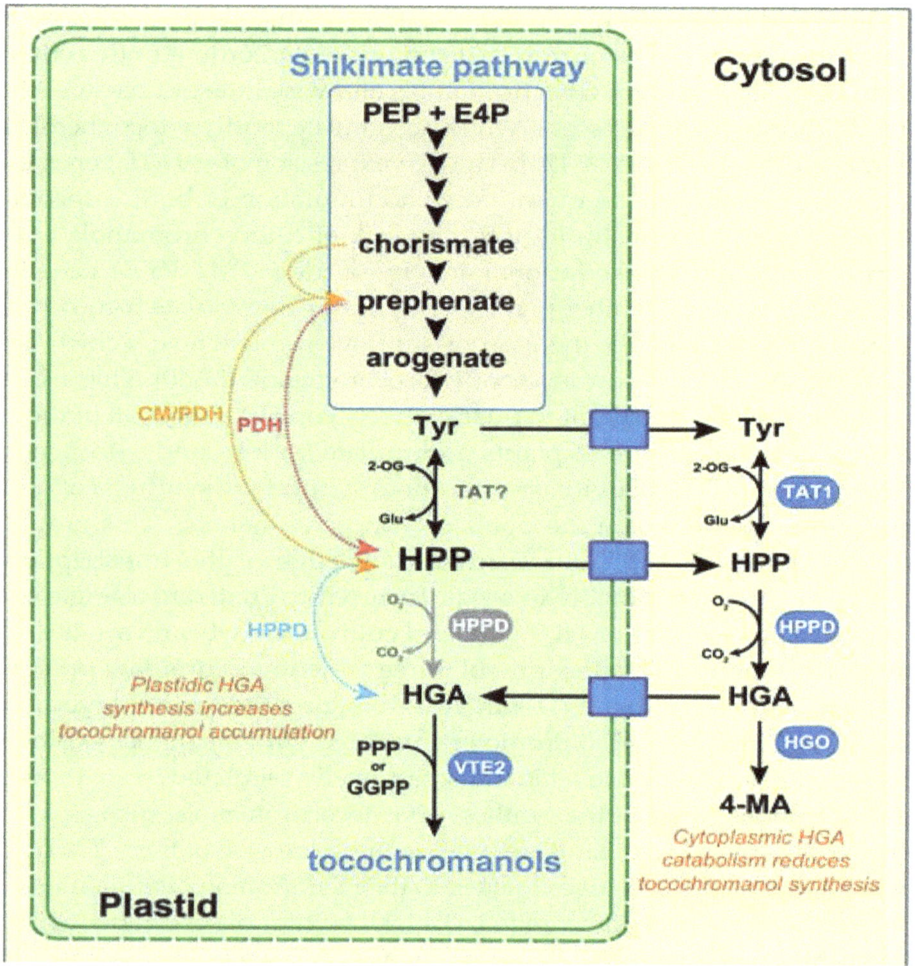

Figure 2. Biosynthesis and transport of homogentisate in plants. Red, orange, and blue dotted lines correspond to transgenic plants overexpressing the coding sequence of yeast *PDH*, bacterial *CM/PDH*, and plant *HPPD*, respectively, all fused to a sequence encoding a chloroplast transit peptide. Biosynthetic enzymes demonstrated to be involved in tocochromanol synthesis are highlighted in blue or gray. In species such as Arabidopsis, HPPD is localized in the cytoplasm. In contrast, in maize, tomato, and cotton, *HPPD* genes exhibit a typical chloroplast transit signal, suggesting that this enzyme is localized in the chloroplasts of these species (HPPD in grey). In soybean, HPPD have been localized in both compartments. Plant species in which HGA biosynthesis is localized in the cytosol must have chloroplast membrane transporters (blue boxes) exporting Tyr and HPP into the cytosol, and importing HGA back into chloroplasts. Abbreviations: CM/PDH, bacterial bi-functional chorismate mutase/prephenate dehydrogenase; E4P, erythrose 4-phosphate; GGPP, geranylgeranyl pyrophosphate; Glu, glutamate; HGA, homogentisate; HGO, homogentisate dioxygenase; HPP, 4-hydroxyphenylpyruvate; HPPD, 4-hydroxyphenylpyruvate dioxygenase; 4-MA, 4-maleylacetoacetate; 2-OG, 2-oxoglutarate; PDH, prephenate dehydrogenase; PEP, phosphoenolpyruvate; PPP, phytyl pyrophosphate; TAT, tyrosine aminotransferase; Tyr, L-tyrosine.

In addition, *HPPD* genes isolated from barley, carrot, and coleus also lack chloroplast transit peptide sequences [62]. Collectively, these demonstrate that HGA biosynthesis, at least in these species, is exclusively localized in the cytoplasm. This data has major consequences regarding the regulation of tocochromanol biosynthesis in these species, since the cytoplasmic HGA biosynthesis implies the existence of chloroplast membrane transporters that export L-tyr/HPP into the cytoplasm, and other one(s) that import HGA back into chloroplasts (Figure 2). Thus, beyond HGA biosynthesis *per se*, these chloroplast membrane transporters might constitute additional levels of regulation of plastidic HGA availability, and thus determine the final amount of tocochromanol produced by a given tissue.

Genetic data obtained from soybean further illustrate how the cytoplasmic HGA biosynthesis and the exchanges of tocochromanol biosynthetic precursors between chloroplasts and the cytoplasm participate in the regulation of tocochromanol biosynthesis in plants. In this species, the HPPD activity is encoded by a single gene that exhibits two transcription start sites. It has been shown that the long transcript encodes a polypeptide imported into the chloroplast, while the short one encodes a polypeptide that remains in the cytoplasm [63]. This indicates that soybean HPPD activity is localized in both the cytoplasm and chloroplasts. In addition, seeds of the soybean *hgo1* mutant, which carries a mutated *HOMOGENTISATE DIOXYGENASE 1* gene encoding an enzyme that catabolizes HGA into 4-maleylacetoacetate (Figure 2), exhibits higher amounts of both HGA and tocochromanols [64]. Interestingly, the HGO1 activity catabolizing HGA is localized in the cytoplasm of soybean cells, indicating that the cytoplasmic HGA catabolism negatively impacts tocochromanol biosynthesis in this species. Similarly, the Arabidopsis HGO gene (At5g54080) encodes a protein expected to be localized in the cytoplasm, according to the The Arabidopsis Information Resource website. Collectively, these data demonstrate that the cytoplasmic HGA synthesis and catabolism in species such as Arabidopsis and soybean are two mechanisms that determine the final amount of tocochromanols in seeds. Moreover, they reveal that yet-unknown chloroplast membrane transporters exporting L-tyr/HPP into the cytoplasm, and other one(s) importing HGA back into chloroplasts, are potentially limiting factors for tocochromanol accumulation. To date, neither the membrane chloroplast transporters exporting L-tyr and HPP in the cytoplasm, nor the one importing HGA back into chloroplasts, have been identified in Arabidopsis. In contrast, a cationic amino acid transporter localized in the chloroplast membrane and capable of exporting phenylalanine, tryptophan, and L-tyr from the stroma into the cytosol has been identified in petunia [65].

The major role of plastidic HGA availability and its transport from the cytoplasm into plastids in the regulation of tocochromanol biosynthesis can be deduced from four metabolic engineering studies that aimed at increasing plant vitamin E activity. In higher plants, HPP derives from the sequential catabolism of L-tyr into chorismate, prephenate, and arogenate (Figure 2). In plants, L-tyr restricts its own biosynthesis, and thus the one of tocochromanols, by feedback inhibition of both arogenate dehydrogenase and prephenate dehydrogenase [20]. In contrast, prokaryotes and yeast produce HPP directly from chorismate via bi-functional chorismate mutase (CM)/prephenate dehydrogenase (PDH) activity, and from prephenate via PDH activity, respectively (Figure 2). It has been previously shown that the overexpression of bacterial *CM/PDH* or yeast *PDH* genes in transgenic plants, including Arabidopsis, strongly increases the accumulation of both HGA and tocochromanols [20,56,66]. Interestingly, both *CM/PDH* and *PDH* coding sequences were fused to a sequence encoding a chloroplast transit peptide and expressed in combination with *HPPD* genes that were also fused to a sequence encoding a chloroplast transit peptide. Collectively, these studies demonstrate that bypassing the plant L-tyr feedback inhibition and functionalizing chloroplasts with the HPPD activity significantly stimulate tocochromanol metabolism in plants.

Interestingly, the overexpression of bacterial *CM/PDH* or yeast *PDH* genes alone is more effective in terms of tocochromanol biosynthesis in Arabidopsis leaves than when these genes are co-expressed in combination with *HPPD* [20,36]. Compared with transgenic Arabidopsis overexpressing *CM/PDH* alone, the lower tocochromanol accumulation in transgenic Arabidopsis leaves carrying both transgenes (*CM/PDH* or *PDH* with *HPPD*) correlates with a much higher accumulation of free HGA [20]. This indicates that whereas HGA availability is limiting for tocochromanol accumulation, a high HGA concentration likely inhibits their biosyntheses. In addition to revealing the potentially toxic effect of HGA on tocochromanol metabolism, these two later studies indicate that the HPPD activity and HPP/HGA trafficking across chloroplast membranes are both not limiting in Arabidopsis leaves. Indeed, the overaccumulation of tocochromanols resulting from the sole overexpression of *CM/PDH* or *PDH* in chloroplasts implies that HPP is efficiently exported into the cytosol where the HPPD activity is localized, and that the cytoplasmic HGA is imported back into chloroplasts to sustain tocochromanol biosynthesis (Figure 2). Since tocochromanol biosynthesis is strongly increased by the overexpression of a bacterial *CM/PDH* gene alone in Arabidopsis leaves, one can conclude that the endogenous HPPD activity (cytoplasmic) and HPP/HGA trafficking are both not so limiting for leaf tocochromanol metabolism in Arabidopsis. In contrast to this, the situation seems very different in tobacco leaves; while the overexpression of the yeast *PDH* gene does not significantly alter tocochromanol accumulation in transgenic tobacco leaves, its overexpression in combination with *HPPD* fused to a chloroplast targeting sequence strongly increases tocochromanol accumulation [66]. The reasons explaining these differences between Arabidopsis and tobacco leaves are currently unknown but suggest that HPPD activity and/or HPP/HGA trafficking in tobacco is limiting compared to Arabidopsis leaves.

In Arabidopsis seeds, re-analysis of previously published data indicates that HPP/HGA trafficking across the chloroplast membranes is much less efficient than in leaves despite the significant tocochromanol metabolism in this tissue. Co-expression of *CM/PDH* in combination with *HPPD* in Arabidopsis stimulates seed tocochromanol accumulation, whereas the expression of *CM/PDH* alone does not significantly alter it (construct pMON36596 versus pMON36520 in the Supplementary data of Karunanandaa et al. [56], 2005, respectively). In this study, a sequence encoding a chloroplast transit peptide was fused to both *CM/PDH* and *HPPD* sequences as well, showing that seed tocochromanol might be enhanced in seeds if seed chloroplasts are functionalized with both activities. This indicates that the endogenous HPPD activity and/or HPP/HGA trafficking is much less efficient in Arabidopsis seeds than in leaves. However, the *HPPD* gene is strongly expressed in Arabidopsis seeds, a tissues in which *HPPD* expression is among its highest during plant development (Figure 3).

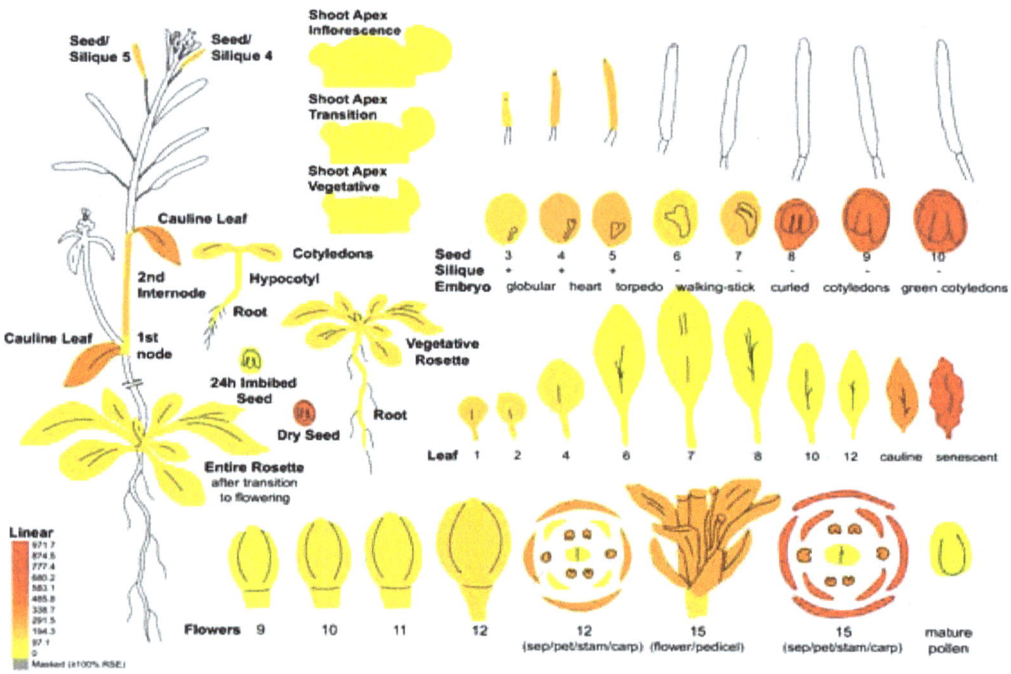

Figure 3. *HPPD* expression pattern during Arabidopsis development. The expression of the Arabidopsis *HPPD* gene (At1g06570) was assessed with ePlant (http://bar.utoronto.ca/eplant). *HPPD* expression level is equal to 697.5 in green cotyledons (SD = 36.3; n = 3), and is the third highest *HPPD* expression after sepals (level = 971.7; SD = 84.2; n = 3) and senescent leaves (level = 797.7; SD = 6.9; n = 3).

This indicates that HPPD activity is likely not limiting tocochromanol metabolism in Arabidopsis seeds, and that in contrast, HPP/HGA trafficking restricts tocochromanol biosynthesis in these tissues. This novel interpretation of old data also suggests that HPP/HGA trafficking across the chloroplast membrane is likely a target of choice to increase tocochromanol biosynthesis in seeds.

The tocochromanol patterns of transgenic plants expressing bacterial *CM/PDH* and yeast *PDH* alone or in combination with *HPPD* vary according to the plant species, organ, and developmental stage. Thus, while young tobacco and Arabidopsis leaves overexpressing *CM/PDH* or *PDH* genes overaccumulate primarily tocotrienols, mature Arabidopsis transgenic leaves expressing these constructs accumulate mostly tocopherols [20,36,66]. In contrast to leaves, Arabidopsis and soybean transgenic seeds expressing *CM/PDH* or *PDH* genes primarily overaccumulate tocotrienols [56]. Since the type of tocochromanol results from the polyprenyl pyrophosphate substrate, these results indicate that the tocopherol precursor PPP is likely limiting in seeds and young leaf tissues, whereas GGPP is not.

5. Regulation of Polyprenyl Pyrophosphate Availability

Since the type of tocochromanol (tocopherol, tocotrienol, PC-8, tocomonoenol) is determined by the polyprenyl pyrophosphate substrate condensed to HGA, the biosynthetic pathways producing the lipophilic tocochromanol precursors (PPP, GGPP, SPP, and THGGPP) are key components in the regulation of tocochromanol biosynthesis. To date, although the tocotrienol biosynthetic pathway is well characterized, and key tocotrienol biosynthetic genes have been identified in plants, there are currently no data describing the mechanisms regulating the biosynthesis of GGPP used for tocotrienol biosynthesis [32]. This may result from the fact that the wild accessions of the genetic model Arabidopsis do not accumulate the tocotrienols that are mostly prevalent in the seeds of Poaceae. As the GGPP that is used for tocotrienol synthesis likely originates from the plastidic methyl erythritol phosphate pathway (MEP), one can assume that the regulation of tocotrienol biosynthesis might be directly linked to this pathway. In addition, the mapping of the tocotrienol QTLs identified in maize and barley grains might improve our understanding of the mechanisms regulating its accumulation [67,68]. It is known that tocotrienols accumulate in plants or tissues that do not usually produce them when HGA is overaccumulated, such as in transgenic Arabidopsis plants expressing *CM/PDH* or *PDH* genes, or in the leaves of transgenic tobacco carrying similar constructs [20,36,56,66]. The current interpretation of these data is that GGPP is likely not limiting in these species or tissues, and that HGA overaccumulation alters the specificity of the tocopherol prenyltransferase. These results might indicate that HGA availability in Poaceae seeds might contribute to the regulation of tocotrienol biosynthesis in these species.

The biosynthesis of PC-8 and its solanesyl benzoquinone precursor plastoquinone-9 (PQ-9) is initiated by the homogentisate solanesyltransferase-dependent condensation of HGA with SPP that comes from the preferential concatenation of GGPP and isopentenyl pyrophosphate [25,69–71]. To date, four genes have been found to specifically regulate PQ-9/PC-8 accumulation in plants. The *Nicotinamide Adenine Dinucleotide Phosphate* (*NADPH*) *dehydrogenase C1* (*NDC1*; AT5G08740) is a type II NAD(P)H quinone oxidoreductase that reduces PQ-9 into PQH_2-9, using ferredoxin as an electron donor [72]. This enzyme is localized in plastoglobuli together with prenyl quinones/quinols and tocochromanols such as PC-8. In Arabidopsis *ndc1* mutants, the leaf PQ pool is more oxidized than in wild-type controls, while PC-8 amounts are reduced by ca 66% [72]. In contrast, leaf tocopherol levels were not affected by the mutation. The proposed model explaining the role of NDC1 in PC-8 accumulation is based on tocopherol cyclase—the enzyme that notably catalyzes the cyclization of PQH_2-9 into PC-8—preferentially using reduced prenyl quinones [73]. Two ABC1 atypical kinases, *ABC1K1* (AT4G31390) and *K3* (AT1G79600), have been shown to regulate PQ-9/PC-8 metabolism in Arabidopsis [74–76]. Both kinases are abundant in plastoglobuli, and single and double *abc1k1* and *abc1k3* mutants exhibit altered PQ-9/PC-8 metabolism. Although the function of these atypical kinases in PQ-9/PC-8 metabolism has been clearly demonstrated, their mode(s) of action remains to be determined. It has been shown that both ABC1K1 and K3 phosphorylate the tocopherol cyclase VTE1. Since the biosynthesis of tocopherols, which requires VTE1 activity as well, was not affected in *abc1k3* leaves, it is unlikely that the ABC1K3 mode of action is mediated by VTE1 phosphorylation. In contrast, tocopherol amounts were significantly reduced in *abc1k1* leaves, suggesting that the ABC1K1 mode of action might involve the regulation of the tocopherol cyclase activity. The role of ABC1K1 and K3 in tocochromanol metabolism might also be mediated by the synthesis of fribrillin, a group of lipid-associated proteins that are localized in chloroplasts and essential for the biosynthesis of PQ-9, and thus PC-8 [77,78]. Indeed, Arabidopsis *fibrillin-5* mutants exhibit lower PQ-9/PC-8 amounts, and it was shown that mutation in *abc1k3* strongly reduces the accumulation of fibrillin proteins [74,77].

Regarding the regulation of tocopherol biosynthesis, it is known that the availability of phytol is a major parameter governing the final amount of tocopherols in a plant tissue. It has been shown, for instance, that the supplementation of plant cell suspensions with free phytol is sufficient to significantly increase tocopherol accumulation in these cells [54–56]. Moreover, feeding Arabidopsis seedlings with radiolabeled phytol has been associated with the biosynthesis of radiolabeled α-tocopherol, thus suggesting that free phytol is likely recycled into tocopherols [79]. The first genetic evidence supporting this biosynthetic model was provided by the Arabidopsis *vte5* that lacks 80% and 65% of the tocopherols in seeds and leaves, respectively [80]. Recently, the VTE5-dependent biosynthesis of tocopherols has also been reported in tomato leaves and fruits [81]. VTE5 is a phytol kinase that phosphorylates the free phytol that is released during chlorophyll catabolism into phytyl phosphate [80]. The chlorophyll-dependent tocopherol biosynthesis is further supported by genetic data provided by the Arabidopsis *g4/chlsyn1* mutant, which carries a mutated chlorophyll synthase that esterifies geranylgeranyl pyrophosphate on chlorophyllide *a* [82]. The leaves of this mutant grown in vitro on a media supplemented with sucrose are albino, and do not accumulate tocopherols. In addition, *g4/chlsyn1* seeds lack 75% of the tocopherols, thus indicating that tocopherol biosynthesis is also mostly chlorophyll-dependent in Arabidopsis seeds as well. Collectively, these data demonstrate that the PPP used for tocopherol biosynthesis primarily originates from the recycling of phytol released during chlorophyll catabolism in both leaves and seeds. This biosynthetic model, including details about enzymes such as Mg-dechelatase, chlorophyllases, and pheophytinase, has been very recently reviewed, and will not be developed here [17].

If one can easily understand the origin of PPP in the seeds of chloroembryophytes such Arabidopsis or rapeseed, which accumulate significant amounts of chlorophylls in developing embryos, how do leucoembryophyte seeds produce tocopherols, since they *a priori* do not synthetize chlorophylls? A comprehensive analysis of vitamin E natural variation in maize grain recently provided an unexpected answer to this puzzling question. Among the 52 QTLs identified for maize grain tocochromanols, QTL5 and QTL24 exhibited scores for phenotypic variance explained among the highest of all identified QTLs [68]. Interestingly, DNA loci covered by QTL5 andQTL24 both carry a gene encoding protochlorophyllide reductase, an enzyme of the chlorophyll biosynthetic pathway [68]. This result suggests that despite their lack of green coloration, leucoembryophyte seeds such as maize grain might produce chlorophylls that, once degraded and recycled, might provide PPP for tocopherol biosynthesis. A biochemical analysis of developing maize grain showed that, whereas they lack any macroscopic green coloration, embryos accumulate very low but detectable traces of the chlorophyll immediate precursor chlorophyllide *a*, of chlorophylls *a* and *b*, and of the first chlorophyll catabolite that lacks the Mg atom pheophytin *a*. In addition, endosperm also accumulated detectable traces of chlorophyll *a*. Although further studies—notably with genetic evidence—are required to definitively link chlorophyll metabolism and tocopherol biosynthesis in leucoembryophyte seeds, these data indicate that leucoembryophyte seeds might produce tocopherols *via* the same mechanism originally described in chloroembryophyte seeds [80,83]. This exiting perspective would definitively link tocopherol metabolism to the one of chlorophylls in plants, and open news questions regarding tocopherol metabolism in non-photosynthetic organisms such as in *Plasmodium falciparum* [14–16].

Although the chlorophyllic origin of tocopherols is clearly established in the seeds and leaves of chloroembryophyte species such as Arabidopsis, little is known about the regulation of PPP biosynthesis linked to tocopherol accumulation. Recently, two novel Arabidopsis ethane methylsulfonate mutants, the *enhanced vitamin e* (*eve*) *1* and *4* mutants, have been isolated by forward genetics [21]. The seeds of *eve1* and *eve4* mutants overaccumulate tocopherols, PC-8, and γ-tocomonoenol, a monounsaturated form of tocochromanols. Interestingly, both *eve1* and *4* seeds did not accumulate any tocotrienols, such as transgenic Arabidopsis plants overaccumulating HGA, suggesting that although HGA metabolism is likely increased in these mutants to sustain tocochromanol metabolism, HGA overaccumulation is not the primary source of its enhancement. In addition, γ-tocomonoenol accumulation has never been reported in Arabidopsis HGA overaccumulating lines, further suggesting that the misregulation of HGA biosynthesis is likely not the primary source of the enhancement of tocochromanol accumulation in *eve1* and *eve4* seeds. The fact that all tocochromanol forms are overaccumulated in *eve1* and *eve4* seeds likely suggests that both mutations affect the chloroplastic isoprenoid metabolism produced by the methyl erythritol phosphate pathway (Figure 4). The mutation responsible for the *eve1* seed phenotype affects the *WRINKLED1* gene that encodes for a transcription factor containing two APETALA2/ethylene response element DNA-binding proteins [84]. This gene is mostly expressed during seed development, although moderate expression has been also detected in roots and flowers [85,86].

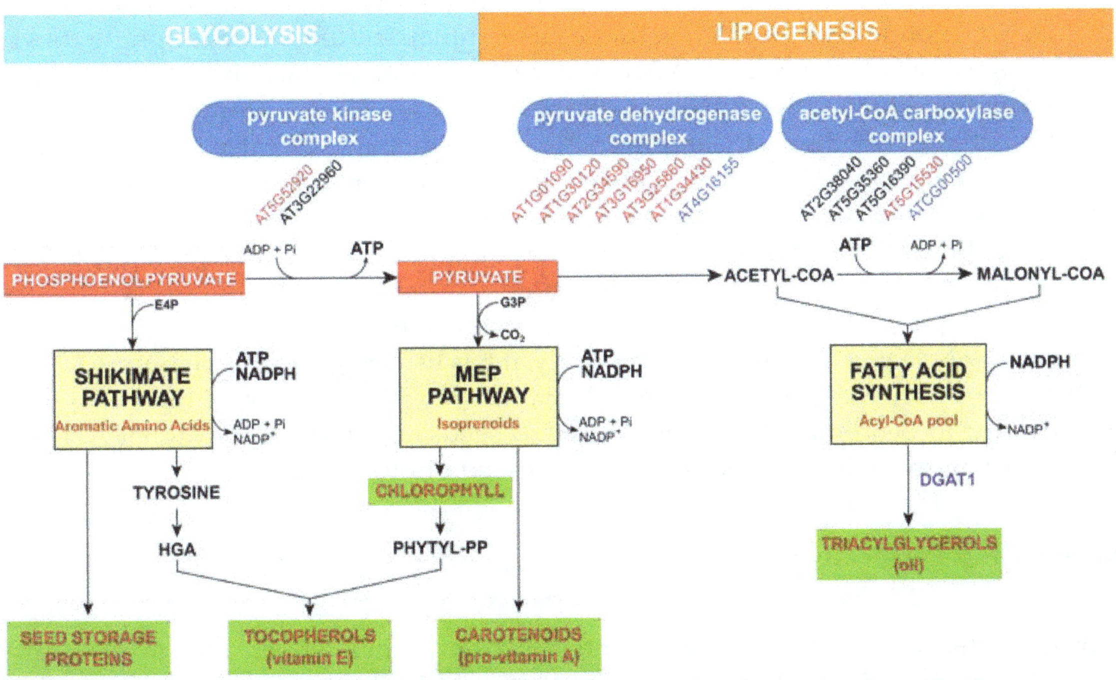

Figure 4. Plastidic intersection of the shikimate pathway, the methyl erythritol phosphate pathway, and lipogenesis. The shikimate pathway, methyl erythritol phosphate (MEP) pathway, and fatty acid synthesis are localized in plastids, and share phosphoenolpyruvate and pyruvate as common biosynthetic precursors. The biosynthesis of triacylglycerols occurs in the endoplasmic reticulum. Arabidopsis Genome Initiative numbers in red indicate that the corresponding gene is downregulated in Arabidopsis *wri1* developing embryos, or upregulated in transgenic plants constitutively expressing the *WRI1* transcription factor. AGI numbers in black indicate that the expression of the corresponding gene is WRI1-independent. AGI numbers in blue indicate that no transcriptomic data was available. Abbreviations: DGAT1, acylCoA:diacylglycerol acyltransferase 1; E4P, erythrose 4-phosphate; G3P, glyceraldehyde 3-phosphate; phytyl-PP, phytyl pyrophosphate.

Targets of the WRI1 transcription factor in plant genomes have been investigated by transcriptomic studies and in vitro enzymatic assays in developing Arabidopsis *wri1* embryos [85–88], in the leaves of transgenic maize lines overexpressing the *ZmWRI1a* gene [89], and in *Nicotiana benthamiana* leaves agroinfiltrated with Arabidopsis, potato, poplar, oat, and nutsedge *WRI1* orthologs [90]. The transcription factor WRI1 regulates the expression of several key biosynthetic genes involved in late glycolysis, fatty acid synthesis, and lipid assembly [85–89]. Thus, WRI1 pushes carbon into fatty acid/lipid metabolism by upregulating key lipid biosynthetic genes. It is interesting to note that the genes encoding almost all of the subunits of the plastidial pyruvate dehydrogenase complex are either downregulated in *wri1* developing embryos or upregulated in transgenic plants overexpressing *WRI1* (Figure 4). Interestingly, tocochromanols are synthetized in chloroplasts as well, and the biosynthetic pathways providing both tocochromanol precursors, i.e., the MEP pathway and the shikimate pathway, use the same biosynthetic precursors, i.e., pyruvate and phosphoenolpyruvate, as those used for fatty acid/lipid synthesis (Figure 4). These suggest that tocochromanol and lipid biosyntheses might compete for these biosynthetic precursors.

Another model explaining the enhancement of tocochromanol metabolism in *wri1* seeds might be considered as well. The transient *WRI1* expression performed in *Nicotiana benthamiana* leaves revealed a novel aspect of WRI1 transcriptome that has not been described neither in transgenic lines constitutively expressing *WRI1* nor in *wri1* seeds. Numerous genes encoding chlorophyll biosynthetic enzymes such as protochlorophyllide oxidoreductase and Mg chelatase, chlorophyll-binding proteins, subunits of the light harvesting complexes, and ATP generation complex subunits were strongly downregulated in tobacco leaves transiently expressing *WRI1* constructs (Supplementary file 6 of Grimberg et al. [90]). The authors concluded that the transient expression of *WRI1* is strongly associated with the downregulation of photosynthesis, including energy and reducing equivalent production, respectively. Interestingly, the endogenous *WRI1* gene is not constitutively expressed in Arabidopsis plants; instead, it is transiently expressed in the developing Arabidopsis embryo [85]. This indicates that the *WRI1* expression in the developing Arabidopsis embryo also might downregulate photosynthesis, and thus the production of ATP, as well as reduce equivalents in embryos. Now, the MEP pathway that produces the building blocks for chloroplastic isoprenoids is strongly dependent on ATP and reducing equivalents such as NADPH (Figure 4). Interestingly, it has been suggested that both ATP and NADPH might be key regulatory components of the MEP pathway [91]. This hypothesis suggests that the enhancement of the tocochromanol metabolism in *wri1* seeds might reflect the higher ATP and NADPH production resulting from the reduced repression of seed photosynthesis.

6. Conclusions and Perspectives

From the first purification of α-tocopherol from wheat germ oil to the latest model of the tocochromanol biosynthetic pathways introducing tocomonoenol biosynthetic genes, our understanding of vitamin E biosynthesis in plants has been considerably enriched [3,21]. In contrast, much less is known about the mechanisms regulating vitamin E biosynthesis in plants. The fact that tocochromanol biosynthesis mobilizes two distinct biosynthetic pathways, the shikimate pathway and the MEP pathway, requires the degradation of two compounds such as L-tyr and chlorophylls, involves a yet-unknown transport system between the cytoplasm and the stroma in plant species in which HGA biosynthesis is localized in the cytoplasm, and is interconnected to fatty acid biosynthesis in plastids, render the understanding of its regulation particularly challenging. Indeed, understanding the regulation of vitamin E biosynthesis will imply that we take up the challenges to understand the regulation of each of these numerous events. Beyond understanding the regulation of vitamin E biosynthesis in plants, it seems important that medical scientists assess the sanitary consequences of the significant vitamin E deficiency independently detected in human populations, including in developed countries. The fundamental role of this vitamin in human reproduction and its benefit in current widespread diseases such as high cholesterol and neurodegenerative pathologies makes it a candidate of choice to improve human health.

Acknowledgments: I am grateful to the University of Fribourg and to the Foundation of Research in Biochemistry and on Vitamins (Epalinges, Switzerland) represented by Claude Bron for supporting the research developed in my laboratory.

References

1. Mène-Saffrané, L.; Pellaud, S. Current strategies for vitamin E biofortification of crops. *Curr. Opin. Biotechnol.* **2017**, *44*, 189–197. [CrossRef] [PubMed]
2. Evans, H.M.; Bishop, K.S. On the existence of a hitherto unrecognized dietary factor essential for reproduction. *Science* **1922**, *56*, 650–651. [CrossRef] [PubMed]
3. Evans, H.M.; Emerson, O.H.; Emerson, G.A. The isolation from wheat germ oil of an alcohol, α-tocopherol, having the properties of vitamin E. *J. Biol. Chem.* **1936**, *113*, 319–332. [CrossRef]
4. Galli, F.; Azzi, A.; Birringer, M.; Cook-Mills, J.M.; Eggersdorfer, M.; Frank, J.; Cruciani, G.; Lorkowski, S.; Katar Özer, N. Vitamin E: Emerging aspects and new directions. *Free Radic. Biol. Med.* **2017**, 16–36. [CrossRef] [PubMed]
5. Li, G.X.; Lee, M.J.; Liu, A.B.; Yang, Z.; Lin, Y.; Shih, W.J.; Yang, C.S. δ-tocopherol is more active than α- or γ-tocopherol in inhibiting lung tumorigenesis in vivo. *Cancer Prev. Res.* **2011**, *4*, 404–413. [CrossRef] [PubMed]
6. La Fata, G.; Weber, P.; Mohajeri, M.H. Effects of vitamin E on cognitive performance during ageing and in Alzheimer's disease. *Nutrients* **2014**, *6*, 5453–5472. [CrossRef] [PubMed]
7. Qureshi, A.A.; Burger, W.C.; Peterson, D.M.; Elson, C.E. The structure of an inhibitor of cholesterol biosynthesis isolated from barley. *J. Biol. Chem.* **1986**, *261*, 10544–10550. [PubMed]
8. Qureshi, A.A.; Sami, S.A.; Salser, W.A.; Khan, F.A. Dose-dependent suppression of serum cholesterol by tocotrienol-rich fraction (TRF25) of rice bran in hypercholesterolemic humans. *Atherosclerosis* **2002**, *161*, 199–207. [CrossRef]
9. Maras, J.E.; Bermudez, O.I.; Qiao, N.; Bakun, P.J.; Boody-Alter, E.L.; Tucker, K.L. Intake of α-tocopherol is limited among US adults. *J. Am. Diet. Assoc.* **2004**, *104*, 567–575. [CrossRef] [PubMed]
10. Polito, A.; Intorre, F.; Andriollo-Sanchez, M.; Azzini, E.; Raguzzini, A.; Meunier, N.; Ducros, V.; O'Connor, J.M.; Coudray, C.; Roussel, A.M.; et al. Estimation of intake and status of vitamin A, vitamin E and folate in older European adults: The ZENITH. *Eur. J. Clin. Nutr.* **2005**, *59*, S42–S47. [CrossRef] [PubMed]
11. Kim, Y.N.; Cho, Y.O. Vitamin E status of 20- to 59-year-old adults living in the Seoul metropolitan area of South Korea. *Nutr. Res. Pract.* **2015**, *9*, 192–198. [CrossRef] [PubMed]
12. Shamim, A.A.; Schulze, K.; Merrill, R.D.; Kabir, A.; Christian, P.; Shaikh, S.; Wu, L.; Ali, H.; Labrique, A.B.; Mehra, S.; et al. Tocopherols are associated with risk of miscarriage in rural Bangladesh. *Am. J. Clin. Nutr.* **2015**, *101*, 294–301. [CrossRef] [PubMed]
13. Péter, S.; Friedel, A.; Roos, F.F.; Wyss, A.; Eggersdorfer, M.; Hoffmann, K.; Weber, P. A Systematic review of global alpha-tocopherol status as assessed by nutritional intake levels and blood serum concentrations. *Int. J. Vitam. Nutr. Res.* **2016**, 1–21. [CrossRef] [PubMed]
14. Sussmann, R.A.C.; Angeli, C.B.; Peres, V.J.; Kimura, E.A.; Katzin, A.M. Intraerythrocytic stages of *Plasmodium falciparum* biosynthesize vitamin E. *FEBS Lett.* **2011**, *585*, 3985–3991. [CrossRef] [PubMed]
15. Sussman, R.A.C.; Fotoran, W.L.; Kimura, E.A.; Katzin, A.M. *Plasmodium falciparum* uses vitamin E to avoid oxidative stress. *Parasit. Vectors* **2017**, *10*, 461. [CrossRef] [PubMed]
16. Cassera, M.B.; Gozzo, F.C.; D'Alexandri, F.L.; Merino, E.F.; del Portillo, H.A.; Peres, V.J.; Almeida, I.C.; Eberlin, M.N.; Wunderlich, G.; Wiesner, J.; et al. The methylerythritol phosphate pathway is functionally active in all intraerythrocytic stages of *Plasmodium falciparum*. *J. Biol. Chem.* **2004**, *279*, 51749–51759. [CrossRef] [PubMed]
17. Pellaud, S.; Mène-Saffrané, L. Metabolic origins and transport of vitamin E biosynthetic precursors. *Front. Plant Sci.* **2017**, *8*, 1959. [CrossRef] [PubMed]
18. Collakova, E.; DellaPenna, D. Isolation and functional analysis of homogentisate phytyltransferase from *Synechocystis* sp. PCC 6803 and Arabidopsis. *Plant Physiol.* **2001**, *127*, 1113–1124. [CrossRef] [PubMed]
19. Savidge, B.; Weiss, J.D.; Wong, Y-H.H.; Lassner, M.W.; Mitky, T.A.; Shewmaker, C.K.; Post-Beittenmiller, D.; Valentin, H.E. Isolation and characterization of homogentisate phytyltransferase genes from *Synechocystis* sp. PCC 6803 and Arabidopsis. *Plant Physiol.* **2002**, *129*, 321–332. [CrossRef] [PubMed]
20. Zhang, C.; Cahoon, R.E.; Hunter, S.C.; Chen, M.; Han, J.; Cahoon, E.B. Genetic and biochemical basis for alternative routes of tocotrienol biosynthesis for enhanced vitamin E antioxidant production. *Plant J.* **2013**, *73*, 628–639. [CrossRef] [PubMed]

21. Pellaud, S.; Bory, A.; Chabert, V.; Romanens, J.; Chaisse-Leal, L.; Doan, A.V.; Frey, L.; Gust, A.; Fromm, K.M.; Mène-Saffrané, L. WRINKLED1 and ACYL-COA:DIACYLGLYCEROL ACYLTRANSFERASE1 regulate tocochromanol metabolism in Arabidopsis. *New Phytol.* **2018**, *217*, 1–16. [CrossRef] [PubMed]
22. Yang, W.; Cahoon, R.E.; Hunter, S.C.; Zhang, C.; Han, J.; Borgschulte, T.; Cahoon, E.B. Vitamin E biosynthesis: Functional characterization of the monocot homogentisate geranylgeranyl transferase. *Plant J.* **2011**, *65*, 206–217. [CrossRef] [PubMed]
23. Mène-Saffrané, L.; Jones, A.D.; DellaPenna, D. Plastochromanol-8 and tocopherols are essential lipid-soluble antioxidants during seed desiccation and quiescence in *Arabidopsis*. *Proc. Natl. Acad. Sci. USA* **2010**, *107*, 17815–17820. [CrossRef] [PubMed]
24. Sadre, R.; Gruber, J.; Frentzen, M. Characterization of homogentisate prenyltransferases involved in plastoquinone-9 and tocochromanol biosynthesis. *FEBS Lett.* **2006**, *580*, 5357–5362. [CrossRef] [PubMed]
25. Tian, L.; DellaPenna, D.; Dixon, R.A. The *pds2* mutation is a lesion in the Arabidopsis homogentisate solanesyltransferase gene involved in plastoquinone biosynthesis. *Planta* **2007**, *226*, 1067–1073. [CrossRef] [PubMed]
26. Cheng, Z.; Sattler, S.; Maeda, H.; Sakuragi, Y.; Bryant, D.A.; DellaPenna, D. Highly divergent methyltransferases catalyze a conserved reaction in tocopherol and plastoquinone synthesis in Cyanobacteria and photosynthetic Eukaryotes. *Plant Cell* **2003**, *15*, 2343–2356. [CrossRef] [PubMed]
27. Van Eenennaam, A.L.; Lincoln, K.; Durrett, T.P.; Valentin, H.E.; Shewmaker, C.K.; Thorne, G.M.; Jiang, J.; Baszis, S.R.; Levering, C.K.; Aasen, E.D.; et al. Engineering vitamin E content: From Arabidopsis mutant to soy oil. *Plant Cell* **2003**, *15*, 3007–3019. [CrossRef] [PubMed]
28. Porfirova, S.; Bergmüller, E.; Tropf, S.; Lemke, R.; Dörmann, P. Isolation of an Arabidopsis mutant lacking vitamin E and identification of a cyclase essential for all tocopherol biosynthesis. *Proc. Natl. Acad. Sci. USA* **2002**, *99*, 12495–12500. [CrossRef] [PubMed]
29. Sattler, S.E.; Gilliland, L.U.; Magallanes-Lundback, M.; Pollard, M.; DellaPenna, D. Vitamin E is essential for seed longevity and for preventing lipid peroxidation during germination. *Plant Cell* **2004**, *16*, 1419–1432. [CrossRef] [PubMed]
30. Shintani, D.; DellaPenna, D. Elevating the vitamin E content of plants through metabolic engineering. *Science* **1998**, *282*, 2098–2100. [CrossRef] [PubMed]
31. Bergmüller, E.; Porfirova, S.; Dörmann, P. Characterization of an Arabidopsis mutant deficient in γ-tocopherol methyltransferase. *Plant Mol. Biol.* **2003**, *52*, 1181–1190. [CrossRef] [PubMed]
32. Cahoon, E.B.; Hall, S.E.; Ripp, K.G.; Ganzke, T.S.; Hitz, W.D.; Coughlan, S.J. Metabolic redesign of vitamin E biosynthesis in plants for tocotrienol production and increased antioxidant content. *Nat. Biotechnol.* **2003**, *21*, 1082–1087. [CrossRef] [PubMed]
33. Hosomi, A.; Arita, M.; Sato, Y.; Kiyose, C.; Ueda, T.; Igarashi, O.; Arai, H.; Inoue, K. Affinity of alpha-tocopherol transfer protein as a determinant of the biological activities of vitamin E analogs. *FEBS Lett.* **1997**, *409*, 105–108. [CrossRef]
34. Aeschimann, W.; Staats, S.; Kammer, S.; Olieric, N.; Jeckelmann, J.M.; Fotiadis, D.; Netscher, T.; Rimbach, G.; Cascella, M.; Stocker, A. Self-assembled α-tocopherol transfer protein nanoparticles promote vitamin E delivery across an endothelial barrier. *Sci. Rep.* **2017**, *7*, 4970. [CrossRef] [PubMed]
35. Zbierzak, A.M.; Kanwischer, M.; Wille, C.; Vidi, P.A.; Giavalisco, P.; Lohmann, A.; Briesen, I.; Porfirova, S.; Bréhélin, C.; Kessler, F.; et al. Intersection of the tocopherol and plastoquinol metabolic pathways at the plastoglobule. *Biochem. J.* **2010**, *425*, 389–399. [CrossRef] [PubMed]
36. Tzin, V.; Malitsky, S.; Aharoni, A.; Galili, G. Expression of a bacterial bi-functional chorismate mutase/prephenate dehydratase modulates primary and secondary metabolism associated with aromatic amino acids in Arabidopsis. *Plant J.* **2009**, *60*, 156–167. [CrossRef] [PubMed]
37. Jiang, J.; Jia, H.; Feng, G.; Wang, Z.; Li, J.; Gao, H.; Wang, X. Overexpression of *Medicago sativa TMT* elevates the α-tocopherol content in *Arabidopsis* seeds, alfalfa leaves, and delays dark-induced leaf senescence. *Plant Sci.* **2016**, *249*, 93–104. [CrossRef] [PubMed]
38. Endrigkeit, J.; Wang, X.; Cai, D.; Zhang, C.; Long, Y.; Meng, J.; Jung, C. Genetic mapping, cloning, and functional characterization of the *BnaX.VTE4* gene encoding a γ-tocopherol methyltransferase from oilseed rape. *Theor. Appl. Genet.* **2009**, *119*, 567–575. [CrossRef] [PubMed]

39. Tang, S.; Hass, C.G.; Knapp, S.J. *Ty3/gypsy*-like retrotransposon knockout of a 2-methyl-6-phytyl-1,4-benzoquinone methyltransferase is non-lethal, uncovers a cryptic paralogous mutation, and produces novel tocopherol (vitamin E) profiles in sunflower. *Theor. Appl. Genet.* **2006**, *113*, 783–799. [CrossRef] [PubMed]
40. Lampi, A.M.; Nurmi, T.; Ollilainen, V.; Piironen, V. Tocopherols and tocotrienols in wheat genotypes in the HEALGRAIN diversity screen. *J. Agric. Food Chem.* **2008**, *56*, 9716–9721. [CrossRef] [PubMed]
41. Goffman, F.D.; Velasco, L.; Thies, W. Quantitative determination of tocopherols in single seeds of rapeseed (*Brassica napus* L.). *Lipid* **1999**, *101*, 142–145. [CrossRef]
42. Xu, S.T.; Zhang, D.L.; Cai, Y.; Zhou, Y.; Shah, T.; Ali, F.; Li, Q.; Li, Z.G.; Wang, W.D.; Li, J.S.; et al. Dissecting tocopherols content in maize (*Zea mays* L.), using two segregating populations and high-density single nucleotide polymorphism markers. *BMC Plant Biol.* **2012**, *12*, 201–214. [CrossRef]
43. Lipka, A.E.; Gore, M.A.; Magallanes-Lundback, M.; Mesberg, A.; Lin, H.; Tiede, T.; Chen, C.; Buell, C.R.; Buckler, E.S.; Rocheford, T.; et al. Genome-wide association study and pathway-level analysis of tocochromanol levels in maize grain. *G3 (Bethesda)* **2013**, *3*, 1287–1299. [CrossRef] [PubMed]
44. Ujiie, A.; Yamada, T.; Fujimoto, K.; Endo, Y.; Kitamura, K. Identification of soybean varieties with high α-tocopherol content. *Breed. Sci.* **2005**, *55*, 123–125. [CrossRef]
45. Dwiyanti, M.S.; Yamada, T.; Sato, M.; Abe, J.; Kitamura, K. Genetic variation of γ-tocopherol methyltransferase gene contributes to elevated α-tocopherol content in soybean seeds. *BMC Plant Biol.* **2011**, *11*, 152–168. [CrossRef] [PubMed]
46. Gilliland, L.U.; Magallanes-Lundback, M.; Hemming, C.; Supplee, A.; Koornneef, M.; Bentsink, L.; DellaPenna, D. Genetic basis for natural variation in seed vitamin E levels in *Arabidopsis thaliana*. *Proc. Natl. Acad. Sci. USA* **2006**, *103*, 18834–18841. [CrossRef] [PubMed]
47. Li, H.; Wang, Y.; Han, Y.; Teng, W.; Zhao, X.; Li, Y.; Li, W. Mapping quantitative trait loci (QTLs) underlying seed vitamin E content in soybean with main, epistatic and QTL × environment effects. *Plant Breed.* **2016**, *135*, 208–214. [CrossRef]
48. Shaw, E.J.; Rajcan, I. Molecular mapping of soybean seed tocopherols in the cross 'OAC Bayfield' × 'OAC Shire'. *Plant Breed.* **2017**, *136*, 83–93. [CrossRef]
49. Chander, S.; Guo, Y.Q.; Yang, X.H.; Yan, J.B.; Zhang, Y.R.; Song, T.M.; Li, J.S. Genetic dissection of tocopherol content and composition in maize grain using quantitative trait loci analysis and the candidate gene approach. *Mol. Breed.* **2008**, *22*, 353–365. [CrossRef]
50. Li, Q.; Yang, X.; Xu, S.; Cai, Y.; Zhang, D.; Han, Y.; Li, L.; Zhang, Z.; Gao, S.; Li, J.; et al. Genome-wide association studies identified three independent polymorphisms associated with α-tocopherol content in maize kernels. *PLoS ONE* **2012**, *7*, e36807. [CrossRef] [PubMed]
51. Marwede, V.; Gül, M.K.; Becker, H.C.; Ecke, W. Mapping of QTL controlling tocopherol content in winter oilseed rape. *Plant Breed.* **2005**, *124*, 20–26. [CrossRef]
52. Wang, X.; Zhang, C.; Li, L.; Fritsche, S.; Endrigkeit, J.; Zhang, W.; Long, Y.; Jung, C.; Meng, J. Unraveling the genetic basis of seed tocopherol content and composition in rapeseed (*Brassica napus* L.). *PLoS ONE* **2012**, *7*, e50038. [CrossRef] [PubMed]
53. Oliver, R.E.; Islamovic, E.; Obert, D.E.; Wise, M.L.; Herrin, L.L.; Hang, A.; Harrison, S.A.; Ibrahim, A.; Marshall, J.M.; Miclaus, K.J.; et al. Comparative systems biology reveals allelic variation modulating tocochromanol profiles in barley (*Hordeum vulgare* L.). *PLoS ONE* **2014**, *9*, e96276. [CrossRef] [PubMed]
54. Furuya, T.; Yoshikawa, T.; Kimura, T.; Kaneko, H. Production of tocopherols by cell culture of safflower. *Phytochemistry* **1987**, *26*, 2741–2747. [CrossRef]
55. Caretto, S.; Speth, E.B.; Fachechi, C.; Gala, R.; Zacheo, G.; Giovinazzo, G. Enhancement of vitamin E production in sunflower cell cultures. *Plant Cell Rep.* **2004**, *23*, 174–179. [CrossRef] [PubMed]
56. Karunanandaa, B.; Qi, Q.; Hao, M.; Baszis, S.R.; Jensen, P.K.; Wong, Y.H.H.; Jiang, J.; Venkatramesh, M.; Gruys, K.J.; Moshiri, F.; et al. Metabolically engineered oilseed crops with enhanced seed tocopherol. *Metab. Eng.* **2005**, *7*, 384–400. [CrossRef] [PubMed]
57. Prabhu, P.R.; Hudson, A.O. Identification and partial characterization of an L-tyrosine aminotransferase (TAT) from *Arabidopsis thaliana*. *Biochem. Res. Int.* **2010**, 549572. [CrossRef]
58. Grossmann, K.; Hutzler, J.; Tresch, S.; Christiansen, N.; Looser, R.; Ehrhardt, T. On the mode of action of the herbicides cinmethylin and 5-benzyloxymethyl-1,2-isoxyzolines: Putative inhibitors of plant tyrosine aminotransferase. *Pest Manag. Sci.* **2012**, *68*, 482–492. [CrossRef] [PubMed]

59. Riewe, D.; Koohi, M.; Lisec, J.; Pfeiffer, M.; Lippmann, R.; Schmeichel, J.; Willmitzer, L.; Altmann, T. A tyrosine aminotransferase involved in tocopherol synthesis in Arabidopsis. *Plant J.* **2012**, *71*, 850–859. [CrossRef] [PubMed]
60. Wang, M.; Toda, K.; Maeda, H.A. Biochemical properties and subcellular localization of tyrosine aminotransferases in *Arabidopsis thaliana*. *Phytochemistry* **2016**, *132*, 16–25. [CrossRef] [PubMed]
61. Garcia, I.; Rodgers, M.; Pepin, R.; Hsieh, T.Z.; Matringe, M. Characterization and subcellular compartmentation of recombinant 4-hydroxyphenylpyruvate dioxygenase from Arabidopsis in transgenic tobacco. *Plant Physiol.* **1999**, *119*, 1507–1516. [CrossRef] [PubMed]
62. Falk, J.; Krauss, N.; Dähnhardt, D.; Krupinska, K. The senescence associated gene of barley encoding 4-hydroxyphenylpyruvate dioxygenase is expressed during oxidative stress. *J. Plant. Physiol.* **2002**, *159*, 1245–1253. [CrossRef]
63. Siehl, D.L.; Tao, Y.; Albert, H.; Dong, Y.; Heckert, M.; Madrigal, A.; Lincoln-Cabatu, B.; Lu, J.; Fenwick, T.; Bermudez, E.; et al. Broad 4-hydroxyphenylpyruvate dioxygenase inhibitor herbicide tolerance in soybean with an optimized enzyme and expression cassette. *Plant Physiol.* **2014**, *166*, 1162–1176. [CrossRef] [PubMed]
64. Stacey, M.G.; Cahoon, R.E.; Nguyen, H.T.; Cui, Y.; Sato, S.; Nguyen, C.T.; Phoka, N.; Clark, K.M.; Liang, Y.; Forrester, J.; et al. Identification of homogentisate dioxygenase as a target for vitamin E biofortification in oilseeds. *Plant Physiol.* **2016**, *172*, 1506–1518. [CrossRef] [PubMed]
65. Widhalm, J.R.; Gutensohn, M.; Yoo, H.; Adebesin, F.; Qian, Y.; Guo, L.; Jaini, R.; Lynch, J.H.; McCoy, R.M.; Shreve, J.T.; et al. Identification of a plastidial phenylalanine exporter that influences flux distribution through the phenylalanine biosynthetic network. *Nat. Commun.* **2015**, *6*, 8142–8152. [CrossRef] [PubMed]
66. Rippert, P.; Scimemi, C.; Dubald, M.; Matringe, M. Engineering plant shikimate pathway for production of tocotrienol and improving herbicide resistance. *Plant Physiol.* **2004**, *134*, 92–100. [CrossRef] [PubMed]
67. Graebner, R.C.; Wise, M.; Cuesta-Marcos, A.; Geniza, M.; Blake, T.; Blake, V.C.; Butler, J.; Chao, S.; Hole, D.J.; Horsley, R.; et al. Quantitative trait loci associated with the tocochromanol (vitamin E) pathway in barley. *PLoS ONE* **2015**, *10*, e0133767. [CrossRef] [PubMed]
68. Diepenbrock, C.H.; Kandianis, C.B.; Lipka, A.E.; Magallanes-Lundback, M.; Vaillancourt, B.; Góngora-Castillo, E.; Wallace, J.G.; Cepela, J.; Mesberg, A.; Bradbury, P.J.; et al. Novel loci underlie natural variation in vitamin E levels in maize grain. *Plant Cell* **2017**, *29*, 2374–2392. [CrossRef] [PubMed]
69. Block, A.; Fristedt, R.; Rogers, S.; Kumar, J.; Barnes, B.; Barnes, J.; Elowsky, C.G.; Wamboldt, Y.; Mackenzie, S.A.; Redding, K.; et al. Functional modelling identifies paralogous solanesyl-diphosphate synthases that assemble the side chain of plastoquinone-9 in plastids. *J. Biol. Chem.* **2013**, *288*, 27594–27606. [CrossRef] [PubMed]
70. Hirooka, K.; Bamba, T.; Fukusaki, E.-I.; Kobayashi, A. Cloning and kinetic characterization of Arabidopsis thaliana solanesyl diphosphate synthase. *Biochem. J.* **2003**, *370*, 679–686. [CrossRef] [PubMed]
71. Hirooka, K.; Izumi, Y.; An, C.-I.; Nakazawa, Y.; Fukusaki, E.-I.; Kobayashi, A. Functional analysis of two solanesyl diphosphate synthases from Arabidopsis thaliana. *Biosci. Biotechnol. Biochem.* **2005**, *69*, 592–601. [CrossRef] [PubMed]
72. Eugeni Piller, L.; Besagnia, C.; Ksas, B.; Rumeau, D.; Bréhélin, C.; Glauser, G.; Kessler, F.; Havaux, M. Chloroplast lipid droplet type II NAD(P)H quinone oxidoreductase is essential for prenylquinone metabolism and vitamin K1 accumulation. *Proc. Natl. Acad. Sci. USA* **2011**, *108*, 14354–14359. [CrossRef] [PubMed]
73. Grütter, C.; Alonso, E.; Chougnet, A.; Woggon, W.D. A biomimetic chromanol cyclization leading to α-tocopherol. *Angew. Chem. Int. Ed.* **2006**, *45*, 1126–1130. [CrossRef] [PubMed]
74. Martinis, J.; Glauser, G.; Valimareanu, S.; Kessler, F. A chloroplast ABC1-like kinase regulates vitamin E metabolism in Arabidopsis. *Plant Physiol.* **2013**, *162*, 652–662. [CrossRef] [PubMed]
75. Martinis, J.; Glauser, G.; Valimareanu, S.; Stettler, M.; Zeeman, S.C.; Yamamoto, H.; Shikanai, T.; Kessler, F. ABC1K1/PGR6 kinase: A regulatory link between photosynthetic activity and chloroplast metabolism. *Plant J.* **2014**, *77*, 269–283. [CrossRef] [PubMed]
76. Lundquist, P.K.; Poliakov, A.; Giacomelli, L.; Friso, G.; Appel, M.; McQuinn, R.P.; Krasnoff, S.B.; Rowland, E.; Ponnala, L.; Sun, Q.; et al. Loss of plastoglobule kinases ABC1K1 and ABC1K3 causes conditional degreening, modified prenyl-lipids, and recruitment of the jasmonic acid pathway. *Plant Cell* **2013**, *25*, 1818–1839. [CrossRef] [PubMed]
77. Kim, E.-H.; Lee, Y.; Kim, H.U. Fibrillin 5 is essential for plastoquinone-9 biosynthesis by binding to solanesyl diphosphate synthases in Arabidopsis. *Plant Cell* **2015**, *27*, 2956–2971. [CrossRef] [PubMed]

78. Kim, E.-H.; Lee, D-W.; Lee, K-R.; Jung, S-J.; Jeon, J-S.; Kim, H.U. Conserved function of fibrillin5 in the plastoquinone-9 biosynthetic pathway in Arabidopsis and rice. *Front. Plant Sci.* **2017**, *8*, 1197. [CrossRef] [PubMed]
79. Ischebeck, T.; Zbierzak, A.M.; Kanwischer, M.; Dormann, M. A salvage pathway for phytol metabolism in Arabidopsis. *J. Biol. Chem.* **2006**, *281*, 2470–2477. [CrossRef] [PubMed]
80. Valentin, H.; Lincoln, K.; Moshiri, F.; Jensen, P.K.; Qi, Q.; Venkatesh, T.V.; Karunanandaa, B.; Baszis, S.R.; Norris, S.R.; Savidge, B.; et al. The Arabidopsis *vitamin E pathway gene5-1* mutant reveals a critical role for phytol kinase in seed tocopherol biosynthesis. *Plant Cell* **2006**, *18*, 212–224. [CrossRef] [PubMed]
81. Almeida, J.; da Silva Azevedo, M.; Spicher, L.; Glauser, G.; vom Dorp, K.; Guyer, L.; del Valle Carranza, A.; Asis, R.; Pereira de Souza, A.; Buckeridge, M.; et al. Down-regulation of tomato PHYTOL KINASE strongly impairs tocopherol biosynthesis and affects prenyllipid metabolism in an organ-specific manner. *J. Exp. Bot.* **2016**, *67*, 919–934. [CrossRef] [PubMed]
82. Zhang, C.; Zhang, W.; Ren, G.; Li, D.; Cahoon, R.E.; Chen, M.; Zhou, Y.; Yu, B.; Cahoon, E.B. Chlorophyll synthase under epigenetic surveillance is critical for vitamin E synthesis, and altered expression affects tocopherol levels in Arabidopsis. *Plant Physiol.* **2015**, *168*, 1503–1511. [CrossRef] [PubMed]
83. Vom Dorp, K.; Hölzl, G.; Plohmann, C.; Eisenhut, M.; Abraham, M.; Weber, A.P.M.; Hanson, A.D.; Dörmann, P. Remobilization of phytol from chlorophyll degradation is essential for tocopherol synthesis and growth of Arabidopsis. *Plant Cell* **2015**, *27*, 2846–2859. [CrossRef] [PubMed]
84. Cernac, A.; Benning, C. *WRINKLED1* encodes an AP2/EREB domain protein involved in the control of storage compound biosynthesis in Arabidopsis. *Plant J.* **2004**, *40*, 575–585. [CrossRef] [PubMed]
85. Baud, S.; Santos Mendoza, M.; To, A.; Harscoët, E.; Lepiniec, L.; Dubreucq, B. WRINKLED1 specifies the regulatory action of LEAFY COTYLEDON2 towards fatty acid metabolism during seed maturation in Arabidopsis. *Plant J.* **2007**, *50*, 825–838. [CrossRef] [PubMed]
86. Focks, N.; Benning, C. *wrinkled1*: A novel, low-seed-oil mutant of Arabidopsis with a deficiency in the seed-specific regulation of carbohydrate metabolism. *Plant Physiol.* **1998**, *118*, 91–101. [CrossRef] [PubMed]
87. Ruuska, S.A.; Girke, T.; Benning, C.; Ohlrogge, J.B. Contrapuntal networks of gene expression during Arabidopsis seed filling. *Plant Cell* **2002**, *14*, 1191–1206. [CrossRef] [PubMed]
88. Maeo, K.; Tokuda, T.; Ayame, A.; Mitsui, N.; Kawai, T.; Tsukagoshi, H.; Ishiguro, S.; Nakamura, K. An AP2-type transcription factor, WRINKLED1, of *Arabidopsis thaliana* binds to the AW-box sequence conserved among proximal upstream regions of genes involved in fatty acid synthesis. *Plant J.* **2009**, *60*, 476–487. [CrossRef] [PubMed]
89. Pouvreau, B.; Baud, S.; Vernoud, V.; Morin, V.; Py, C.; Gendrot, G.; Pichon, J.-P.; Rouster, J.; Paul, W.; Rogowsky, P.M. Duplicate maize *Wrinkled1* transcription factors activate target genes involved in seed oil biosynthesis. *Plant Physiol.* **2011**, *156*, 674–686. [CrossRef] [PubMed]
90. Grimberg, Å.; Carlsson, A.S.; Marttila, S.; Bhalerao, R.; Hofvander, P. Transcriptional transitions in *Nicotiana benthamiana* leaves upon induction of oil synthesis by WRINKLED1 homologs from diverse species and tissues. *BMC Plant Biol.* **2015**, *15*, 192. [CrossRef] [PubMed]
91. Banerjee, A.; Sharkey, T.D. Methylerythritol 4-phosphate (MEP) pathway metabolic regulation. *Nat. Prod. Rep.* **2014**, *31*, 1043–1055. [CrossRef] [PubMed]

8

Phylloquinone and Menaquinone-4 Tissue Distribution at Different Life Stages in Male and Female Sprague–Dawley Rats Fed Different VK Levels Since Weaning or Subjected to a 40% Calorie Restriction since Adulthood

Guylaine Ferland [1,*], Isabelle Doucet [1,2] and Dominique Mainville [1,3]

1 Département de nutrition, Université de Montréal, Montréal, QC H3C 3J7, Canada; isadoucet@me.com (I.D.); dominique.mainville@hotmail.com (D.M.)
2 Hôpital de la Cité-de-la-Santé, Laval, QC H7M 3L9, Canada
3 CIUSSS du Centre-Sud-de-l'Île-de-Montréal, Centre de réadaptation Lucie-Bruneau, Montréal, QC H2H 2N8, Canada
* Correspondence: guylaine.ferland@umontreal.ca

Abstract: Whether through the vitamin K-dependent proteins or the individual K vitamers, vitamin K (VK) is associated with a number of age-related conditions (e.g., osteoporosis, atherosclerosis, insulin resistance, cognitive decline). In light of this, we investigated the influence of lifetime dietary VK exposure on the tissue distribution of phylloquinone (K_1) and menaquinone-4 (MK-4) vitamers in 3-, 12- and 22-month-old male and female rats fed different K_1 diets since weaning or subjected to a 40% calorie restricted diet (CR) since adulthood. Dietary K_1 intakes around the minimal amount required for normal blood coagulation had no significant influence on body weights of both male and female rats at different life stages. Tissue contents of the K vitamers differed according to organs, were generally higher in females than in males, and increased with K_1 intake. The MK-4/total VK ratios tended to be increased in old age possibly reflecting an increased physiological demand for MK-4 during aging. Our study also confirmed the greater susceptibility of male rats to low VK containing diet, notably at a younger age. Despite lifelong higher K_1 intakes per unit body weight, tissue K_1 and MK-4 contents at 20 months were generally lower in CR rats compared to their *ad libitum* (*AL)* counterparts. Whether the lower tissue MK-4 content is the result of lower synthesis from K_1 or greater tissue utilization remains to be determined. However, the more youthful coagulation profile observed in old CR rats (*vs. AL* rats) tends to support the notion that CR is associated with greater utilization of the K vitamers to sustain physiological functions.

Keywords: phylloquinone; menaquinone-4; tissue distribution; sex; age; diet; caloric restriction

---

1. Introduction

As a unique cofactor to the gamma-glutamyl carboxylase (GGCX), an enzyme that converts specific glutamic acid residues to gamma-carboxyglutamic acid in precursor proteins, vitamin K (VK) *i.e.*, all K vitamers, participates in the biological activation of several proteins. The vitamin K-dependent proteins (VKDPs) are notably involved in hemostasis, the calcification process (*i.e.*, bone matrix and vasculature), brain function, and glucose metabolism [1–4]. Compounds with VK activity all have a common 2-methyl-1,4-naphtoquinone ring but differ in structure at the 3-position. Phylloquinone (K_1), derived from plants, is the main dietary form, while the menaquinones, which are of bacterial origin, form a family of compounds with unsaturated isoprenyl side chains of various lengths [5].

One of the menaquinones, menaquinone-4 (MK-4), is not a common product of bacterial synthesis but is synthesized from phylloquinone with menadione as an intermediate [6–8]. In recent years, the human UbiA prenyltransferase containing 1 (UBIAD1) enzyme was shown to be responsible for the MK-4 biosynthesis [9,10].

In addition to its role as enzymatic cofactor in the carboxylation reaction, there is evidence to support other specific actions for VK notably, the K_1 and MK-4 vitamers. Specifically, both vitamers have been involved in the synthesis of sphingolipids, a group of complex lipids present in brain cell membranes and which possess important cell signaling properties [11]. Recent studies also point to protective roles for K_1 and MK-4 against oxidative stress and inflammatory processes. *In vitro*, both vitamers were shown to limit the production of interleukin-6 (IL-6) and other proinflammatory cytokines through the inhibtion of nuclear factor kappaB [12–14] whereas, *in vivo*, MK-4 limited inflammation in encephalomyelitis [15]. Both K_1 and MK-4 have also been shown to prevent glutathione depletion-mediated oxidative injury and cell death in primary culture of oligodendrocyte precursors and immature fetal cortical neurons [16,17]. Menaquinone-4 specifically has also been shown to possess potent anticancer properties, inducing apoptosis in several types of tumor cells [18] and inhibiting growth of hepatocarcinoma cells [19]. At the molecular level, MK-4 is a ligand for the steroid xenobiotic receptor [20,21] and promotes protein kinase A (PKA) activation [22–24], a signaling pathway that has also been associated with enhanced testosterone production in rats [25].

Tissue concentrations of the K vitamers have been investigated in various rat strains and shown to vary according to organs [6–8], dietary intake [7,26–28], and sex [29,30]. The role of age on diet-induced changes in tissue VK distribution was also investigated in animals of various ages (*i.e.*, 3, 12, 24 months) fed different VK diets for short periods of time (about one month) [28,29]. Collectively, these studies have provided essential information on the factors that influence the tissue contents of the K vitamers in rats, and the mechanisms underlying the biotransformation of K_1 to MK-4. However, to our knowledge, no studies have reported on lifetime VK dietary exposure on tissue distribution at distinct life stages.

Aging is a complex process that negatively impacts the development of the different systems and their ability to function. Age-related diseases include cancer, cardiovascular disease, diabetes, osteoporosis, and neurodegenerative diseases such as dementia and Alzheimer's disease [31]. Caloric restriction (CR) is a well-established experimental model, which has been shown to increase longevity and delay the onset of age-related diseases in various experimental models (*i.e.*, invertebrate model organisms, rodents, primates). In rodents, this dietary regimen has been shown to extend lifespan by up to 50% [32,33].

Whether through the VKDPs or the specific actions of K_1 and MK-4, VK is associated with numerous age-associated conditions including osteoporosis, diabetes, cardiovascular disease and cognitive decline [1,2]. In light of this, we endeavoured to investigate the influence of lifetime dietary VK exposure on the tissue distribution of the K_1 and MK-4 vitamers in two models of aging. In the first study (Study 1), we report the tissue VK distribution in 3-, 12- and 22-month-old male and female rats fed different K_1 diets since weaning. In the second study (Study 2), we report the VK tissue distribution in 20-month-old male and females rats, which were fed *ad libitum* (*AL*) throughout their lives or were subjected to a 40% calorie restricted diet (CR) since adulthood.

2. Methods and Materials

2.1. Animals and Diets

Protocols for both studies were approved by the Animal Care Committee of the Université de Montréal in compliance with the guidelines of the Canadian Council on Animal Care.

Study 1. A total of 120 rats were used for this study. 4-week-old male and female Sprague–Dawley rats were obtained from Charles Rivers Canada Inc. (St Constant, QC, Canada) and housed 3 per cage in suspended stainless steel wire-bottom cages (to prevent coprophagy) in a room kept at 22 °C with a 12 h light-dark cycle. Rats were kept in the same housing conditions and rat facility throughout the experimental period (22 months). For one week, animals had free access to a semi-synthetic powdered diet prepared according to the Teklad control diet (#TD 89248) which consisted of 22% casein (vitamin free), 48.5% sucrose, 15% corn starch, 5% corn oil, 4.6% fiber (cellulose), 3.9% mineral mix and 1% vitamin mix (Teklad Test Diets, Madison, WI, USA). After this acclimatization period, rats were randomly assigned to a diet containing either low (L; ~100 μg/kg diet), adequate (A; ~500 μg/kg diet) or high (H; ~1500 μg/kg diet) levels of K_1. These diets compared to the Teklad control diet (#TD 89248) except for vitamin K, where menadione was replaced by K_1 (Sigma Chemicals, St-Louis, MO, USA). The powder diets were prepared in our laboratory and K_1 concentrations evaluated by HPLC analysis were: Mean ± SEM, $n = 8$; 104 ± 9 μg/kg diet, 433 ± 13 μg/kg diet, and 1668 ± 9 μg/kg diet, respectively. These dietary concentrations of K_1 were chosen to provide rats with a range of intakes around the minimal amount required for normal coagulation activity namely 500 μg K_1/kg diet [34]. Rats had free access to water and food. Food intake and body weights were recorded every 2 weeks, and the health of the rats was monitored regularly by a veterinarian throughout the experimental period. Distinct groups of male and female rats from each dietary group were killed at 3, 12 and 22 months of age (n = 5–7/sex/age/diet), after having been food deprived overnight prior to the day of the experiment.

Study 2. A total of 48 rats were used for this study. 4-week-old male and female Sprague–Dawley rats were obtained from Charles Rivers Canada, Inc. (St Constant, QC, Canada). Animals were individually housed in wire-bottom cages under constant temperature of 22 °C and a 12 h light/12 h dark cycle. After one week of acclimatization, rats were given free access to the Teklad control diet (#TD 89248) (described above) where menadione was replaced by K_1 (Sigma Chemicals, St-Louis, MO, USA) at a concentration of ~500 μg/kg diet (Mean ± SEM, $n = 8$; 479 ± 13 μg K_1/kg diet by analysis). At 8 months of age, 16 male and 16 female rats were randomized in two dietary groups: one group was given free access to food (*ad libitum* (*AL*)) while the second group was subjected to a 20% reduction in daily caloric intake for two weeks, and 40% (CR) thereafter based on the mean intake of *AL* rats. A gradual approach to CR was adopted to minimize stress on the animals. Diet fed the CR rats was adjusted for vitamins (including K_1) and minerals, so that intakes of micronutrients were identical to those of *AL* animals: 22% casein (vitamin free), 48.5% sucrose, 15% corn starch, 5% corn oil, 4.6% fiber (cellulose), 5.85% mineral mix, 1.67% vitamin mix (Teklad Test Diets, Madison, WI, USA), and 835 μg K_1/kg diet. Eight males and eight females aged three months and fed *AL* since weaning, served as the "young" control group. All animals had free access to water. Food intake and body weights were assessed weekly and every two weeks respectively, and health of the rats was monitored regularly by a veterinarian throughout the study. Distinct groups of male and female rats were killed at 3 and 20 (*AL* and CR) months of age (n = 6–8/group, after having been food deprived overnight prior to the day of the experiment.

2.2. Sacrifice Procedure (Applies to Both Studies)

On the day of sacrifice, rats were anesthesized with sodium pentobarbital (45 mg/Kg body weight, ip), blood was withdrawn from the abdominal aorta and collected in a vacutainer containing 9:1, v/v trisodium citrate (Becton Dickinson Co, Rutherford, NJ, USA), and plasma was immediately separated by a 10-min centrifugation (500× g at 4 °C). The liver, heart, kidneys, spleen, brain, ovaries or testis were harvested, washed in 0.9% saline solution, weighed and stored at −80 °C until analysis.

2.3. Analytical Procedure (Applies to Both Studies)

Phylloquinone and MK-4 were quantified by HPLC as previously described [35]. Briefly, tissue samples were pulverized in anhydrous Na_2SO_4 (10 times tissue weight) and extracted for 1 h in 10 mL of acetone containing an internal standard (2 ng/50 μL 2-Methyl-3-(3,7,11,15,19-pentamethyl-2-eicosenyl)-1,4-naphthalenedione—also referred to as (K_1(25)) (GL Synthesis Inc., Worcester, MA, USA). Extracts were centrifuged (500× g at 4 °C for 10 min), dried under nitrogen at 45 °C and the solid residue was reextracted with 6 mL of hexane and 2 mL of water for 3 min. After centrifugation, the top hexane layer was dried under nitrogen and redissolved in 2 mL of hexane for solid phase extraction on 3 mL silica gel columns (JT Baker Inc., Phillipsburg, NJ, USA). The K_1 and MK-4 fraction was eluted with 8 mL of hexane:diethyl ether (97:3, v/v), evaporated under nitrogen and the residue dissolved in 0.02 mL of dimethyl chloride and 0.180 mL methanol containing aqueous phase (10 mmol/L zinc chloride, 10 mmol/L acetic acid and 5 mmol/L sodium acetate; 5 mL aqueous phase was added to 1 L methanol). Quantitative analysis of the vitamers was performed by reverse-phase HPLC using a C-18 reverse phase column and fluorescence detection. The calibration standard consisted of a mixture of K_1, MK-4 and K_1(25) at 2 ng/50 μL. The percent recovery for the samples was calculated from the internal standard and found to be 85%–90%. Tissue concentrations are expressed relative to wet weight. Plasma K_1 and MK-4 concentrations were quantified using the same HPLC technique as previously described [36,37].

Prothrombin times (PT) and activated partial thromboplastin times (APTT) were performed on an AC/100 Automated Clot Timer (Fisher Scientific Ltd, Montreal, QC, Canada) using thromboplastin and cephalin reagents (Sigma Chemical, St-Louis, MO, USA).

2.4. Statistical Analysis

All data are expressed as the mean ± SEM. Study 1. Body weight, food intake, K_1 intake, PT, APTT, plasma and tissue K_1 and MK-4 were analysed with respect to diet, sex and age, by three-way ANOVA (main effects) followed by pairwise multiple comparisons (Holm–Sidak method). Homogeneity of variance for ANOVA was assessed using the Shapiro–Wilk test and variables that were not normally distributed were log-transformed prior to the analysis. The effect of diet was further tested within each sex and age group by conducting distinct one-way ANOVA's followed by Tukey's *post hoc* tests. Tissue K_1 and MK-4 concentration differences were tested in 12-month-old male and female rats fed the adequate diet (as reference groups), using one-way ANOVA's followed by Tukey's *post hoc* tests. Study 2. Body weight, food intake, K_1 intake, PT, APTT, plasma and tissue K_1 and MK-4 were assessed in males and females with respect to age and diet, with distinct one-way ANOVA's followed by Tukey's post hoc tests. Homogeneity of variance for ANOVA was assessed using the Shapiro-Wilk test and variables that were not normally distributed were log-transformed prior to the analysis. Student' t-test was used to further assess the effect of CR at 20 months, and that of sex for given age and diet groups. Differences were considered significant at $p < 0.05$. Three-way analyses of variance were conducted using SigmaPlot version 12.0 (Systat Software, Inc., San Jose, CA, USA) whereas one-way analyses of variance and t-tests were conducted using GraphPad Prism6 version 6.01 (GraphPad Software, Inc., La Jolla, CA, USA).

3. Results

3.1. Study 1

3.1.1. Body Weights, Food, and K_1 Intakes

Mean body weights (BW) of male (M) and female (F) rats at 3, 12, and 22 months of age are presented in Figure 1 for the low (L), adequate (A) and high (H) dietary groups, respectively. Body weights increased with age in both males and females ($p < 0.001$). At all ages, body weights were higher in males than in females ($p < 0.001$) but were not affected by diet.

Daily food (g) and K_1 (μg) intakes expressed per 100 g· BW are presented in Table 1 for 3-, 12-, and 22-month-old male and female rats fed the L, A or H diets. Food intakes decreased with age in both males and females ($p < 0.001$) and were higher in females than in males at 3- and 12- but not at 22-months of age ($p < 0.001$). Food intakes did not vary among the dietary groups in males at any age in contrast to females where, at 3 months, food intakes were significantly higher in the H than in the L and A groups ($p < 0.05$). Phylloquinone intakes decreased with age irrespective of diet in both males and females ($p < 0.001$), and were higher in females than in males at 3 and 12 but not at 22 months of age ($p < 0.001$). As expected, K_1 intakes were significantly different between each dietary group, in both sexes ($p < 0.001$).

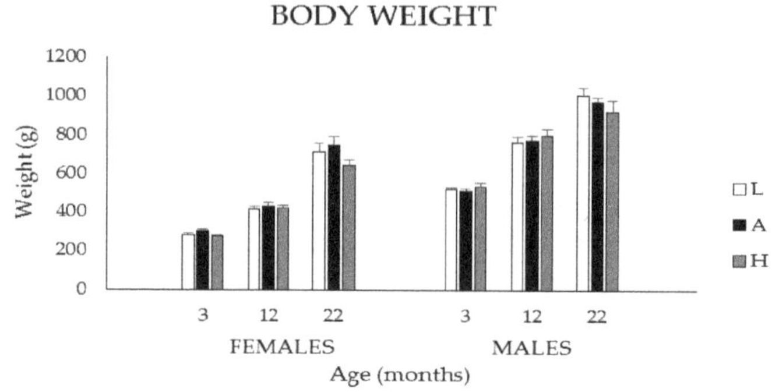

Figure 1. Mean body weights of 3-, 12-, and 22-month-old male (M) and female (F) Sprague–Dawley rats fed the L, A or H diets throughout their lives. Based on the 3-way ANOVA analysis, body weights increased with age in both M and F ($p < 0.001$). At all ages, body weights were higher in M than in F ($p < 0.001$) but were not affected by diet ($p = 0.258$), a finding confirmed by the individual one-way ANOVAs conducted at the group level. Values are expressed as mean ± SEM. (3 months F: n = 16/diet gp (group); M: n = 16/diet gp; 12 months F: n = 15–16/diet gp; M: n = 16/diet gp; 22 months F: n = 6–7/diet gp; M: n = 7–9/diet gp).

Table 1. Daily food (g/100 g body weight (BW)) and K_1 (μg/100 g· BW) intakes of 3-, 12-, and 22-month-old male (M) and female (F) Sprague–Dawley rats fed the low (L), adequate (A) or high (H) diets throughout their lives.

Age (Months)	Diet	Food Intake (g/100 BW/Day)		K_1 Intake (μg/100 g· BW/Day)	
		F	M	F	M
3	L	5.7 ± 0.2	4.5 ± 0.1	562.6 ± 15.9	444.6 ± 9.4
	A	5.6 ± 0.2	4.5 ± 0.1	2780.4 ± 83.0 ^{c}	2204.8 ± 56.2 ^{c}
	H	6.3 ± 0.1 ^{a,b}	4.7 ± 0.2	9433.2 ± 164.3 ^{a,b}	7022.3 ± 217.7 ^{a,b}
12	L	4.2 ± 0.2	3.0 ± 0.1	414.9 ± 15.3	297.2 ± 11.6
	A	4.2 ± 0.2	3.2 ± 0.1	2063.6 ± 101.2 ^{c}	1574.8 ± 51.4 ^{c}
	H	3.8 ± 0.2	3.0 ± 0.1	5987.3 ± 174.2 ^{a,b}	4386.0 ± 165.9 ^{a,b}
22	L	2.6 ± 0.2	2.7 ± 0.1	253.6 ± 14.4	268.9 ± 9.9
	A	2.5 ± 0.2	2.6 ± 0.1	1231.5 ± 85.6^{c}	1281.9 ± 43.5 ^{c}
	H	2.8 ± 0.2	2.7 ± 0.2	4141.4 ± 245.1 ^{a,b}	3954.1 ± 229.3 ^{a,b}

Based on the 3-way ANOVA analysis, food intakes decreased with age in both sexes ($p < 0.001$) and were higher in F than in M at 3 and 12 but not at 22 months of age ($p < 0.001$). Food intakes did not vary according to diet in M in contrast to F where, at 3 months, food intakes were significantly higher in the H than L and A groups ($p < 0.05$). Phylloquinone intakes decreased with age irrespective of diet in both sexes ($p < 0.001$) and were higher in F than in M at 3 and 12 but not at 22 months of age ($p < 0.001$). Phylloquinone intakes were significantly different between each dietary group, in both sexes ($p < 0.001$). The effect of diet was further tested within each sex and age group by one-way ANOVA's followed by Tukey's *post hoc* tests; ^{a}: $p < 0.05$ between H and L group same age and sex; ^{b}: $p < 0.05$ between H and A group same age and sex; ^{c}: $p < 0.05$ between A and L group same age and sex. Values are expressed as mean ± SEM; n for each group are as in Figure 1.

3.1.2. Plasma and Tissue K_1, MK-4, and Total VK (K_1 + MK-4) Concentrations, and MK-4/Total VK Ratios

Plasma and tissue (the liver, heart, kidneys, spleen, brain, ovaries and testes) K_1, MK-4 and total VK (K_1 + MK-4) concentrations are presented in Table 2. In plasma, there were no main sex or age effects but in most groups, K_1 concentrations increased with dietary K_1 (F:H *vs.* A and L in all age groups; M:H *vs.* A and L at 12 months, H *vs.* L at 3 and 22 months ($p < 0.05$). No MK-4 could be detected in plasma hence group differences for total VK values are as those for K_1.

Table 2. Plasma and tissue (liver, heart, kidneys, spleen, brain, ovaries and testes) K_1, MK-4 and total (K_1 + MK-4) vitamin K (VK) concentrations of 3-, 12-, and 22-month-old M and F Sprague–Dawley rats fed the L, A or H diets throughout their lives.

Organ (Months)	VK Diet (μg)	K1 F	K1 M	MK-4 F	MK-4 M	K1 + MK4 F	K1 + MK4 M
		pmol/g or L Plasma					
Plasma							
3	L	0.14 ± 0.11	0.04 ± 0.09	nd	nd	0.14 ± 0.11	0.04 ± 0.09
	A	0.21 ± 0.08	0.27 ± 0.17	nd	nd	0.21 ± 0.08	0.27 ± 0.17
	H	0.67 ± 0.35 ^{a,b}	0.41 ± 0.30 ^{a}	nd	nd	0.67 ± 0.35 ^{a,b}	0.41 ± 0.30 ^{a}
12	L	0.36 ± 0.29	0.21 ± 0.08	nd	nd	0.36 ± 0.29	0.21 ± 0.08
	A	0.44 ± 0.08	0.15 ± 0.08	nd	nd	0.44 ± 0.08	0.15 ± 0.08
	H	1.83 ± 0.53 ^{a,b}	0.76 ± 0.43 ^{a,b}	nd	nd	1.83 ± 0.53 ^{a,b}	0.76 ± 0.43 ^{a,b}
22	L	0.96 ± 0.35	0.84 ± 0.97	nd	nd	0.96 ± 0.35	0.84 ± 0.97
	A	1.83 ± 0.58	1.19 ± 0.42	nd	nd	1.83 ± 0.58	1.19 ± 0.42
	H	4.60 ± 1.63 ^{a,b}	2.29 ± 1.08 ^{a}	nd	nd	4.60 ± 1.63 ^{a,b}	2.29 ± 1.08 ^{a}
Liver							
3	L	46.4 ± 4.9	43.0 ± 13.9	26.7 ± 2.6	16.4 ± 3.5	73.1 ± 6.3	59.5 ± 16.4
	A	49.8 ± 7.7	68.6 ± 25.7	37.4 ± 7.2	10.2 ± 3.2	87.2 ± 12.5	78.8 ± 27.3
	H	199.6 ± 30.0 ^{a,b}	73.3 ± 19.5	135.5 ± 14.6 ^{a,b}	14.5 ± 2.9	335.1 ± 32.7 ^{a,b}	87.8 ± 17.7
12	L	71.5 ± 14.3	33.7 ± 7.8	35.8 ± 7.4	23.6 ± 7.7	107.3 ± 20.7	57.4 ± 11.3
	A	171.9 ± 43.8 ^{c}	44.3 ± 6.8	68.4 ± 10.9	31.9 ± 7.6	240.3 ± 41.5 ^{c}	76.2 ± 12.7
	H	410.3 ± 13.9 ^{a,b}	122.5 ± 37.6 ^{a}	142.7 ± 10.9 ^{a}	38.9 ± 11.8	553.0 ± 22.4 ^{a}	161.5 ± 43.4 ^{a}
22	L	34.7 ± 2.9	25.6 ± 5.4	65.0 ± 9.3	57.5 ± 8.8	99.7 ± 8.1	83.1 ± 13.7
	A	69.2 ± 12.6 ^{c}	52.6 ± 8.5	81.0 ± 17.9	58.8 ± 7.8	150.2 ± 21.7	111.4 ± 8.3
	H	191.1 ± 14.3 ^{a,b}	79.1 ± 19.1 ^{a}	104.4 ± 18.0	61.7 ± 16.0	295.4 ± 29.9 ^{a}	140.8 ± 25.8
Heart							
3	L	13.2 ± 1.7	9.5 ± 0.3	19.5 ± 2.2	9.7 ± 1.6	32.7 ± 3.2	19.2 ± 1.7
	A	32.1 ± 2.1 ^{c}	31.2 ± 1.9 ^{c}	25.0 ± 2.4	26.6 ± 5.2 ^{c}	57.1 ± 2.9 ^{c}	57.7 ± 5.6 ^{c}
	H	300.4 ± 74.4 ^{a,b}	188.1 ± 42.1 ^{a,b}	265.9 ± 60.2 ^{a,b}	59.9 ± 11.5 ^{a,b}	566.2 ± 134.4 ^{a,b}	248.0 ± 52.6 ^{a,b}
12	L	16.3 ± 0.7	15.6 ± 5.3	17.7 ± 2.7	34.7 ± 20.9	34.0 ± 3.4	50.2 ± 26.0
	A	41.5 ± 6.4 ^{c}	32.1 ± 4.0 ^{c}	27.7 ± 4.3	15.7 ± 3.6	69.2 ± 10.4 ^{c}	47.7 ± 7.4
	H	225.6 ± 32.0 ^{a,b}	213.9 ± 42.6 ^{a,b}	165.9 ± 24.6 ^{a,b}	79.6 ± 11.4 ^{a,b}	391.5 ± 51.9 ^{a,b}	293.4 ± 52.9 ^{a,b}
22	L	30.8 ± 4.7	30.1 ± 2.8	56.9 ± 3.5	43.5 ± 3.8	87.6 ± 5.1	73.6 ± 3.1
	A	54.9 ± 7.3 ^{c}	47.1 ± 7.7	62.5 ± 7.7	42.0 ± 8.1	117.4 ± 12.1	89.1 ± 15.4
	H	106.3 ± 14.4 ^{a,b}	100.9 ± 39.0 ^{a}	104.0 ± 24.1	89.7 ± 25.8	210.2 ± 37.1 ^{a,b}	190.6 ± 56.1

Table 2. *Cont.*

Organ (Months)	VK Diet (µg)	K1 F	K1 M	MK-4 F	MK-4 M	K1 + MK4 F	K1 + MK4 M
		pmol/g or L Plasma					
Kidneys							
3	L	2.8 ± 0.5	4.7 ± 0.6	17.6 ± 3.2	11.9 ± 3.5	20.4 ± 3.6	16.6 ± 3.2
	A	9.3 ± 4.3	6.5 ± 1.4	29.9 ± 2.9	14.7 ± 3.7	39.2 ± 4.9	21.1 ± 3.1
	H	18.7 ± 4.7	10.2 ± 2.2	176.7 ± 24.6 [a]	34.9 ± 9.2	195.4 ± 28.1 [a,b]	45.1 ± 10.9 [a]
12	L	4.3 ± 1.1	3.7 ± 0.8	28.5 ± 8.8	12.1 ± 3.8	32.8 ± 9.5	15.8 ± 4.4
	A	6.0 ± 1.2	6.6 ± 1.1	32.6 ± 8.4	22.1 ± 5.8	38.6 ± 9.6	28.8 ± 6.8
	H	32.0 ± 4.6 [a,b]	6.4 ± 1.8	154.1 ± 34.8 [a,b]	32.2 ± 8.5 [a]	186.1 ± 30.3 [a,b]	38.6 ± 8.9 [a]
22	L	7.7 ± 0.9	3.6 ± 0.5	30.8 ± 4.5	26.3 ± 3.0	38.5 ± 4.7	30.0 ± 3.1
	A	11.6 ± 1.1	7.8 ± 0.6 [c]	52.4 ± 7.1	38.9 ± 3.7	63.9 ± 7.6 [c]	46.7 ± 4.2
	H	30.6 ± 9.8 [a,b]	20.3 ± 5.5 [a,b]	42.3 ± 8.6	19.4 ± 8.4	72.9 ± 13.3 [a]	39.7 ± 12.8
Spleen							
3	L	16.7 ± 1.5	16.6 ± 2.3	17.2 ± 3.2	8.6 ± 1.9	33.9 ± 4.0	25.1 ± 3.3
	A	24.9 ± 4.4	28.0 ± 3.4 [c]	23.6 ± 6.8	17.1 ± 3.9	48.5 ± 9.6	45.1 ± 4.7
	H	80.1 ± 17.8 [a,b]	49.4 ± 6.0 [a,b]	73.1 ± 15.3 [a,b]	37.6 ± 4.2 [a,b]	153.2 ± 28.7 [a,b]	86.9 ± 5.1 [a]
12	L	15.5 ± 1.8	15.5 ± 6.8	17.5 ± 3.5	11.4 ± 4.4	33.0 ± 5.2	26.8 ± 10.6
	A	30.4 ± 4.5 [c]	31.8 ± 10.4	50.9 ± 11.9	47.2 ± 17.1	81.3 ± 15.2	79.0 ± 26.6
	H	110.9 ± 17.7 [a,b]	38.2 ± 7.0	66.8 ± 8.7	35.7 ± 12.5	177.6 ± 22.8 [a]	73.8 ± 18.2 [a]
22	L	18.8 ± 3.9	22.7 ± 6.0	43.1 ± 10.6	56.3 ± 14.4	61.8 ± 10.8	79.0 ± 19.4
	A	28.4 ± 4.7	26.1 ± 3.8	67.1 ± 8.9	48.3 ± 7.8	95.5 ± 13.2	74.3 ± 11.1
	H	91.9 ± 14.9 [a,b]	126.7 ± 17.2 [a,b]	101.5 ± 21.1 [a]	120.6 ± 22.1	193.4 ± 31.1 [a,b]	247.2 ± 35.9 [a,b]
Brain							
3	L	2.0 ± 0.7	2.3 ± 0.4	54.2 ± 7.1	21.1 ± 1.6	56.2 ± 7.3	23.4 ± 1.3
	A	4.3 ± 0.8	3.7 ± 0.6	64.5 ± 4.8	47.2 ± 5.6 [c]	68.8 ± 5.1	51.0 ± 5.7 [c]
	H	8.0 ± 0.7 [a,b]	8.4 ± 0.9 [a,b]	197.5 ± 7.6 [a,b]	144.3 ± 12.0 [a,b]	205.4 ± 8.0 [a,b]	152.6 ± 12.7 [a,b]
12	L	1.6 ± 0.3	2.6 ± 1.2	47.1 ± 4.1	46.9 ± 18.9	48.7 ± 4.0	49.5 ± 20.1
	A	4.2 ± 0.4 [c]	3.3 ± 0.5	71.9 ± 7.1 [c]	40.6 ± 3.9	76.1 ± 7.3 [c]	43.9 ± 4.4
	H	7.4 ± 1.2 [a,b]	9.1 ± 2.3 [a]	187.2 ± 20.8 [a,b]	157.6 ± 10.5 [a,b]	194.6 ± 20.7 [a,b]	166.7 ± 12.4 [a,b]
22	L	2.2 ± 0.3	3.9 ± 0.2	53.5 ± 5.9	56.8 ± 11.9	55.7 ± 6.0	60.6 ± 11.8
	A	3.2 ± 0.2	3.4 ± 0.4	66.7 ± 7.9	85.5 ± 4.1	70.0 ± 8.0	88.9 ± 4.2
	H	4.4 ± 0.8 [a]	5.4 ± 1.7	70.0 ± 8.5	63.3 ± 20.5	74.4 ± 9.0	68.7 ± 21.9

Table 2. *Cont.*

Organ (Months)	VK Diet (μg)	K1 F	K1 M	MK-4 F	MK-4 M	K1 + MK4 F	K1 + MK4 M
		pmol/g or L Plasma					
Ovaries							
3	L	89.1 ± 35.9		190.6 ± 39.1		279.7 ± 34.4	
	A	133.3 ± 19.2		296.1 ± 100.0		429.5 ± 98.5	
	H	267.6 ± 42.4 [a]		616.4 ± 48.2 [a]		884.0 ± 89.7 [a,b]	
12	L	60.0 ± 22.1		187.1 ± 39.9		247.1 ± 54.7	
	A	218.2 ± 9.2 [c]		517.2 ± 93.4 [c]		735.4 ± 99.8 [c]	
	H	424.4 ± 46.6 [a]		762.1 ± 67.3 [a]		1186.5 ± 111.2 [a]	
22	L	183.9 ± 32.3		516.2 ± 72.2		700.1 ± 99.4	
	A	307.8 ± 50.2		706.6 ± 90.7		1014.4 ± 138.4	
	H	416.6 ± 46.7		656.7 ± 49.6		1073.3 ± 51.8	
Testes							
3	L		13.4 ± 4.5		63.8 ± 7.2		77.3 ± 6.6
	A		7.2 ± 1.4		134.5 ± 15.8 [c]		141.6 ± 16.3 [c]
	H		11.8 ± 3.6		292.4 ± 30.0 [a,b]		304.1 ± 28.6 [a,b]
12	L		9.9 ± 4.8		83.4 ± 28.3		93.3 ± 29.4
	A		20.9 ± 12.8		258.7 ± 43.6 [c]		279.7 ± 51.4 [c]
	H		22.0 ± 11.8		299.1 ± 52.3 [a]		321.1 ± 45.0 [a]
22	L		4.5 ± 0.6		64.3 ± 8.1		68.8 ± 8.2
	A		6.8 ± 0.6		96.3 ± 8.3 [c]		103.1 ± 8.7 [c]
	H		13.3 ± 1.9 [a,b]		81.4 ± 9.5		94.7 ± 9.7

Main sex, diet and age effects were assessed by conducting 3-way ANOVAs followed by pairwise multiple comparisons; results for these analyses are presented in the text (Section 3.1.2). The effect of diet on plasma and tissue K_1, MK-4 and total VK concentrations were further tested within each sex and age group by one-way ANOVA's followed by Tukey's *post hoc* tests; [a]: $p < 0.05$ between H and L groups same age and sex, [b]: $p < 0.05$ between H and A groups same age and sex, [c]: $p < 0.05$ between A and L groups same age and sex. Values are expressed as mean ± SEM; n = 5–7/sex/age/diet groups. MK-4: menaquinone-4. nd: non-detectable.

Tissue K_1 concentrations were highest in ovaries and liver and lowest in the brain and kidneys, other tissues presenting intermediate levels ($p < 0.001$). A main sex effect was seen for the liver, kidneys, and heart, females showing higher K_1 concentrations than males ($p < 0.001$). The 3-way ANOVA also revealed a main diet effect for most organs ($p < 0.001$), differences being more frequently observed between the L and H, and the A and H groups ($p < 0.05$); dietary group differences (one-way ANOVA) are detailed in Table 2. A significant main effect was observed for age in the liver, heart, kidneys, and ovaries but differences varied according to organs and dietary groups ($p < 0.001$). Specifically, in the liver, K_1 concentrations increased between 3 and 12 months and were decreased at 22 months ($p < 0.05$). In the heart and kidneys, K_1 concentrations at 3 and 12 months were generally similar and were increased at 22 months, the extent of the change varying according to sex and dietary groups ($p < 0.05$). Finally, in ovaries, concentrations were observed to increase throughout life in all dietary groups ($p < 0.05$).

Tissue MK-4 concentrations were highest in ovaries and testes followed by the brain, the lowest amounts being seen in the heart and kidneys ($p < 0.001$). A main sex effect was observed for the liver, heart, kidneys, and the brain with females showing higher concentrations than males ($p < 0.001$). In most cases, the sex effect was observed at all ages and tended to be more pronounced in the H group ($p < 0.05$).

As for K_1, MK-4 tissue concentrations varied as a function of diet, differences being mainly observed between the L and H, and the A and H groups ($p < 0.05$); dietary group differences (one-way ANOVA) are detailed in Table 2. The 3-way ANOVA also revealed a main age effect in all organs, differences varying according to organs, sex (when applicable), and dietary groups ($p < 0.001$). In liver and ovary, concentrations increased throughout life in all dietary groups ($p < 0.05$) whereas in the heart, kidneys, spleen, and the brain, the extent of age-associated increases varied according to sex and dietary groups. In testes, concentrations were comparable at 3 and 12 months (for a given dietary group), and were significantly decreased at 22 months, mainly due to the lower concentrations of rats fed the A and H diets ($p < 0.05$).

Tissue total VK (K_1 + MK-4) concentrations were highest in ovaries followed by testes and liver, concentrations in other organs being statistically similar ($p < 0.001$). Except for the spleen, a main sex effect was observed in all organs, females showing higher total VK concentrations than males ($p < 0.001$). In the liver, the sex effect was observed at all ages and in most dietary groups while in the heart, kidneys and the brain, sex effect was more pronounced at 3 and 12 months in the H diet ($p < 0.05$). A main diet effect was also seen in most organs ($p < 0.001$), differences being mainly observed between the L and H, and the A and H groups ($p < 0.05$); dietary group differences (one-way ANOVA) are detailed in Table 2. The 3-way ANOVA also revealed a significant main effect for age in all organs, differences varying according to organs, sex (when applicable), and dietary groups ($p < 0.001$).

Specifically, in the liver, total VK concentrations increased between 3 and 12 months and decreased in the second year of life, the age effect being more pronounced in females fed the A and H diets ($p < 0.05$). In spleen, total VK concentrations were increased at 22 months compared to 3 and 12 months, the effect being particularly marked in males fed the H diet ($p < 0.05$). In brain, in both sexes, concentrations were comparable at 3 and 12 months (for a given dietary group) and were decreased at 22 months, largely due to the lower concentrations of rats fed the H diet ($p < 0.05$). In ovaries, total VK contents increased throughout life, the extent and time of change depending on the dietary groups ($p < 0.05$). Finally, in testes, total VK concentrations were comparable at 3 and 12 months (for a given dietary group), and were significantly decreased at 22 months, mainly due to the lower concentrations of rats fed the A and H diets ($p < 0.05$).

In light of the growing importance of MK-4 in various physiological functions, tissue MK-4 relative to total VK was computed for each organ in all animals as the ratio MK-4/total VK (Figure 2) (In plasma, MK-4 could not be detected hence no ratios were computed for this variable). In contrast to what is observed for K_1, MK-4, and total VK, the MK-4/total VK ratios were much less affected by sex, diet, and age. Furthermore, MK-4 represents the main K vitamer in a number of organs. This is notably the case for the brain where the MK-4/total VK ratios are close to one irrespective of sex, diet and age. Menaquinone-4 is also the preferred K vitamer in testes and kidneys while ovaries, spleen, heart, and liver present more of a mixture of the two vitamers ($p < 0.001$). The 3-way ANOVA revealed a main sex effect in the heart, kidneys, and brain ($p < 0.001$), females showing higher ratios than males, ($p < 0.05$). The main diet effects were seen in all organs except for spleen ($p < 0.001$), ratios tending to be higher in the L diet groups ($p < 0.05$); dietary group differences (one-way ANOVA) are detailed in Figure 2. Finally, the 3-way ANOVA also revealed an age effect in liver, heart and spleen ($p < 0.001$). Specifically, in liver and spleen, ratios were increased at 22 months (*vs.* 3 and 12 months) notably in rats fed the L and A diets ($p < 0.05$). In the heart, ratios were increased at 22 months (*vs.* 3 and 12 months) especially in rats fed the A and H diets ($p < 0.05$).

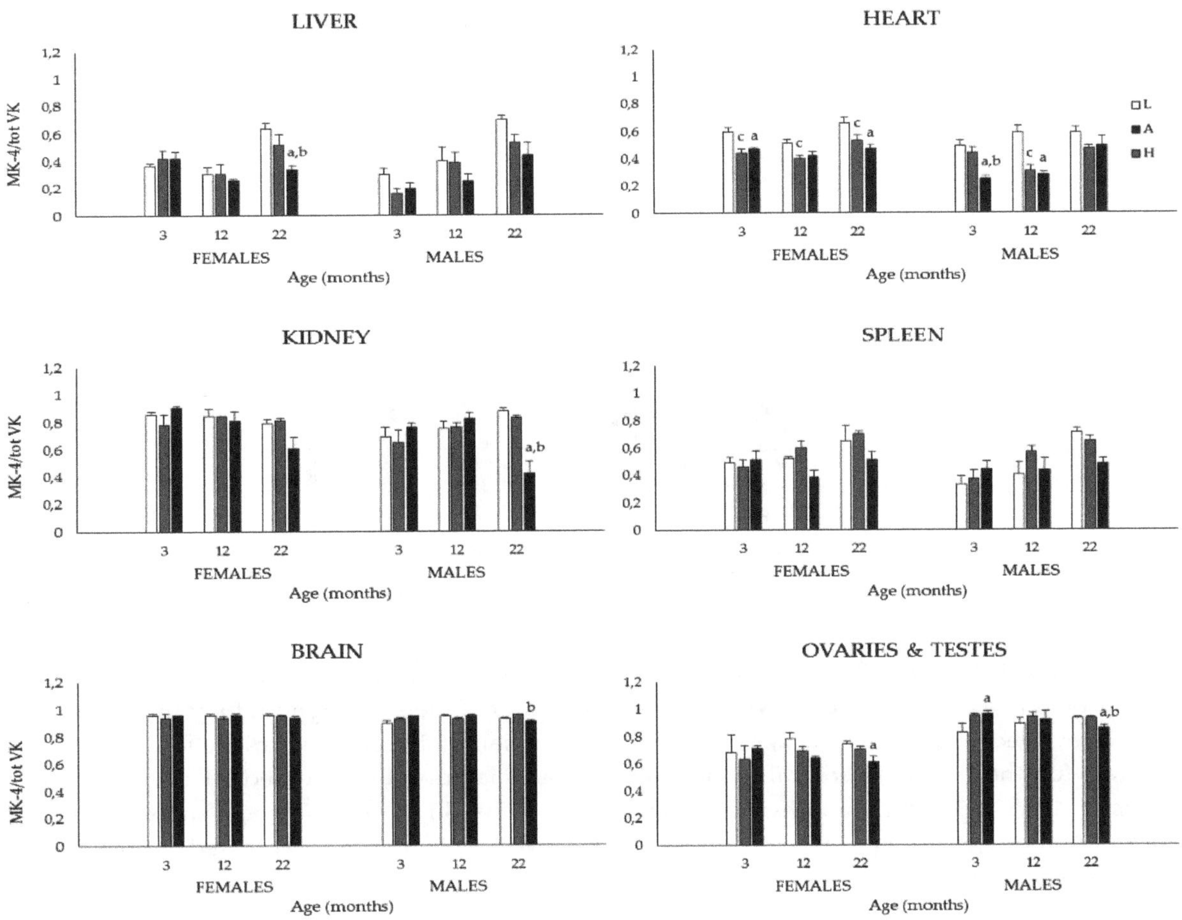

Figure 2. Tissue MK-4/total VK ratios of 3-, 12-, and 22-month-old M and F Sprague–Dawley rats fed the L, A or H diets throughout their lives. No ratios were computed for plasma as MK-4 could not be detected. Main sex, diet and age effects were assessed by conducting 3-way ANOVAs followed by pairwise multiple comparisons; results for these analyses are presented in the text (Section 3.1.2). The effect of diet on tissue MK-4/total VK ratios were further tested within each sex and age group by one-way ANOVA's followed by Tukey's *post hoc* tests; [a]: $p < 0.05$ between H and L group same age and sex; [b]: $p < 0.05$ between H and A group same age and sex; [c]: $p < 0.05$ between A and L group same age and sex. Values are expressed as mean ± SEM; n = 5–7/sex/age/diet groups.

3.1.3. Prothrombin and Activated Partial Thromboplastin Times

Results for prothrombin (PT) and activated partial thromboplastin (APTT) times are presented in Figure 3. The 3-way ANOVA revealed no main sex and age effects for either variable. However, dietary K_1 intakes significantly affected the coagulation times of male rats fed the L diet. Specifically, the low

K_1 containing diet was associated with increased PT in 3-month-old (*vs.* H diet), and increased APTT in 3- (*vs.* A and H diets) and 12-month-old (*vs.* H diet) male rats ($p < 0.05$).

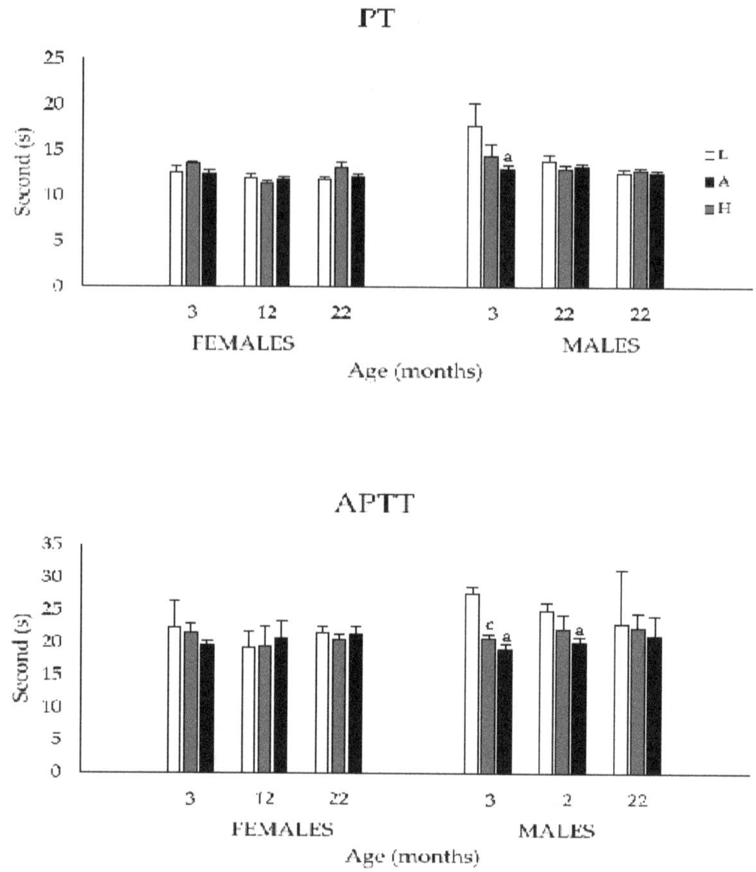

Figure 3. Prothrombin (PT) and activated partial thromboplastin (APTT) times of 3-, 12-, and 22-month-old M and F Sprague–Dawley rats fed the L, A or H diets throughout their lives. The 3-way ANOVA revealed no main sex and age effects for either variables. In contrast, a diet effect was observed in M rats fed the L diet. Specifically, this diet was associated with increased PT at 3 months and increased APTT at 3 and 12 months; [a]: $p < 0.05$ between H and L group same age and sex; [c]: $p < 0.05$ between A and L group same age and sex (one-way ANOVA). Values are expressed as mean ± SEM; n = 4–7/sex/age/diet groups.

3.2. *Study 2*

3.2.1. Body Weights, Food, and K_1 Intakes

Body weights, daily food (g/day and g/100 g· BW/day), and K_1 (µg/day and µg/100 g· BW) intakes of 3- and 20-month-old male and female Sprague–Dawley rats fed an *ad libitum* (*AL*) or calorie restricted (CR) diet are presented in Table 3. In all age and diet groups, body weights were significantly higher in male than female rats ($p < 0.05$). In animals of both sexes fed the *AL* diet, body weights were significantly increased at 20 months compared to 3 months and as expected, were signifiantly lower in the 20 CR than 20 *AL* group ($p < 0.05$).

Table 3. Body weights, daily food (g/day and g/100 g· BW/day), and K_1(μg/day and μg/100 g· BW) intakes of 3- and 20-month-old M and F Sprague–Dawley rats fed an *ad libitum* (*AL*) or calorie restricted (CR) diet.

Age (Months)	Diet	Body Weight (g)		Food Intake (g/Day)		K_1 Intake (μg/Day)		Food Intake (g/100 g· BW/Day)		K_1 Intake (μg/100 g· BW/Day)	
		F	M	F	M	F	M	F	M	F	M
3	*AL*	277 ± 35^{z}	523 ± 73	16.5 ± 1.7^{z}	22.5 ± 1.3	8.3 ± 0.8^{z}	11.2 ± 0.6	6.0 ± 0.5^{z}	4.3 ± 0.4	3.0 ± 0.2^{z}	2.2 ± 0.2
20	*AL*	$647 \pm 171^{y,z}$	939 ± 132^{y}	18.0 ± 3.5^{z}	27.1 ± 3.8^{y}	9.0 ± 1.8	13.6 ± 9.3	2.9 ± 0.5^{y}	2.9 ± 0.4^{y}	1.4 ± 0.2^{y}	1.4 ± 0.2^{y}
	CR	$281 \pm 29^{z,*}$	$484 \pm 37^{*}$	$11.0^{x,z,*}$	$16.0^{x,*}$	9.2^{z}	13.3	$4.6^{x,z,*}$	3.9^{*}	$3.8^{x,z,*}$	$3.3^{x,*}$

In all age and diet groups, body weights were higher in M than F ($p < 0.05$). In both sexes fed the *AL* diet, body weights were significantly increased at 20 months (*vs.* 3 months) and significantly decreased in 20 CR rats (*vs.* 20 *AL*) ($p < 0.05$). Food intakes expressed as g/day were significantly higher in M than F in all age and diet groups, and were higher in 20 *AL* *vs.* 3 groups ($p < 0.05$). As expected, food intakes were lower in the 20 CR than in 20 *AL* groups (both sexes; $p < 0.05$). Phylloquinone intakes μg/day were significantly higher in M than F (3 and 20 CR) but were similar among age and diet groups ($p < 0.05$). When expressed per 100 g· BW, food and K_1 intakes (μg/100 g· BW/day) were higher in F than M (3 and 20 CR groups), were lower in older animals fed the *AL* diet (*vs.* 3 months), and were higher in the 20 CR *vs.* 20 *AL* groups ($p < 0.05$); ^{x}: $p < 0.05$ between 20 CR and 3-month group, same sex; ^{y}: $p < 0.05$ between 20 *AL* and 3-month group, same sex; ^{z}: $p < 0.05$ between M and F, same age and diet; *: $p < 0.05$ between 20 *AL* and 20 CR, same sex. Values are expressed as mean ± SEM; n = 6–8/sex/age/diet groups.

Food intakes expressed as g/day were significantly higher in males than in females in all age and diet groups, and were higher in 20 *AL vs.* 3-month-old groups ($p < 0.05$). In both sexes and, as expected, food intakes of 20 CR rats were lower than those of the 20 *AL* group and also of the 3-month-old groups ($p < 0.05$). Phylloquinone (K_1) intakes expressed as µg/day were significantly higher in males than in females (3 and 20 CR groups; ($p < 0.05$) but did not differ among age and diet groups.

Given the impact of the CR model on body weights, food (g) and K_1 (µg) intakes are also reported per 100 g· BW. When expressed in this manner, food intakes were significantly higher in females than in males in the 3-month and 20 CR groups ($p < 0.05$), and were significantly lower in older animals (F: 20 *AL vs.* 3 months, 20 CR *vs.* 3 months; M: 20 *AL vs.* 3 months, $p < 0.05$). In addition, and in both sexeses, were lower in the 20 *AL vs.* 3-month-old group ($p < 0.05$).

Finally, when expressed as µg/100 g· BW/day, K_1 intakes were significantly higher in females than in males in the 3-month and 20 CR groups ($p < 0.05$), and in both sexes, were lower in the 20 *AL vs.* 3-month-old group ($p < 0.05$). As mentioned previously, the diet fed the CR rats was adjusted to contain similar amounts of vitamins (including K_1) and minerals as that fed the *AL* group. However, due to their lower body weights at 20 months, in both sexeses, K_1 intakes (µg/100 g· BW/day) of CR rats were significantly higher than those fed the *AL* diet ($p < 0.05$).

3.2.2. Plasma and Tissue K_1, MK-4, and Total VK (K_1 + MK-4) Concentrations, and MK-4/Total VK Ratios

Plasma and tissue (the liver, heart, kidneys, spleen, brain, ovaries and testes) K_1, MK-4 and total VK (K_1 + MK-4) concentrations of 3- and 20-month-old male and female Sprague–Dawley rats fed an *AL* or CR diet are presented in Table 4. In both sexes, plasma K_1 concentrations were significantly increased at 20 (*AL* and CR) compared to 3 months, and were significantly higher in females than males ($p < 0.05$). A diet effect was also observed in both sexeses at 20 months, rats fed the CR diet showing decreased K_1 concentrations compared to those of the respective *AL* groups ($p < 0.05$). Menaquinone-4 was undetectable in plasma, hence group differences for total VK values are as those for K_1.

Table 4. Plasma and tissue (the liver, heart, kidneys, spleen, brain, ovaries and testes) K_1, MK-4 and total VK (K_1 + MK-4) concentrations of 3- and 20-month-old M and F Sprague–Dawley rats fed an *AL* or CR diet.

Diet		K1		MK-4		K1 + MK4	
		F	M	F	M	F	M
		pmol/g or L Plasma		pmol/g or L Plasma		pmol/g or L Plasma	
				Plasma			
3	*AL*	0.21 ± 0.03	0.25 ± 0.08	nd	nd	0.21 ± 0.03	0.25 ± 0.08
20	*AL*	1.73 ± 0.15 ^{y,z}	1.12 ± 0.11 ^{y}	nd	nd	1.73 ± 0.15 ^{y,z}	1.12 ± 0.11 ^{y}
	CR	1.35 ± 0.10 ^{x,z,*}	0.85 ± 0.07 ^{x,*}	nd	nd	1.35 ± 0.10 ^{x,*}	0.85 ± 0.07 ^{x,*}
				Liver			
3	*AL*	54.2 ± 8.1	48.4 ± 17.9	43.4 ± 3.6 ^{z}	18.5 ± 2.1	97.6 ± 7.7	56.9 ± 20.0
20	*AL*	71.2 ± 7.9	50.7 ± 6.1	66.6 ± 12.0	54.5 ± 6.1 ^{y}	137.8 ± 17.9	105.2 ± 7.2 ^{y}
	CR	49.0 ± 5.7 *	50.6 ± 6.6	61.6 ± 8.2	48.6 ± 5.6 ^{x}	110.6 ± 10.5	99.2 ± 7.3 ^{x}
				Heart			
3	*AL*	32.1 ± 2.1	31.2 ± 1.9	24.7 ± 2.4	26.2 ± 5.1	56.7 ± 2.9	57.4 ± 5.5
20	*AL*	47.2 ± 6.4	46.9 ± 5.1	55.5 ± 5.6 ^{y}	43.3 ± 5.6	102.8 ± 10.2 ^{y}	90.2 ± 9.6 ^{y}
	CR	32.7 ± 6.8	41.5 ± 5.8	53.6 ± 4.8 ^{x,z}	38.7 ± 4.6	86.3 ± 9.0	80.2 ± 7.4
				Kidney			
3	*AL*	9.3 ± 4.3	5.6 ± 1.4	29.5 ± 2.8 ^{z}	12.0 ± 3.3	38.7 ± 4.9 ^{z}	17.6 ± 3.5
20	*AL*	11.8 ± 1.1 ^{z}	7.6 ± 0.4	54.5 ± 4.7 ^{y,z}	35.0 ± 3.9 ^{y}	66.3 ± 5.1 ^{y,z}	42.6 ± 4.3 ^{y}
	CR	10.1 ± 1.0 ^{z}	6.2 ± 0.4 *	45.3 ± 4.7 ^{z}	33.2 ± 1.6 ^{x}	55.4 ± 5.0 ^{z}	39.4 ± 1.5 ^{x}

Table 4. *Cont.*

Diet		K1		MK-4		K1 + MK4	
		F	M	F	M	F	M
		pmol/g or L Plasma		pmol/g or L Plasma		pmol/g or L Plasma	
Spleen							
3	*AL*	23.6 ± 5.1	25.1 ± 2.3	17.0 ± 3.0	19.7 ± 3.7	40.6 ± 7.0	44.8 ± 5.3
20	*AL*	26.9 ± 3.2	23.5 ± 2.2	64.0 ± 7.2 ^{y,z}	41.1 ± 4.4 ^{y}	90.9 ± 8.9 ^{y,z}	64.6 ± 6.3
	CR	24.2 ± 3.0	23.0 ± 3.0	53.7 ± 6.0 ^{x}	42.8 ± 5.7 ^{x}	77.9 ± 7.8 ^{x}	65.7 ± 7.2
Brain							
3	*AL*	4.3 ± 0.8	3.7 ± 0.6	63.6 ± 4.7 ^{z}	46.6 ± 5.5	67.9 ± 5.0 ^{z}	50.3 ± 5.6
20	*AL*	3.5 ± 0.4	3.6 ± 0.4	69.9 ± 5.6	66.3 ± 7.3	73.4 ± 5.8	70.0 ± 7.3
	CR	4.6 ± 0.4	3.9 ± 0.4	52.9 ± 5.8 *	54.8 ± 7.2	57.4 ± 5.9	58.7 ± 7.4
Ovaries							
3	*AL*	133.7 ± 19.6		426.5 ± 114.9		560.2 ± 133.1	
20	*AL*	278.5 ± 27.4 ^{y}		636.3 ± 58.5		914.8 ± 76.7 ^{y}	
	CR	240.5 ± 28.0 ^{x}		453.4 ± 42.1 *		693.9 ± 65.0 *	
Testes							
3	*AL*		6.1 ± 1.0		131.8 ± 19.0		137.9 ± 19.6
20	*AL*		6.1 ± 0.6		110.4 ± 7.8		116.5 ± 7.8
	CR		4.6 ± 0.3		123.6 ± 8.9		128.2 ± 8.7

Age and diet effects were determined in M and F by conducting distinct one-way ANOVA's followed by Tukey's *post hoc* tests. Student' *t*-test was used to further assess the effect of CR at 20 months, and that of sex *i.e.*, given age and diet group. ^{x}: $p < 0.05$ between 20 CR and 3-months, same sex; ^{y}: $p < 0.05$ between 20 *AL* and 3 months, same sex; ^{z}: $p < 0.05$ between M and F, same age and diet; *: $p < 0.05$ between 20 *AL* and 20 CR, same sex. Values are expressed as mean ± SEM; n = 6–8/sex/age/diet groups.

Tissue K_1, MK-4, and total VK content profiles were similar to those reported in Study 1. Ovaries contained the highest amounts of total VK with high levels of both K vitamers ($p < 0.001$). Similarly, organs differed in their relative K_1 and MK-4 contents (Table 4) with much higher MK-4/total VK ratios in organs such as the brain, testes, and kidneys (*i.e.*, 0.8–0.95) than in the liver and heart (*i.e.*, ~0.5).

Regarging K_1, there was a general trend for concentrations to be higher in females than in males, this difference reaching statistical significance in kidneys ($p < 0.05$). In both sexes and for most organs, K_1 concentrations were similar at 3 and 20 months except for ovaries where concentrations were significantly increased at 20 compared to 3 months ($p < 0.05$). Finally, and although differences reached statistical significance only in the liver (F) and kidneys (M) ($p < 0.05$), K_1 concentrations at 20 months tended to be lower in the CR than in the *AL* groups (Table 4).

In contrast to K_1, MK-4 concentrations were much more affected by sex with females showing higher concentrations than males in the liver (3 months), heart (20 CR), kidneys (all groups), spleen (20 *AL*), and the brain (3 months) ($p < 0.05$). In a number of organs, MK-4 concentrations also increased as a function of age, the effect being particularly marked in the liver (M: 20 *AL*, 20 CR), heart (F: 20 *AL*, 20 CR), kidneys (M: 20 *AL*, 20 CR; F: 20 *AL*), and spleen (M and F: 20 *AL*, 20 CR), ($p < 0.05$). Finally, as observed for K_1, MK-4 concentrations tended to be lower in rats fed the CR regimen, differences reaching statistical significance in brain (F) and ovaries ($p < 0.05$) (Table 4).

As for the individual K vitamers, females generally presented higher tissue total VK concentrations than males, differences reaching statistical significance in kidney (all groups), spleen (20 *AL*), and brain (3 months) ($p < 0.05$). Similarly, total VK was generally increased at 20 months when compared to tissue concentrations at 3 months, the effect being more often observed in old rats fed the *AL* regimen liver (M: 20 *AL*, 20 CR), heart (M and F: 20 *AL*), kidney (M: 20 *AL*, 20 CR; F: 20 *AL*), spleen (F: 20 *AL*, 20 CR), and ovaries (20 *AL*). Finally, as oberved for individual K vitamers, the CR regimen was associated, at 20 months, with lower total VK concentrations, differences reaching statistical significance in ovaries ($p < 0.05$) (Table 4).

Finally, MK-4/total VK ratios were little affected by sex although they were significantly higher in females than males in liver (3 months) and heart (20 CR) ($p < 0.05$) (Figure 4). As observed in study 1, ratios were increased at 20 months in the liver (M: 20 *AL*, 20 CR), heart (F: 20 CR), kidneys (M: 20 *AL*, 20 CR), and spleen (M and F: 20 *AL*, 20 CR) ($p < 0.05$). Finally, MK-4/total VK ratios at 20 months were largely unaffected by the CR regimen with only the ratio for brain (F) being statistically decreased in CR compared to that in the *AL* group ($p < 0.05$).

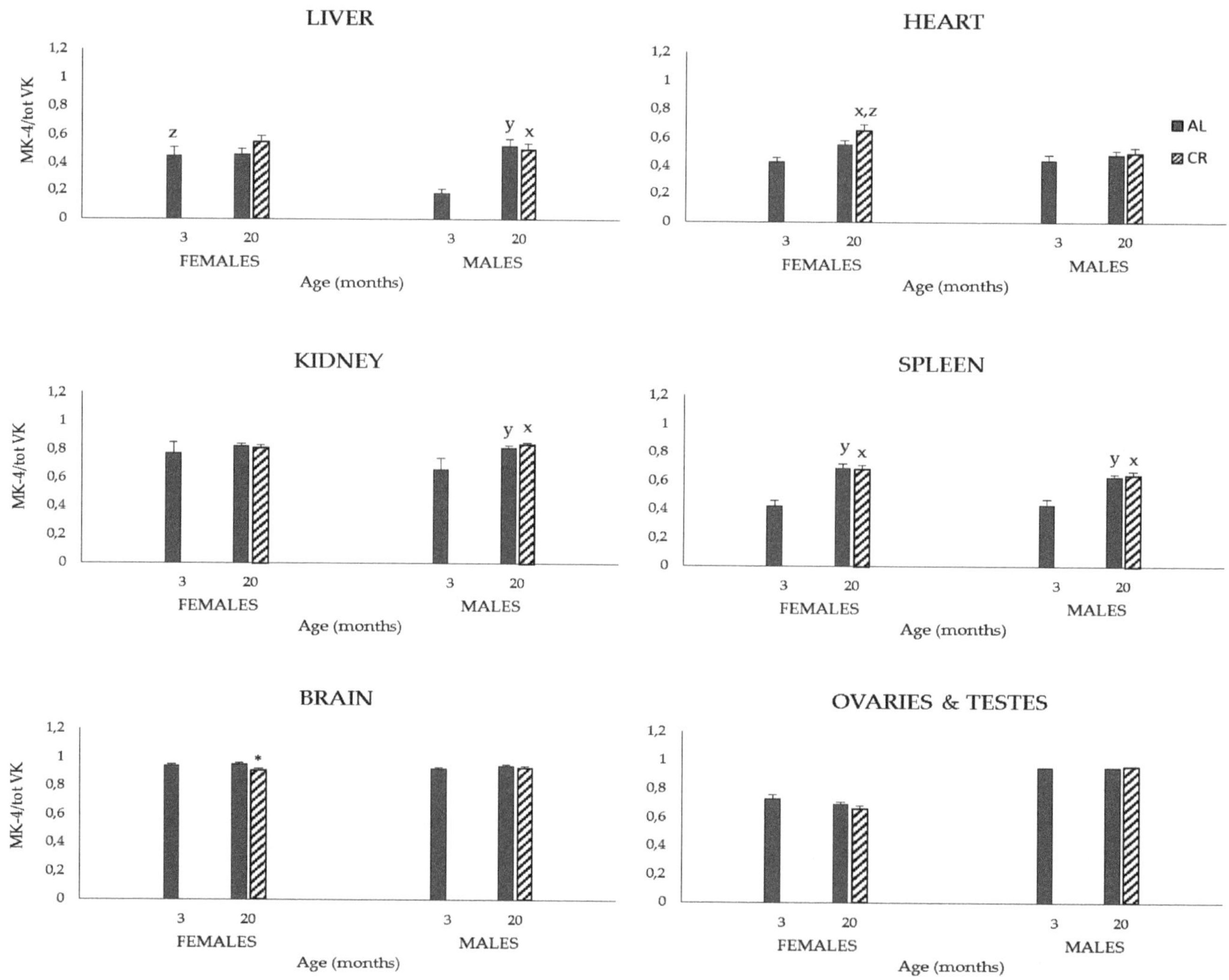

Figure 4. Tissue MK-4/total VK ratios of 3- and 20-month-old M and F Sprague–Dawley rats fed an *AL* or CR diet. Age and diet effects were determined in M and F by conducting distinct one-way ANOVA's followed by Tukey's *post hoc* tests. Student' *t*-test was used to further assess the effect of CR at 20 months, and that of sex *i.e.*, given age and diet group. ^{x}: $p < 0.05$ between 20 CR and 3 months, same sex; ^{y}: $p < 0.05$ between 20 *AL* and 3 months, same sex; ^{z}: $p < 0.05$ between M and F, same age and diet; *: $p < 0.05$ between 20 *AL* and 20 CR, same sex. Values are expressed as mean ± SEM; n = 6–8/sex/age/diet groups.

3.2.3. Prothrombin and Activated Partial Thromboplastin Times

Results for prothrombin (PT) and activated partial thromboplastin (APTT) times are presented in Table 5. At 20 months of age, a diet effect was observed in male rats, the mean PT value of CR rats being statistically increased compared to that of *AL* animals ($p < 0.05$), and comparable to that of rats aged 3 months. A sex effect was also observed for PT in 20-month-old rats fed the CR diet, males showing a statistically higher mean value than females ($p < 0.05$).

Table 5. Prothrombin (PT) and activated partial thromboplastin (APTT) times of 3- and 20-month-old M and F Sprague–Dawley rats fed an *AL* or CR diet.

Age (Months)	Diet	PT		APTT	
		(s)			
		M	F	M	F
3	*AL*	14.5 ± 1.2	13.5 ± 0.3	20.8 ± 1.2	21.6 ± 1.3
20	*AL*	12.8 ± 0.2	12.8 ± 0.3	21.7 ± 1.4	20.0 ± 1.6
	CR	14.0 ± 0.4 ^{z,*}	12.9 ± 0.2	23.3 ± 1.6	20.3 ± 1.1

At 20 months, the mean PT value of M fed the CR diet was statistically higher than that of the 20 *AL* group ($p < 0.05$), and comparable to that of male rats aged 3 months. A sex effect was observed in 20-month-old rats fed the CR diet, M showing a statistically higher mean value than F ($p < 0.05$). ^{x}: $p < 0.05$ between 20 CR and 3-months, same sex; ^{y}: $p < 0.05$ between 20 *AL* and 3 months, same sex; ^{z}: $p < 0.05$ between M and F, same age and diet; *: $p < 0.05$ between 20 *AL* and 20 CR, same sex. Values are expressed as mean ± SEM; n = 6–8/sex/age/diet groups.

4. Discussion

All K vitamers classically serve as cofactors in a carboxylation reaction that results in the conversion of specific glutamic acid residues to gamma-carboxyglutamic acid in precursor proteins *i.e.*, VKDPs. In addition, there is increasing evidence that K_1 and MK-4 have additional actions outside their role as enzymatic cofactor, e.g., inflammation, oxidative stress. In recent years, VK has been associated with a number of age-related conditions such as osteoporosis [1], the calcification process [3], insulin resistance [4,38], cancer [39], and cognitive decline [11]. This report aimed to investigate the influence of lifetime dietary VK exposure on the tissue content and distribution of the K_1 and MK-4 vitamers at different life stages in male and female rats fed different diets since weaning, or subjected to caloric restriction, a life-prolonging model.

4.1. Study 1

In the first study, conducted in 3-, 12- and 22-month-old male and female rats fed different K_1 diets since weaning, body weights were found to increase with age in both sexes but were not significantly affected by lifetime K_1 intakes. Body weights have been shown to increase during aging in rodents and our results concur with previous studies [40,41]. The lack of effect of K_1 intakes on body weights is of interest given the recently proposed role of VK in energy metabolism. In a series of studies using murine models, a specific form of the VKDP osteocalcin has been shown to modulate glucose and insulin metabolism, energy expenditure, and fat mass [4]. Although the endocrine role of osteocalcin remains an intense subject of debate, other studies conducted in rats [42] and humans [38,43] point to potential beneficial effects of increased VK intakes on metabolic profile and body weights. The trend towards lower body weights observed at 22 months in both males and females fed the H diet goes along those lines.

Plasma K_1 increased as a function of diet in both sexes, however, no MK-4 could be detected under our experimental conditions. The presence of MK-4 in the circulation in response to K_1 intake has been variable, some studies reporting low [6,27,28] or undetectable [8] values. Tissue contents and distribution of the K vitamers were found to differ, with K_1 as the predominant vitamer in some organs *i.e.*, the liver, heart, and MK-4 in others *i.e.*, testes and brain. Such differential distributions of the K vitamers were observed in previous short-term studies [6,8,26,29]. One notable finding of the present study, however, is the large amount of total VK observed in ovaries, this organ being rich in both K_1 and MK-4 vitamers. High levels of VK have been reported in a previous study [29], although levels were significantly lower than those reported here. Differences in strain (Brown–Norway *vs.* Sprague–Dawley) and VK content of the diets could explain the differences between the two studies. However, the high VK content of ovaries is intriguing as this organ is not known to be particularly rich in either of the known VKDPs. Whether the K vitamers possess actions in the ovary beyond their role in the carboxylation reaction remains to be determined; however, in a series of older studies, VK was shown to possess estrogenic activity. Specifically, treatment of castrate mice with either K_1 and menadione resulted in increases in uterine weights and cornification of the vaginal epithelium [44].

Increasing K_1 intake generally resulted in higher tissue K_1 and MK-4, differences being mainly observed between the L and H, and the A and H groups suggesting that intakes >500 μg K_1/kg diet are needed for tissue accumulation. These results are in line with those of previous studies conducted in normal [26] and germ-free [45] rats. In the great majority of organs, total VK tissue contents were higher in females than in males, the effect being mainly seen at 3 and 12 months of age. This finding has been observed by others [29,30] and is likely explained by the facilitatory action of estrogens on the intestinal absorption of K_1 [46]. As discussed below, this estrogenic effect on VK absorption could contribute to the greater resistance of female rats to VK deficiency. Concentrations of the K vitamers and total VK were also affected by age in a number of organs (*i.e.*, the liver, spleen, brain, ovaries and testes), differences varying according to organs, sex (when applicable), and dietary groups. Except for ovaries for which VK contents increased throughout life, total VK concentrations either increased between 3 and 12 months or were comparable, and decreased in the second year of life. In 3-, 12- and 24-months old Brown–Norway rats which had been fed a nonpurified diet (NIH 31 M), liver K_1 was found to be increased and MK-4 to be decreased in the heart, kidneys, lung, and cerebellum of old animals [29]. In a more recent study conducted in Fisher 344 male rats aged two, 12, and 24 months, a 28-day administration of a low K_1 containing diet (~200 μg K_1/kg diet) was associated with higher MK-4 concentrations in the liver, spleen, kidneys, heart, and cortex (myelin) in 24- compared to two-month-old rats; the opposite effect was observed for testes [28]. Divergent results among studies could be explained by differences in experimental design *i.e.*, VK contents of the diets, duration of exposure, *etc.*, and strain of animals.

In light of the growing importance of MK-4 in various physiological functions and given that the aging process can affect enzymatic activities [32,47] which could include those involved in the K_1 to MK-4 conversion, we assessed the relative MK-4 to total VK tissue content (MK-4/total VK) in all organs. In contrast to what was observed for K_1, MK-4, and total VK, the MK-4/total VK ratios were much less affected by sex, diet, and age. Regarding the latter, an interesting trend was observed. In high MK-4 containing organs such as the brain, testes, kidneys and ovaries, the high MK-4/total VK ratios were maintained in old age, this finding being observed for both sexes and in most dietary groups. In organs with lower MK-4 contents *i.e.*, liver, heart and spleen, MK-4/total VK ratios tended to increase with age in both sexes and dietary groups. Hence, irrespective of an organ's usual MK-4 content, the proportion of this vitamer relative to total VK appears to increase with age. Whether this trend reflects an increased physiological demand for MK-4 in handling age-related conditions such as inflammation and oxidative stress remains to be established, but such hypothesis should be pursued in future studies.

Male rats have long been shown to be less resistant to VK deficiency compared to females [30,48,49]. The increased PT and APTT observed in young male rats fed the L diet corroborate these observations and confirm earlier findings that diets containing <500 μg K_1/kg diet are insufficient to maintain normal coagulation [34]. It should be mentioned that, despite their increased coagulation times, no rat presented signs of bleeding or died due to hemorrhage.

4.2. Study 2

By virtue of its nature, the CR dietary regimen resulted in significantly lower body weights in old CR compared to *AL* groups. As a corollary to this and because the diet fed the CR rats was adjusted to contain equimolar amounts of vitamins and minerals as that fed the *AL* group, K_1 intakes of CR rats were significantly higher than those fed the *AL* diet when expressed per unit body weight (Table 3). As shown in Table 4, the dietary regimen had no impact on the K vitamer profile in plasma and tissues, organs rich in K_1 (*i.e.*, liver, heart) and MK-4 (*i.e.*, brain, testes) being those observed in study 1. Likewise, ovaries were found to contain high quantities of both K vitamers and the highest

VK content of all organs. The general trend for higher VK tissue concentrations in females than in males was also observed, the effect being particularly marked for the MK-4 vitamer. Age had little effect on K_1 tissue contents in contrast to MK-4, which were generally increased at 20 months compared to 3 months. Interestingly, despite the fact that rats fed the CR regimen consumed more K_1 per unit body weight than their *AL* counterparts since adulthood, their tissue K_1 and MK-4 contents at 20 months tended to be decreased when compared to those of the *AL* group. Lower tissue MK-4 content could be the result of lower synthesis from K_1 or greater tissue utilization. Although assessing the activity of the UBIAD1 enzyme would have provided useful information regarding tissues' synthetic capacities, this hypothesis is unlikely given that the MK-4/total VK ratios at 20 months were largely unaffected by CR. The second hypothesis probably represents a more plausible explanation as the aging process is characterized by molecular and cellular events that leads to impaired function and increased vulnerability to death [47,50]. In fact, a study conducted in 4-, 19- and 28-month-old rats aiming at assessing the impact of CR on α-tocopherol tissue distribution point in this direction. Compared to tissues of 19-month-old *AL* rats, α-tocopherol concentrations in CR rats were found to be lower by 48% in plasma, 30% in kidneys, 60% in the liver, and 44% in the heart homogenate. These results were interpreted as reflecting a greater utilization of tissue α-tocopherol in limiting the age-induced oxidative damage to membranes [51].

Finally, in this study, coagulation times were increased in old male rats fed the *AL* diet (PT, $p < 0.05$; trend for APTT). The fact that animals subjected to CR were able to maintain a more youthful coagulation profile *i.e.*, similar to that of 3-month-old animals, supports the notion that this dietary regimen is associated with a greater utilization of the K vitamers.

5. Conclusions

Dietary K_1 intakes around the minimal amount required for normal blood coagulation had no significant influence on body weights of both male and female rats at different life stages. Tissue contents of the K vitamers differed according to organs, were generally higher in females than in males, and increased with K_1 intake. The MK-4/total VK ratios tended to increase with age, possibly reflecting an increased physiological demand for MK-4 during aging. Our study also confirmed the greater susceptibility of male rats to VK insufficiency, notably at a younger age.

Despite lifelong higher K_1 intakes per unit body weight, tissue K_1 and MK-4 contents at 20 months were generally lower in CR rats compared to their *AL* counterparts. Whether the lower tissue MK-4 content is the result of lower synthesis from K_1 or greater tissue utilization remains to be determined. However, the more youthful coagulation profile observed in old CR rats (*vs. AL* rats) tends to support the notion that CR is associated with greater utilization of the K vitamers to sustain physiological functions.

Acknowledgments: This work was supported by the Natural Sciences and Engineering Research Council of Canada (NSERC). The authors wish to thank Mses Sylvie Roy, Bouchra Ouliass, and Elisabeth Bélanger for their valuable assistance in the preparation of this manuscript.

Author Contributions: Guylaine Ferland designed the studies. Isabelle Doucet and Dominique Mainville conducted the experimental work and analyses. All 3 authors contributed to interpretation of the data and writing of the manuscript. All authors reviewed the final manuscript.

References

1. Booth, S.L. Roles for vitamin K beyond coagulation. *Annu. Rev. Nutr.* **2009**, *29*, 89–110. [CrossRef] [PubMed]
2. Ferland, G. The discovery of vitamin K and its clinical applications. *Ann. Nutr. Metab.* **2012**, *61*, 213–218. [CrossRef] [PubMed]
3. Beulens, J.W.; Booth, S.L.; van den Heuvel, E.G.; Stoecklin, E.; Baka, A.; Vermeer, C. The role of menaquinones (vitamin K_2) in human health. *Br. J. Nutr.* **2013**, *110*, 1357–1368. [CrossRef] [PubMed]

4. Ferron, M.; Lacombe, J. Regulation of energy metabolism by the skeleton: Osteocalcin and beyond. *Arch. Biochem. Biophys.* **2014**, *561*, 137–146. [CrossRef] [PubMed]
5. Shearer, M.J.; Newman, P. Recent trends in the metabolism and cell biology of vitamin K with special reference to vitamin K cycling and mk-4 biosynthesis. *J. Lipid Res.* **2014**, *55*, 345–362. [CrossRef] [PubMed]
6. Thijssen, H.H.; Drittij-Reijnders, M.J. Vitamin K distribution in rat tissues: Dietary phylloquinone is a source of tissue menaquinone-4. *Br. J. Nutr.* **1994**, *72*, 415–425. [CrossRef] [PubMed]
7. Thijssen, H.H.; Drittij-Reijnders, M.J.; Fischer, M.A. Phylloquinone and menaquinone-4 distribution in rats: Synthesis rather than uptake determines menaquinone-4 organ concentrations. *J. Nutr.* **1996**, *126*, 537–543. [PubMed]
8. Al Rajabi, A.; Booth, S.L.; Peterson, J.W.; Choi, S.W.; Suttie, J.W.; Shea, M.K.; Miao, B.; Grusak, M.A.; Fu, X. Deuterium-labeled phylloquinone has tissue-specific conversion to menaquinone-4 among fischer 344 male rats. *J. Nutr.* **2012**, *142*, 841–845. [CrossRef] [PubMed]
9. Hirota, Y.; Tsugawa, N.; Nakagawa, K.; Suhara, Y.; Tanaka, K.; Uchino, Y.; Takeuchi, A.; Sawada, N.; Kamao, M.; Wada, A.; *et al.* Menadione (vitamin K_3) is a catabolic product of oral phylloquinone (vitamin K_1) in the intestine and a circulating precursor of tissue menaquinone-4 (vitamin K_2) in rats. *J. Biol. Chem.* **2013**, *288*, 33071–33080. [CrossRef] [PubMed]
10. Nakagawa, K.; Sawada, N.; Hirota, Y.; Uchino, Y.; Suhara, Y.; Hasegawa, T.; Amizuka, N.; Okamoto, T.; Tsugawa, N.; Kamao, M.; *et al.* Vitamin K2 biosynthetic enzyme, UBIAD1 is essential for embryonic development of mice. *PLoS ONE* **2014**, *9*, e104078. [CrossRef] [PubMed]
11. Ferland, G. Vitamin K, an emerging nutrient in brain function. *Biofactors* **2012**, *38*, 151–157. [CrossRef] [PubMed]
12. Reddi, K.; Henderson, B.; Meghji, S.; Wilson, M.; Poole, S.; Hopper, C.; Harris, M.; Hodges, S.J. Interleukin 6 production by lipopolysaccharide-stimulated human fibroblasts is potently inhibited by naphthoquinone (vitamin K) compounds. *Cytokine* **1995**, *7*, 287–290. [CrossRef] [PubMed]
13. Ohsaki, Y.; Shirakawa, H.; Hiwatashi, K.; Furukawa, Y.; Mizutani, T.; Komai, M. Vitamin K suppresses lipopolysaccharide-induced inflammation in the rat. *Biosci. Biotechnol. Biochem.* **2006**, *70*, 926–932. [CrossRef] [PubMed]
14. Ohsaki, Y.; Shirakawa, H.; Miura, A.; Giriwono, P.E.; Sato, S.; Ohashi, A.; Iribe, M.; Goto, T.; Komai, M. Vitamin K suppresses the lipopolysaccharide-induced expression of inflammatory cytokines in cultured macrophage-like cells via the inhibition of the activation of nuclear factor κB through the repression of IKKalpha/beta phosphorylation. *J. Nutr. Biochem.* **2010**, *21*, 1120–1126. [CrossRef] [PubMed]
15. Moriya, M.; Nakatsuji, Y.; Okuno, T.; Hamasaki, T.; Sawada, M.; Sakoda, S. Vitamin K_2 ameliorates experimental autoimmune encephalomyelitis in lewis rats. *J. Neuroimmunol.* **2005**, *170*, 11–20. [CrossRef] [PubMed]
16. Li, J.; Lin, J.C.; Wang, H.; Peterson, J.W.; Furie, B.C.; Furie, B.; Booth, S.L.; Volpe, J.J.; Rosenberg, P.A. Novel role of vitamin K in preventing oxidative injury to developing oligodendrocytes and neurons. *J. Neurosci.* **2003**, *23*, 5816–5826. [PubMed]
17. Li, J.; Wang, H.; Rosenberg, P.A. Vitamin K prevents oxidative cell death by inhibiting activation of 12-lipoxygenase in developing oligodendrocytes. *J. Neurosci. Res.* **2009**, *87*, 1997–2005. [CrossRef] [PubMed]
18. Shibayama-Imazu, T.; Aiuchi, T.; Nakaya, K. Vitamin K_2-mediated apoptosis in cancer cells: Role of mitochondrial transmembrane potential. *Vitam. Horm.* **2008**, *78*, 211–226. [PubMed]
19. Ozaki, I.; Zhang, H.; Mizuta, T.; Ide, Y.; Eguchi, Y.; Yasutake, T.; Sakamaki, T.; Pestell, R.G.; Yamamoto, K. Menatetrenone, a vitamin K_2 analogue, inhibits hepatocellular carcinoma cell growth by suppressing cyclin D1 expression through inhibition of nuclear factor κB activation. *Clin. Cancer Res.* **2007**, *13*, 2236–2245. [CrossRef] [PubMed]
20. Tabb, M.M.; Sun, A.; Zhou, C.; Grun, F.; Errandi, J.; Romero, K.; Pham, H.; Inoue, S.; Mallick, S.; Lin, M.; *et al.* Vitamin K_2 regulation of bone homeostasis is mediated by the steroid and xenobiotic receptor SXR. *J. Biol. Chem.* **2003**, *278*, 43919–43927. [CrossRef] [PubMed]
21. Ichikawa, T.; Horie-Inoue, K.; Ikeda, K.; Blumberg, B.; Inoue, S. Steroid and xenobiotic receptor SXR mediates vitamin K_2-activated transcription of extracellular matrix-related genes and collagen accumulation in osteoblastic cells. *J. Biol. Chem.* **2006**, *281*, 16927–16934. [CrossRef] [PubMed]

22. Tsang, C.K.; Kamei, Y. Novel effect of vitamin K_1 (phylloquinone) and vitamin K_2 (menaquinone) on promoting nerve growth factor-mediated neurite outgrowth from PC12D cells. *Neurosci. Lett.* **2002**, *323*, 9–12. [CrossRef]
23. Otsuka, M.; Kato, N.; Shao, R.X.; Hoshida, Y.; Ijichi, H.; Koike, Y.; Taniguchi, H.; Moriyama, M.; Shiratori, Y.; Kawabe, T.; *et al.* Vitamin K_2 inhibits the growth and invasiveness of hepatocellular carcinoma cells via protein kinase A activation. *Hepatology* **2004**, *40*, 243–251. [CrossRef] [PubMed]
24. Ichikawa, T.; Horie-Inoue, K.; Ikeda, K.; Blumberg, B.; Inoue, S. Vitamin K_2 induces phosphorylation of protein kinase A and expression of novel target genes in osteoblastic cells. *J. Mol. Endocrinol.* **2007**, *39*, 239–247. [CrossRef] [PubMed]
25. Ito, A.; Shirakawa, H.; Takumi, N.; Minegishi, Y.; Ohashi, A.; Howlader, Z.H.; Ohsaki, Y.; Sato, T.; Goto, T.; Komai, M. Menaquinone-4 enhances testosterone production in rats and testis-derived tumor cells. *Lipids Health Dis.* **2011**, *10*, 158. [CrossRef] [PubMed]
26. Ronden, J.E.; Thijssen, H.H.; Vermeer, C. Tissue distribution of K-vitamers under different nutritional regimens in the rat. *Biochim. Biophys. Acta* **1998**, *1379*, 16–22. [CrossRef]
27. Sato, T.; Ozaki, R.; Kamo, S.; Hara, Y.; Konishi, S.; Isobe, Y.; Saitoh, S.; Harada, H. The biological activity and tissue distribution of 2′,3′-dihydrophylloquinone in rats. *Biochim. Biophys. Acta* **2003**, *1622*, 145–150. [CrossRef]
28. Booth, S.L.; Peterson, J.W.; Smith, D.; Shea, M.K.; Chamberland, J.; Crivello, N. Age and dietary form of vitamin K affect menaquinone-4 concentrations in male fischer 344 rats. *J. Nutr.* **2008**, *138*, 492–496. [PubMed]
29. Huber, A.M.; Davidson, K.W.; O'Brien-Morse, M.E.; Sadowski, J.A. Tissue phylloquinone and menaquinones in rats are affected by age and gender. *J. Nutr.* **1999**, *129*, 1039–1044. [PubMed]
30. Huber, A.M.; Davidson, K.W.; O'Brien-Morse, M.E.; Sadowski, J.A. Gender differences in hepatic phylloquinone and menaquinones in the vitamin K-deficient and -supplemented rat. *Biochim. Biophys. Acta* **1999**, *1426*, 43–52. [CrossRef]
31. Anton, B.; Vitetta, L.; Cortizo, F.; Sali, A. Can we delay aging? The biology and science of aging. *Ann. N. Y. Acad. Sci.* **2005**, *1057*, 525–535. [CrossRef] [PubMed]
32. Speakman, J.R.; Mitchell, S.E. Caloric restriction. *Mol. Asp. Med.* **2011**, *32*, 159–221. [CrossRef] [PubMed]
33. Fontana, L.; Partridge, L. Promoting health and longevity through diet: From model organisms to humans. *Cell* **2015**, *161*, 106–118. [CrossRef] [PubMed]
34. Kindberg, C.G.; Suttie, J.W. Effect of various intakes of phylloquinone on signs of vitamin K deficiency and serum and liver phylloquinone concentrations in the rat. *J. Nutr.* **1989**, *119*, 175–180. [PubMed]
35. Carrie, I.; Portoukalian, J.; Vicaretti, R.; Rochford, J.; Potvin, S.; Ferland, G. Menaquinone-4 concentration is correlated with sphingolipid concentrations in rat brain. *J. Nutr.* **2004**, *134*, 167–172. [PubMed]
36. Davidson, K.W.; Sadowski, J.A. Determination of vitamin K compounds in plasma or serum by high-performance liquid chromatography using postcolumn chemical reduction and fluorimetric detection. *Methods Enzymol.* **1997**, *282*, 408–421. [PubMed]
37. Wang, L.Y.; Bates, C.J.; Yan, L.; Harrington, D.J.; Shearer, M.J.; Prentice, A. Determination of phylloquinone (vitamin K_1) in plasma and serum by HPLC with fluorescence detection. *Clin. Chim. Acta* **2004**, *347*, 199–207. [CrossRef] [PubMed]
38. Booth, S.L.; Centi, A.J.; Gundberg, C. Bone as an endocrine organ relevant to diabetes. *Curr. Diab. Rep.* **2014**, *14*, 556. [CrossRef] [PubMed]
39. Tokita, H.; Tsuchida, A.; Miyazawa, K.; Ohyashiki, K.; Katayanagi, S.; Sudo, H.; Enomoto, M.; Takagi, Y.; Aoki, T. Vitamin K_2-induced antitumor effects via cell-cycle arrest and apoptosis in gastric cancer cell lines. *Int. J. Mol. Med.* **2006**, *17*, 235–243. [CrossRef] [PubMed]
40. Menard, C.; Quirion, R.; Bouchard, S.; Ferland, G.; Gaudreau, P. Glutamatergic signaling and low prodynorphin expression are associated with intact memory and reduced anxiety in rat models of healthy aging. *Front. Aging Neurosci.* **2014**, *6*, 81. [PubMed]
41. Moyse, E.; Bedard, K.; Segura, S.; Mahaut, S.; Tardivel, C.; Ferland, G.; Lebrun, B.; Gaudreau, P. Effects of aging and caloric restriction on brainstem satiety center signals in rats. *Mech. Ageing Dev.* **2012**, *133*, 83–91. [CrossRef] [PubMed]
42. Sogabe, N.; Maruyama, R.; Baba, O.; Hosoi, T.; Goseki-Sone, M. Effects of long-term vitamin K_1 (phylloquinone) or vitamin K_2 (menaquinone-4) supplementation on body composition and serum parameters in rats. *Bone* **2011**, *48*, 1036–1042. [CrossRef] [PubMed]

43. Knapen, M.H.; Schurgers, L.J.; Shearer, M.J.; Newman, P.; Theuwissen, E.; Vermeer, C. Association of vitamin K status with adiponectin and body composition in healthy subjects: Uncarboxylated osteocalcin is not associated with fat mass and body weight. *Br. J. Nutr.* **2012**, *108*, 1017–1024. [CrossRef] [PubMed]
44. Mellette, S.J. Interrelationships between vitamin K and estrogenic hormones. *Am. J. Clin. Nutr.* **1961**, *9*, 108–116. [PubMed]
45. Ronden, J.E.; Drittij-Reijnders, M.J.; Vermeer, C.; Thijssen, H.H. Intestinal flora is not an intermediate in the phylloquinone-menaquinone-4 conversion in the rat. *Biochim. Biophys. Acta* **1998**, *1379*, 69–75. [CrossRef]
46. Jolly, D.W.; Craig, C.; Nelson, T.E., Jr. Estrogen and prothrombin synthesis: Effect of estrogen on absorption of vitamin K1. *Am. J. Physiol.* **1977**, *232*, H12–H17. [PubMed]
47. Lopez-Otin, C.; Blasco, M.A.; Partridge, L.; Serrano, M.; Kroemer, G. The hallmarks of aging. *Cell* **2013**, *153*, 1194–1217. [CrossRef] [PubMed]
48. Metta, V.A.; Mameesh, M.S.; Johnson, B.C. Vitamin K deficiency in rats induced by the feeding of irradiated beef. *J. Nutr.* **1959**, *69*, 18–22. [PubMed]
49. Gustafsson, B.E.; Daft, F.S.; Mc, D.E.; Smith, J.C.; Fitzgerald, R.J. Effects of vitamin K-active compounds and intestinal microorganisms in vitamin K-deficient germfree rats. *J. Nutr.* **1962**, *78*, 461–468. [PubMed]
50. Kenessary, A.; Zhumadilov, Z.; Nurgozhin, T.; Kipling, D.; Yeoman, M.; Cox, L.; Ostler, E.; Faragher, R. Biomarkers, interventions and healthy ageing. *New Biotechnol.* **2013**, *30*, 373–377. [CrossRef] [PubMed]
51. Kamzalov, S.; Sohal, R.S. Effect of age and caloric restriction on coenzyme q and alpha-tocopherol levels in the rat. *Exp. Gerontol.* **2004**, *39*, 1199–1205. [CrossRef] [PubMed]

9

Recent Advances in our Understanding of Tocopherol Biosynthesis in Plants: An Overview of Key Genes, Functions and Breeding of Vitamin E Improved Crops

Steffi Fritsche [1,*], Xingxing Wang [1,2] and Christian Jung [1]

1 Plant Breeding Institute, Christian-Albrechts-University of Kiel, 24118 Kiel, Germany; wangxingxing@caas.cn (X.W.); c.jung@plantbreeding.uni-kiel.de (C.J.)

2 Institute of Cotton Research of Chinese Academy of Agricultural Sciences, Anyang 455000, China

* Correspondence: steffi.fritsche@scionresearch.com

Abstract: Tocopherols, together with tocotrienols and plastochromanols belong to a group of lipophilic compounds also called tocochromanols or vitamin E. Considered to be one of the most powerful antioxidants, tocochromanols are solely synthesized by photosynthetic organisms including plants, algae, and cyanobacteria and, therefore, are an essential component in the human diet. Tocochromanols potent antioxidative properties are due to their ability to interact with polyunsaturated acyl groups and scavenge lipid peroxyl radicals and quench reactive oxygen species (ROS), thus protecting fatty acids from lipid peroxidation. In the plant model species *Arabidopsis thaliana*, the required genes for tocopherol biosynthesis and functional roles of tocopherols were elucidated in mutant and transgenic plants. Recent research efforts have led to new outcomes for the vitamin E biosynthetic and related pathways, and new possible alternatives for the biofortification of important crops have been suggested. Here, we review 30 years of research on tocopherols in model and crop species, with emphasis on the improvement of vitamin E content using transgenic approaches and classical breeding. We will discuss future prospects to further improve the nutritional value of our food.

Keywords: vitamin E; tocopherol; antioxidant; biofortification; crop breeding

---

1. Introduction

Four tocopherols and four tocotrienols form a group of lipid-soluble antioxidants called tocochromanols, commonly known as vitamin E [1,2]. Their basic structure is simple, comprising a polar chromanol ring and a hydrophobic polyprenyl side chain, products of the shikimate and 1-deoxy-D-xylulose 5-phosphate (DOXP) pathways. Tocochromanols with a fully saturated side chain are called tocopherols and those with an unsaturated side chain tocotrienols. The number of methyl groups in the chromanol ring defines the four natural occurring α, β, γ, and δ-tocopherol and tocotrienol subforms [3]. Vitamin E activity involves scavenging peroxyl radicals and quenching reactive oxygen species (ROS). The most active form of vitamin E is α-tocopherol and thus the most needed form of vitamin E in our diet [4]. It is generally found in high concentrations in vegetable oils such as almond, safflower, or canola oil or in other high-fat sources such as nuts, seeds, or grains [5]. Food-grade canola oil, or 00-type rapeseed oil, has a high-quality nutritional composition similar to that of olive oil, and tocopherols are one of the main nutritionally relevant constituents. Despite vitamin E's importance in the human diet, dietary studies show that the recommended daily allowance is often not met, so, improving its quantity and composition has become a target in crop breeding [6].

In this review, we follow the elucidation of the tocopherol biosynthesis pathway genes over the last 30 years of research, with a particular focus on their function and their involvement in plant processes. We will focus on the biosynthesis bottlenecks detected and the transgenic and non-transgenic breeding efforts that have been undertaken in order to improve the antioxidant and nutritional values of important crops.

2. Biosynthesis and Chemical Function

Tocopherol biosynthesis is initiated in the plant's cytoplasm, but, except for this first step, its biosynthesis takes place in the plastids. Here, the necessary enzymes are localized at the inner envelope or in the plastoglobules [7–9]. The biosynthesis starts through the formation of the aromatic head group homogentisic acid (HGA), which is catalyzed by the enzyme *p*-hydroxyphenylpyruvate and is derived from tyrosine degradation [10,11]. The polyprenyl side chain, phytyl diphosphate (phytyl-PP/PDP), is suggested to originate from the DOXP pathway, as well as from the recycling of free phytol derived from the chlorophyll degradation process [12,13]. In *Arabidopsis thaliana (A. thaliana)*, this step is catalyzed sequentially by two phytol kinases [13,14]. The two substrates, HGA and PDP, are fused together in the following step, mediated by the enzyme homogentisate phytyltransferase (HPT), to 2-methyl-6-phytyl-1,4-benzoquinol (MPBQ). MPBQ, in turn, serves as substrate either for tocopherol cyclase (TC) or MPBQ methyltransferase. MPBQ methyltransferase methylates MPBQ to 2,3-dimethyl-6-phytyl-1,4-benzoquinone (DMPBQ), while tocopherol cyclase transforms both MPBQ and DMPBQ to γ- and δ-tocopherol, respectively. Lastly, the enzyme γ-tocopherol methyltransferase (γ-TMT) catalyzes the conversion of γ- to α-tocopherol and of δ- to β-tocopherol (Figure 1, Table 1).

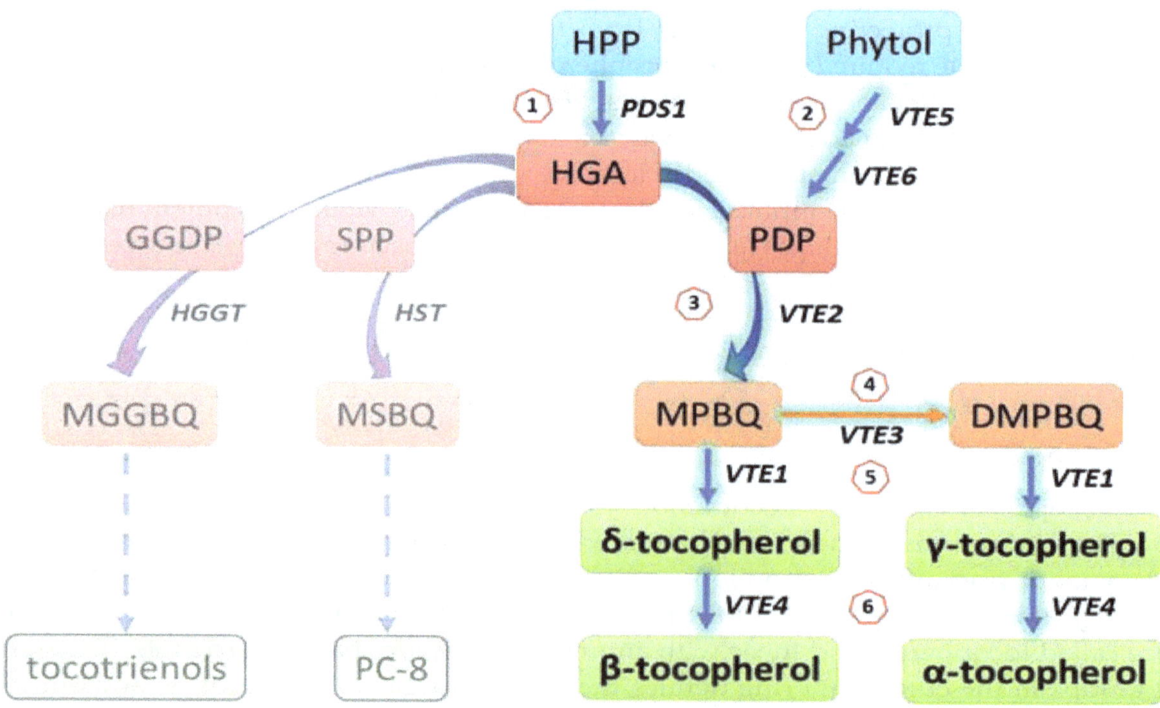

Figure 1. Simplified model of the tocopherol biosynthesis pathway in *A. thaliana* (highlighted branch of the pathway). Compound names are given in the boxes and gene names are indicated in italic. The circled numbers refer to the biosynthesis steps described in detail in Table 1. Adapted from [15]. *HGGT*: homogentisic acid geranylgeranyl transferase; *HST*: homogentisic acid solanesyl transferase; GGDP: geranylgeranyl diphosphate; MGGBQ: 2-methyl-6-geranylgeranyl-1,4-benzoquinol; PC-8: plastochromanol-8; SPP: solanesyl pyrophosphate.

Table 1. Genes and enzymes of the tocopherol biosynthesis in *A. thaliana*.

Biosynthesis Step	Gene	Enzyme	Function	Substrate [1]	Product	At Locus	Reference
1	*PDS1*	HPPD	Head group synthesis	HPP	HGA	AT1G06570	[16–18]
2	*VTE5*	Phytol kinase	Phosphorylation	Phytol + CTP/UTP	Phytyl-P	AT5G04490	[14]
	VTE6	Phytyl -P kinase	Phosphorylation	Phytol-P + CTP	Phytyl-PP(PDP)	AT1G78620	[13]
3	*VTE2*	HPT	Phytylation	HGA + PDP	MPBQ	AT2G18950	[19–23]
4	*VTE3*	MPBQ/ MSBQ MT	Methylation	MPBQ/MSBQ	DMPQ	AT3G63410	[24–26]
5	*VTE1*	TC	Cyclization	MPBQ/DMPQ	γ-tocopherol/ δ-tocopherol	AT4G32770	[27–30]
6	*VTE4*	γ-TMT	Methylation	δ-tocopherol/ γ-tocopherol	α-tocopherol/ β-tocopherol	AT1G64970	[30–33]

[1] Only those compounds related to the tocopherol biosynthesis are mentioned. Genes and their corresponding enzyme names: *PDS1*/HPPD: p-hydroxyphenylpyruvate dioxygenase; *VTE1*/TC: tocopherol cyclase; *VTE2*/HPT: homogentisic acid phytyl transferase; *VTE3*/MT: methyltransferase; *VTE4*/ γ-TMT: γ-tocopherol methyltransferase; *VTE5/VTE6*: phytol kinase. Substrates and products: CTP/UTP: cytidine triphosphate/ uridine triphosphate; DMPBQ: 2,3-dimethyl-6-phytyl-1,4-benzoquinone; HGA: homogentisic acid; HPP: *p*-hydroxyphenylpyruvate; MPBQ: 2-methyl-6-phytyl-1,4-benzoquinol; MSBQ: 2-methyl-6-solanesyl-1,4-benzoquinol; Phytyl-PP/PDP: phytyl diphosphate; PDP: phytyldiphosphate.

Tocopherols are one of the most valuable antioxidants because of their remarkable chemical mode of action. They interact with polyunsaturated acyl groups and protect polyunsaturated fatty acids from lipid peroxidation by scavenging lipid peroxy radicals and quenching ROS produced e.g., by photosystem II and during membrane lipid peroxidation [34,35]. During this process, tocopherols donate their phenolic hydrogen to lipid-free radicals, thus neutralizing the radical, terminating the autocatalytic lipid peroxidation processes and protecting cell membranes [36,37]. The resulting tocopherol radicals are more stable, are less reactive, and, more importantly, can be reconverted to the corresponding tocopherol by reacting with other antioxidants such as ascorbate or glutathione. This allows each tocopherol to participate in many scavenging reactions before being degraded. Collectively, these properties make tocopherols highly efficient as antioxidants [38]. Furthermore, tocopherols are able to deactivate singlet oxygen ($^1O_2$), which oxidizes, amongst others, membrane lipids, proteins, amino acids, nucleic acids, nucleotides, and carbohydrates [39,40]. The chemical reaction of tocopherols with $^1O_2$ results in the corresponding tocopherol quinones (and other derivatives), some of which have been shown to be potent antioxidants [41–43].

3. Tocopherols in Plants and Mammalians

Tocopherols occur in mammalians, photosynthetic bacteria, fungi, algae, and plants, but only photosynthetic organisms are able to synthesize them [2,3]. The content, composition, and presence of tocopherols varies widely in different plant tissues. They can be found in seeds, fruits, roots, and tubers and are usually present in the green parts of higher plants [15,44]. The most abundant form in leaves is α-tocopherol, whereas the dominating tocopherol form in seeds is γ-tocopherol [2,33]. Nevertheless, in some crops, for instance, sunflower, olive, safflower, wild *Euphorbia*, or grape, α-tocopherol is the main tocopherol form in seeds [45–49]. Total tocopherol content and composition strongly changes under conditions of plant oxidative stress including high light, salinity, drought, and low temperatures [3,31,32,50,51]. Both plant growth and development affect the levels of tocopherol content and composition, which changes for example during senescence, chloroplast to chromoplast conversion, fruit ripening, and seed development [51–55].

Since 1922, when the term vitamin E was introduced by Evans and Bishop [56], the role of vitamin E has been extensively studied in mammalian systems and the beneficial effects demonstrated. Their antioxidant and radical scavenging mechanisms have been described in a variety of studies [57–60]. In these studies, tocopherols and tocotrienols are termed vitamin E as they usually occur as a mixture in food. Because vitamin E cannot be synthesized by humans, it is an essential component of our nutrition. A sufficient uptake of vitamin E can help to prevent neurological disorders and chronic diseases, especially those believed to have an oxidative stress component such as atherosclerosis, cataracts, and cancer [60–69]. In recent years, studies focused also on the role of other vitamin E forms such as γ-tocopherol, δ-tocopherol, and γ-tocotrienol as well as on the non-antioxidant molecular mechanisms to explain the regulatory effects of vitamin E on signal transduction and gene expression in mammals [70–72].

According to the German Society for Nutrition (Deutsche Gesellschaft für Ernährung e.V.), the recommended daily amount of vitamin E for an adult between 25 and 51 years is 14 mg/day. Nuts, seeds, and vegetable oils are among the best sources for the dietary uptake but also green leafy vegetables, fruits, and cereals. Soybean, rapeseed, and corn oil are the best dietary sources for γ-tocopherol, whereas the most biologically active form of vitamin E, α-tocopherol, can be found in wheat germ oil, sunflower, and olive oils [34,73]. Of the naturally occurring α-forms, the stereoisomers RRR-α-tocopherols have the highest biological activity. They can be stored and transported in the body due to specific selection by the hepatic α-tocopherol transfer protein (α-TTP) [34]. Thus, the increase in vitamin E content and the enrichment of α-tocopherol in vegetable oils is of particular interest in crop breeding.

4. Studying the Plant Tocopherol Biosynthesis Key Genes

In leaves, tocopherols are located in chloroplast membranes, plastoglobules, and thylakoid membranes and are thus in close proximity to the photosynthetic apparatus. For this reason, it was believed that tocopherols were the most important antioxidants in plants for preventing damage to the apparatus from photosynthesis-derived ROS. However, recent studies indicate that tocopherols only partially contribute to a considerable variety of plant antioxidants such as carotenoids, ascorbates, glutathiones, and flavonoids, which also contribute to photo-protection [74–76]. Nevertheless, tocopherols are crucial for the inhibition of non-enzymatic lipid peroxidation during stress conditions, supporting the germination of seedlings and are needed for the protection of seed storage lipids [15,32,77]. They are involved in a plethora of others functions such as the activation of plant defense responses, intracellular signaling, transcript regulation, and function in membrane stability [32,77–79].

Step 1: Homogentisic Acid Synthesis

The first committed step of the tocopherol biosynthesis is initiated by the gene *PDS1*, known to encode the enzyme p-hydroxyphenylpyruvate dioxygenase (HPPD) and was initially detected in carrot cells [10]. The corresponding *A. thaliana pds1* mutant was devoid of tocopherols and plastoquinones and had a lethal photobleached phenotype, thus showing that *PDS1* is a key gene of the tocopherol biosynthesis pathway [16,17]. In *Escherichia coli* (*E. coli*) expression studies, the protein HPPD catalyzed the accumulation of HGA. The subsequent oxidative polymerization of HGA to an ochronotic pigment resulted in a brownish coloration of the growth medium [10,80–82].

Constitutive expression of *PDS1* in *A. thaliana* plants led to elevated tocopherol concentrations of up to 43% in leaves and 28% in seeds, without a change in tocopherol composition [18]. In other studies, overexpression of the gene in tobacco leaves or in *A. thaliana* seeds resulted only in slightly increased tocopherol concentrations [83–85]. It was reasoned that HGA not only serves as a substrate for tocochromanols synthesis but also for other secondary plant metabolites e.g., plastoquinones [17]. Higher tocopherol concentrations were achieved when *PDS1* was co-expressed with downstream genes within the tocopherol biosynthetic pathway, the tocopherol content in seeds of *A. thaliana*, rapeseed, and corn kernels increased up to 1.8-, 2.0- and 3-fold, respectively [86–88].

The expression of *PDS1* is also linked to fruit ripening as well as leaf senescence in rice and barley [54,81,89]. Both ripening and leaf aging are correlated with an increase in tocopherol concentration, which is thought to be induced by ethylene treatment and oxidative stress [54,81]. This was underlined by sequence motifs for abscisic acid- and ethylene-specific response elements that were found in the promoter region of *PDS1*, indicating that these compounds can affect tocopherol biosynthesis.

Step 2: Polyprenyl Side Chain Synthesis

Uptake experiments of cotyledon-derived soybean suspension cultures with different tocopherol precursors demonstrated that PDP, together with HGA, has a high impact on tocopherol synthesis [86]. PDP, the polyprenyl side chain of tocopherols, can originate from two sources: direct reduction of geranylgeranyl diphosphate (GGDP) and free phytol, a product of chlorophyll degradation [14,90–92]. The latter was detected in experiments where the addition of free phytol in safflower cell cultures resulted in an 18-fold increase in total tocopherol content [93]. Additionally, feeding experiments of *A. thaliana* seedlings with labeled PDP demonstrated the integration of free phytol into tocopherols [92]. Further evidence was the detection of an *A. thaliana vte5*-1 mutant plant, which had a 20% reduced seed tocopherol concentration compared to the wild type and increased amounts of free phytol. The corresponding VTE5 protein had a high homology to a dolichol kinase and was able to catalyze the phosphorylation of free phytol into PDP [14].

Interestingly, tomato plants that have *VTE5*-like knockdown genes and are deficient in leaf and fruit tocopherol displayed multifaceted impacted metabolisms. While the chlorophyll content was not affected, the knockdown resulted in an alteration of the prenyl lipid profile in fruits and in an increase in the fatty acid phytyl ester synthesis in leaves, leading to changes in photosynthesis and sugar partitioning, which in turn affected tomato fruit quality [94].

The long-missing second enzyme of the phosphorylation pathway, phytyl phosphate kinase (VTE6) has recently been discovered using a phylogenetic approach [13]. The transgenic constitutive overexpression of the gene resulted in a 2-fold increase in PDP that led to a higher γ-tocopherol accumulation in seeds. The corresponding Arabidopsis mutant plants were tocopherol-deficient in leaves, and impaired in seed longevity and plant growth [13]. Intriguingly, the authors speculated that the impaired growth of the *vte6* mutants might be an effect of phytol accumulation rather than tocopherol shortage, resulting in a disruption of chlorophyll and galactolipid synthesis in chloroplast membranes. Recent studies also showed that tocopherol levels are indirectly regulated through the contribution of chlorophyll synthases by reducing PDP precursors, thus providing new possible alternative routes for improving tocopherol content [91,95].

Step 3: MPBQ (2-Methyl-6-Phytyl-1,4-Benzoquinol) Synthesis

The condensation of HGA and PDP to MPBQ is catalyzed by the enzyme HPT, which is encoded by the gene *VTE2* [96,97]. *A. thaliana* plants lacking *VTE2* are completely deficient in all tocopherol derivatives and all pathway precursors, indicating that this is a limiting step in tocopherol biosynthesis [98]. Transgenic approaches downregulating *VTE2* mRNA levels by antisense RNA led to a 10-fold reduction of tocopherol content in *A. thaliana* seeds. In contrast, overexpression of *VTE2* resulted in up to a 2-fold increased tocopherol concentration in seeds and up to a 4.4-fold increase in leaves [20,22]. Interestingly, in rapeseed, only minor increases were attained by seed-specific expression of the *VTE2* gene from the bacteria Synechocystis sp. PCC 6803, suggesting species-specific differences in tocopherol biosynthesis regulation [86]. The constitutive expression of the lettuce homolog (*LsHPT*) caused an increase up to 4-fold of the α- and 2.6-fold of γ-tocopherol content in lettuce leaves in comparison to the non-transformed plants [99].

The lack of tocopherols in *A. thaliana vte2* mutants made their functional role particularly apparent in those plants. Seedlings exhibited severe defects during germination and early seedling growth due to high concentrations of non-enzymatic lipid peroxides and hydroxy fatty acids, indicating that tocopherols are crucial for the prevention of lipid oxidation during these important developmental stages. The seedlings were disturbed in root growth and in cotyledon expansion and showed a slowed storage lipid catabolism [21]. Furthermore, the authors showed that seed viability was heavily impacted in *vte2* mutants compared to the wild type, probably due to the non-enzymatic oxidation of storage lipids. The accumulation of lipid peroxidation products in *vte2* mutants was correlated with an increased expression of many defense-related genes, showing another main role of tocopherols in the regulation of plant defense responses by modulating the levels of lipid peroxidation products [21]. The developmental and molecular phenotypes of *vte2* are abolished if tri-unsaturated fatty acids are suppressed as shown in the quadruple mutant *fad3-2fad7-2fad8vte2-1*, proving that there is a *vte2*-specific phenotype [100]. The presence of plastochromanol-8 (PC-8), a homolog of γ-tocotrienol with a C40 prenyl side chain, suppresses the phenotypes associated with lower plant fitness and seed longevity in *vte2* plants [101]. PC-8 has been found in vegetable oils and shown to display antioxidant activity, comparable to that of tocopherols [102,103].

Under normal growth conditions, as well as high light stress, adult *vte2* plants are indistinguishable from wild-type plants, confirming that tocopherols are substitutable by other antioxidants at this developmental stage [21,27,32]. However, if the same plants are subjected to low temperature, severe changes in gene transcription, as well as biochemical and physiological phenotypes, can be observed. The plants are compromised in transfer cell development and photoassimilate export, resulting in growth impairment [32,78,104]. Maeda et al., found that the specific underlying mechanisms need to be further investigated but speculate that plastid-localized tocopherols may have a role in the endoplasmic reticulum (ER) membrane lipid biosynthesis causing these effects [104].

Step 4: DMPBQ (2,3-dimethyl-6-phytyl-1,4-benzoquinone) Synthesis

The enzyme that methylates MPBQ to DMPBQ was first identified in *Synechocystis* sp. PCC 6803 and shares substrate specificities with the corresponding protein in *A. thaliana*, MPBQ methyltransferase [25,26]. The enzyme is encoded by the gene *VTE3* and without the catalysis of the prenylquinol DMPBQ, α- and γ-tocopherol could not be produced. The enzyme is also involved in plastoquinone synthesis and is able to use 2-methyl-6-solanesyl-1,4-benzoquinol (MSBQ) for the formation of plastoquinol-9 (PQ-9).

Several *A. thaliana vte3* mutants were isolated that had different phenotypes according to their origin and the severity of the mutation. Plants with a mutated *vet3-1* allele, derived from ethyl methanesulfonate (EMS) mutagenesis, were found to have a partial loss-of-function of the enzyme. As a result, an altered tocopherol composition along with reduced MPBQ/MSBQ methyltransferase activity was observed. In these plants, both δ- and β-tocopherol concentrations in leaves were increased at the expense of α-tocopherol, whereas γ-tocopherol was replaced by higher δ-tocopherol levels, but PQ amounts were not affected in seeds [25,26]. In contrast, plants with the non-functional *vte3-2* allele or Ds-tagged *A. thaliana* plants, which have a complete gene disruption, were deficient in α- and γ-tocopherol, as well as PQ. These mutants exhibited a pale green phenotype, abnormal chloroplasts and did not survive beyond the seedling stage [24,25].

The overexpression of *VTE3* in *A. thaliana* and soybean did not have a substantial impact on the tocopherol amounts but severely changed the tocopherol composition [26,75]. In seeds of transgenic soybean, increased γ- and α-tocopherol concentrations with simultaneous strong reductions in δ- and β-tocopherols concentrations were observed [26]. The seed-specific co-expression of *A. thaliana VTE3* and *VTE4* (γ-TMT) in soybean seeds shifted the tocopherol composition in favor of α-tocopherol (>90%). This is especially of interest for the genetic engineering of crop plants, in which seeds are naturally enriched in γ-tocopherol (e.g., rapeseed). The nutritional value of those plants could be enhanced by changing the composition towards α-tocopherol.

Step 5: Synthesis of γ-Tocopherol and δ-Tocopherol

Similar to the *vte2* mutant plants, *vte1* mutant plants lack all tocopherol forms due to the absence of a functional tocopherol cyclase (TC) enzyme. They accumulate the intermediate product DMPBQ, the un-cyclized precursor of γ-tocopherol, instead [27]. The expression of *AtVTE1* cDNA in *E. coli* efficiently converted DMPBQ into γ-tocopherol, demonstrating the cyclase activity of the enzyme [4,55,105]. Seed-specific expression of the *VTE1* gene from *A. thaliana* and maize (*Zea mays*) in transgenic rapeseed (*Brassica napus*) increased concentrations of all tocopherol forms in the seed oil of T_1 and T_2 generation plants. However, using different *B. napus VTE1* alleles, only a 1.5-fold increase in seed α-tocopherol was produced [82,105].

Interestingly, expression of the endogenous *VTE1* gene in *A. thaliana* plants under a constitutive promoter resulted in a 7-fold increase of the leaf tocopherol concentration and an extreme shift from α- to γ-tocopherol [28]. The reason for this shift was recently unraveled by Zbierzak et al. (2010). The authors showed that the co-elution of PC-8 with γ-tocopherol during High-performance liquid chromatography (HPLC) separation masked the result of increased γ-tocopherol concentrations [106]. PC-8 shares the same head group with γ-tocopherol and is derived from a cyclization step of PQ-9, the redox component of photosystem II. PQ-9 accumulates in *A. thaliana vte1* mutants, whereas PC-8 accumulates with tocopherols in *VTE1*-overexpressing plants, showing that TC is also able to cycle PQ-9 into PC-8 [105,106]. Accordingly, *AtVTE1* overexpression in rapeseed induces a 2.4-fold increase in PC-8 levels [105]. Nevertheless, the proportion of PC-8 with respect to total tocochromanols only ranged between 5 and 10%, suggesting that the majority of the effects observed in *vte1* mutants are indeed caused due to the absence of tocopherols [106].

The *A. thaliana vte1* mutant is not inhibited in its development, despite being deficient in tocopherols and $^1O_2$ accumulation in chloroplasts [107]. Germination, growth, chlorophyll content, and photosynthetic quantum yield were similar to the wild type and only slightly different in response to photo-oxidative stress and/or low temperatures [21,27,108]. The absence of these phenotypes is explained by the accumulation of the redox-active DMPBQ, whose quinol form can have similar antioxidant properties to tocopherol [21]. Furthermore, the absence of tocopherols in *vte1* mutants resulted in an increase of ascorbate and glutathione, which belong to the most abundant antioxidants in higher plants. This effect was reversed when *VTE1* was overexpressed: their concentrations were reduced to 40–60% relative to wild-type plants [28,75]. It is known that the ascorbate–glutathione cycle is linked to the regeneration of tocopheroxyl radicals, the oxidized forms of tocopherol and the result of the reaction of tocopherols with lipid peroxyl radicals [36]. Hence, ascorbate deficiency in *A. thaliana vte1* mutants caused increased lipid peroxidation in water-stressed plants [109]. Furthermore, the overexpression of *VTE1* led to enhanced tolerance against salt stress in rice and drought stress in tobacco plants, providing evidence that crop species with increased tolerance to environmental stresses as well as high tocopherol content could be developed [110,111].

Intriguingly, another analysis of *A. thaliana vte1* mutants revealed a different role of tocopherols and indicated that α-tocopherol may have an impact on cellular signaling by altering plant hormone levels [112,113]. In these mutants, an age-dependent increase of jasmonic acid levels was detected. The levels were up to 2.4-fold higher compared to the wild type and accompanied by reduced plant growth and increased anthocyanin production. It is suggested that the reaction is indirectly triggered by tocopherols by controlling the extent of lipid peroxidation and therefore the accumulation of lipid hydroperoxides, which, in turn, are used for jasmonic acid synthesis [114]. The role of jasmonic acid, especially during senescence, is associated with the downregulation of housekeeping genes, such as photosynthetic genes, and with the upregulation of defense genes related to biotic and abiotic stress [115,116]. These findings further support the hypothesis that tocopherols may, albeit indirectly, contribute to gene expression regulation [78].

The analysis of the maize gene *sucrose export defective1* (*SXD1*) led to the suggestion that tocopherols might play a role in regulating carbon translocation. The maize *sxd1* mutant has a *vte1* mutant resembling phenotype that is characterized, amongst others, by the leaf-specific accumulation of starch and anthocyanin, and the deposition of callose in phloem parenchyma transfer cells. These characteristics are coincident with a loss of the symplastic transport, as well as a typical increase of the soluble sugar content due to the sucrose export deficiency [117–119]. RNAi inhibition of *StSXD1* expression in potato also induces defects in carbohydrate transport [120], showing that the functions of tocopherols are not assigned to a specific photosynthesis type and may be conserved in monocot and dicot plant species [55].

Step 6: Synthesis of α-Tocopherol and β-Tocopherol

The final step of the tocopherol synthesis is catalyzed by the gene *VTE4* and encodes a key enzyme (γ-TMT) that methylates both δ- and γ-tocopherol to β- and α-tocopherol, respectively (Figure 1). Correspondingly, α-tocopherol was absent in leaves of *vte4 A. thaliana* mutants, whereas high levels of γ-tocopherol accumulated [31]. Development and growth of the mutant plants was similar to that of the wild type, with only slight differences during oxidative stress, e.g., in chlorophyll content and photosynthetic quantum yield. The accumulation of γ-tocopherol had no impact on the amount of fatty acids or on lipid hydrolysis, indicating that γ-tocopherol is able to functionally substitute α-tocopherol [31,32].

VTE4-silenced tobacco plants had a decreased tolerance against salt-induced stress but an increased tolerance towards sorbitol stress and methyl viologen, an inductor of photo-oxidative stress. These findings suggest specific functions for different tocopherol forms with respect to stress, e.g., γ-tocopherol in the desiccation tolerance of seeds [50]. This hypothesis is supported by the fact that γ-tocopherol is the naturally predominant form in most seeds. Sattler et al. (2004) could show that a loss of γ-tocopherol increases the oxidation of polyunsaturated fatty acids and thereby diminishes seed longevity in *A. thaliana* [21]. Intriguingly, only in mature leaves of salt-stressed *vte4* mutant plants transcription levels of jasmonic acid- and ethylene-signaling genes were downregulated, but not in *vte1* mutants, or in wild-type plants. This suggests that γ-tocopherol, rather than α-tocopherol, plays a role in the regulation of these genes during osmotic stress [121].

The exclusive overexpression of the *VTE4* gene in leaves changed both tocopherol composition and content, resulting in elevated α-tocopherol values and up to a 30% increase in total tocopherol content [75]. Seed-specific expression of the gene nearly converted the entire amount of γ-tocopherol into α-tocopherol in soybean and *A. thaliana* [26,33]. Because most plant species accumulate mainly γ-tocopherol in seeds (>95%), γ-TMT activity might be a limiting bottleneck for α-tocopherol synthesis in seeds. This is consistent with the isolation of low α-tocopherol sunflower mutants, the natural wild type of which normally exhibit up to 90% α-tocopherol in kernels [122]. In these sunflower mutants, two *VTE4* paralogues are reduced or disrupted in their expression, leading to the accumulation of γ-tocopherol (>90%). This confirms that *VTE4* expression in sunflower seeds directly regulates the amount of α-tocopherol.

The fact that γ-TMT activity is limiting, becomes particularly clear when plants are exposed to abiotic stress. High levels of γ- and δ-tocopherol levels were observed in stressed leaves of *VTE2* overexpressing plants but not when *VTE2* and *VTE4* were simultaneously expressed [123]. Moreover, the concomitant overexpression of *VTE2* and *VTE4* was additive in *A. thaliana* leaves and seeds. The total tocopherol content increased up to 12-fold, while, at the same time, all of the γ-tocopherol was converted to α-tocopherol [20,75]. Thus, *VTE4* is suggested to be a key gene for metabolic engineering of enhanced α-tocopherol levels in crop plants. Similarly, using a transgenic approach, Endrigkeit et al., showed that a *B. napus VTE4* homolog was able to increase the α-tocopherol content 50-fold in transgenic Arabidopsis seeds, providing a promising candidate for the marker-assisted selection of α-tocopherol content in rapeseed [124].

5. Breeding for Higher Vitamin E Content

Improving vitamin E content in staple crops has been a major aim of crop breeding due to its benefits for health and oil quality [125]. Vitamin E content and composition vary widely in different crops, such as rapeseed, maize, rice, soybean, and barley [126–130]. These variations provide an incentive for breeding varieties that have superior vitamin E content. Quantitative genetic approaches, which map quantitative trait loci (QTLs) onto linkage maps or which detect associations between markers and phenotypes, are powerful methods to dissect complex traits in crops [131]. To date, dozens of QTL and association mapping studies related to vitamin E have been carried out in major crops including rapeseed, maize, soybean, rice, barley, and tomato [95,126,127,129,130,132–134]. As an example, Marwede et al., detected eight QTL-related to tocopherol content and composition in a doubled haploid rapeseed population [135]. However, Wang et al. discovered 33 QTLs and 61 associated loci for rapeseed tocopherol content and composition in a joint QTL, candidate gene, and association mapping study [132]. In another candidate-gene based association analysis, alleles of genes encoding the key enzymes of the core biosynthetic pathway associated with tocopherol content and composition in rapeseed were identified [126]. Intriguingly, the found QTLs explained only a small part of the phenotypic variation in tocopherol content and composition in rapeseed (5–30%). Diepenbrock et al. found 52 QTLs associated with vitamin E content using a 5000 line U.S. nested association mapping (NAM) panel [95]. Surprisingly, of the 14 resolved to individual genes, six novel genes affecting tocochromanols in plants were identified. These included unexpectedly two chlorophyll biosynthetic enzymes being major determinants of tocopherol content in non-photosynthetic maize grains, allowing new insights into tocopherol biosynthesis regulation [95]. Nevertheless, these QTL and association mapping analyses provide the foundation for improving vitamin E content in crops but also indicate that the genetic mechanism of vitamin E biosynthesis in crops remains incomplete and needs more comprehensive research. Some crop species are also facing breeding bottlenecks due to their low genetic inheritance in elite germplasm and have to use introgression from wild species, mutagenesis, or biotech methods to enhance different forms and levels of tocopherol [135–138].

Moreover, Quadrana et al., analyzed *VTE3* alleles and detected that their differential expression is associated with differences in methylation of a short-interspersed nuclear element (SINE) retrotransposon located in the promoter region that is responsible for the regulation of vitamin E content in tomatoes [139]. In another study, it was found that a chlorophyll synthase was able to induce the production of small interfering RNAs, accompanied with an increase in tocopherol levels [91]. These observations indicate that the tocopherol biosynthetic pathway might be regulated epigenetically and could also partially explain the low phenotypic variation found in QTL studies.

The vitamin E biosynthetic pathway has been well elucidated in model species, and select genes have been transformed and overexpressed individually or collectively in various plants to improve vitamin E content and composition [26,87,125,128,140–149]. For oil crops, the enhancement of γ-tocopherol is important in order to prevent oil peroxidation and thus to improve oil quality [150]. Since α-tocopherol is considered to have the highest nutritional value for humans and livestock, breeding crops with high α-tocopherol concentrations and good nutritional value is a target. For example, Yusuf et al., was able to elevate α-tocopherol concentrations 6-fold by overexpressing Arabidopsis *VTE4* in *B. juncea* plants [151]. In another study, α-tocopherol content was increased up to 11 times in soybean by overexpressing *VTE4* [152,153]. Interestingly, by transgenically expressing the *VTE1* gene, rice and tobacco plants with an increased tolerance against salt and drought stress, respectively, and a simultaneously enhanced tocopherol content were developed [110,111]. These findings provide prospects for breeding vitamin E biofortified crops that are even tolerant against environmental stresses through biotechnology methods.

In contrast to attempts to improve α-tocopherol content, it is relatively difficult to significantly increase the total vitamin E content in crops. The most successful attempts at increasing total vitamin E content have occurred in rapeseed and soybean, with a nearly 2.4-fold and 15-fold enhancement, respectively, of total vitamin E content after co-overexpression of several key genes for vitamin E biosynthesis [86,87]. Collectively, these observations indicate that the tocopherol biosynthetic pathway and its regulation are complex. Nevertheless, natural variations and transgenic strategies can be used in vitamin E biofortification breeding.

6. Conclusions and Challenges

Present studies using model plant species demonstrate that vitamin E biosynthesis genes are well understood. The use of mutant plants has helped with the discovery and analysis of the roles of tocopherols in plant processes beyond their antioxidant function. However, open questions remain about the specific functions of the different tocopherol forms as well as their concrete roles in signaling and defense responses. Additionally, plastoquinones and tocotrienols, which are known to be derived from the same head group as tocopherols, have gained attention in recent years but most of their roles still remain elusive [17,55,102,154,155].

Recently, new genes and epigenetic mechanisms have been discovered through investigations of the chlorophyll degradation pathway, transgenic and phylogenetic approaches, or by conducting joint linkage/genome-wide association studies [13,91,95]. Moreover, even in crops with hexaploid genomes, such as oat, the genes of the tocopherol pathway have been identified via deep sequencing and by using the high conservation of the tocopherol biosynthesis genes between plant species [156].

Natural variations of vitamin E content have been investigated and demonstrated wide variations in/among different crops, which suggest a tremendous genetic potential for breeding vitamin E improved crops. On this basis, several QTL/association mapping studies have been carried out and have detected a range of genetic loci associated with vitamin E content and composition, but of which many detected loci cannot pinpoint candidate genes [95,129,130,132,157–159]. Furthermore, epigenetics may be involved in regulating the vitamin E biosynthesis and can partially explain the low phenotypic variation of the detected genetic loci, indicating that vitamin E biosynthesis in crops may be more complex than that in model plants [91,139]. Transgenic approaches have also been used for vitamin E improvement in crops, and an increased α-tocopherol content has been achieved [20]. Elevating vitamin E content, even by stacking candidate genes, is still a challenge, but tocopherol enhancing alleles of the pathway genes have been identified, for example, in *B. napus*, and can now be used for marker-assisted breeding [86,126].

To date, many crops have been sequenced including vitamin E-rich staple crops, such as rapeseed, soybean, maize, and rice [160–163]. These sequences will be used in the process of cloning new genes from QTL and enable us to fully understand the genetic basis of vitamin E variations and biosynthesis. Thanks to the rapid development of biotechnology, many methods for efficient genome-editing have become available [164]. For example, CRISPR/Cas9 (Clustered Regularly Interspaced Short Palindromic Repeats/ CRISPR-associated protein 9), which is one of the most popular genome-editing methods at present, can efficiently and precisely edit gene/genes in mammals and plants. A genome-editing approach based on the cloned genes from QTL in crops and CRISPR/Cas9 can be a promising alternative strategy in breeding vitamin E biofortification crops [165].

Acknowledgments: We are grateful for Kim McGrouter and Michelle Harnett from Scion, Rotorua, as well as the two anonymous reviewers for critically reading the manuscript and suggesting substantial improvements.

References

1. DellaPenna, D.; Pogson, B.J. Vitamin synthesis in plants: Tocopherols and carotenoids. *Annu. Rev. Plant Biol.* **2006**, *57*, 711–738. [CrossRef] [PubMed]
2. Grusak, M.A.; DellaPenna, D. Improving the nutrient composition of plants to enhance human nutrition and health. *Annu. Rev. Plant Biol.* **1999**, *50*, 133–161. [CrossRef] [PubMed]
3. Munné-Bosch, S.; Alegre, L. The function of tocopherols and tocotrienols in plants. *Crit. Rev. Plant Sci.* **2002**, *21*, 31–57. [CrossRef]
4. DellaPenna, D.; Last, R.L. Progress in the dissection and manipulation of plant vitamin E biosynthesis. *Physiol. Plant.* **2006**, *126*, 356–368. [CrossRef]
5. DellaPenna, D. A decade of progress in understanding vitamin E synthesis in plants. *J. Plant Physiol.* **2005**, *162*, 729–737. [CrossRef] [PubMed]

6. Péter, S.; Friedel, A.; Roos, F.F.; Wyss, A.; Eggersdorfer, M.; Hoffmann, K.; Weber, P. A systematic review of global alpha-tocopherol status as assessed by nutritional intake levels and blood serum concentrations. *Int. J. Vitam. Nutr. Res.* **2016**, *14*, 1–21. [CrossRef] [PubMed]

7. Soll, J.; Douce, R.; Schultz, G. Site of biosynthesis of alpha-tocopherol in spinach chloroplasts. *FEBS Lett.* **1980**, *112*, 243–246. [CrossRef]

8. Vidi, P.A.; Kanwischer, M.; Baginsky, S.; Austin, J.R.; Csucs, G.; Dormann, P.; Kessler, F.; Brehelin, C. Tocopherol cyclase (VTE1) localization and vitamin E accumulation in chloroplast plastoglobule lipoprotein particles. *J. Biol. Chem.* **2006**, *281*, 11225–11234. [CrossRef] [PubMed]

9. Soll, J.; Schultz, G.; Joyard, J.; Douce, R.; Block, M.A. Localization and synthesis of prenylquinones in isolated outer and inner envelope membranes from spinach chloroplasts. *Arch. Biochem. Biophys.* **1985**, *238*, 290–299. [CrossRef]

10. Garcia, I.; Rodgers, M.; Lenne, C.; Rolland, A.; Sailland, A.; Matringe, M. Subcellular localization and purification of a *p*-hydroxyphenylpyruvate dioxygenase from cultured carrot cells and characterization of the corresponding cDNA. *Biochem. J.* **1997**, *325 Pt 3*, 761–769. [CrossRef] [PubMed]

11. Riewe, D.; Koohi, M.; Lisec, J.; Pfeiffer, M.; Lippmann, R.; Schmeichel, J.; Willmitzer, L.; Altmann, T. A tyrosine aminotransferase involved in tocopherol synthesis in *Arabidopsis*. *Plant J.* **2012**, *71*, 850–859. [CrossRef] [PubMed]

12. Hortensteiner, S. Chlorophyll degradation during senescence. *Annu. Rev. Plant Biol.* **2006**, *57*, 55–77. [CrossRef] [PubMed]

13. Vom Dorp, K.; Hölzl, G.; Plohmann, C.; Eisenhut, M.; Abraham, M.; Weber, A.P.; Hanson, A.D.; Dörmann, P. Remobilization of phytol from chlorophyll degradation is essential for tocopherol synthesis and growth of *Arabidopsis*. *Plant Cell* **2015**, *27*, 2846–2859. [CrossRef] [PubMed]

14. Valentin, H.E.; Lincoln, K.; Moshiri, F.; Jensen, P.K.; Qi, Q.; Venkatesh, T.V.; Karunanandaa, B.; Baszis, S.R.; Norris, S.R.; Savidge, B.; et al. The Arabidopsis vitamin E pathway gene5-1 mutant reveals a critical role for phytol kinase in seed tocopherol biosynthesis. *Plant Cell* **2006**, *18*, 212–224. [CrossRef] [PubMed]

15. Mene-Saffrane, L.; DellaPenna, D. Biosynthesis, regulation and functions of tocochromanols in plants. *Plant Physiol. Biochem.* **2010**, *48*, 301–309. [CrossRef] [PubMed]

16. Norris, S.R.; Shen, X.; DellaPenna, D. Complementation of the Arabidopsis pds1 mutation with the gene encoding *p*-hydroxyphenylpyruvate dioxygenase. *Plant Physiol.* **1998**, *117*, 1317–1323. [CrossRef] [PubMed]

17. Norris, S.R.; Barrette, T.R.; DellaPenna, D. Genetic dissection of carotenoid synthesis in Arabidopsis defines plastoquinone as an essential component of phytoene desaturation. *Plant Cell* **1995**, *7*, 2139–2149. [CrossRef] [PubMed]

18. Tsegaye, Y.; Shintani, D.K.; DellaPenna, D. Overexpression of the enzyme *p*-hydroxyphenolpyruvate dioxygenase in *Arabidopsis* and its relation to tocopherol biosynthesis. *Plant Physiol. Biochem.* **2002**, *40*, 913–920. [CrossRef]

19. Schwab, R.; Palatnik, J.F.; Riester, M.; Schommer, C.; Schmid, M.; Weigel, D. Specific effects of microRNAs on the plant transcriptome. *Dev. Cell* **2005**, *8*, 517–527. [CrossRef] [PubMed]

20. Collakova, E.; DellaPenna, D. Homogentisate phytyltransferase activity is limiting for tocopherol biosynthesis in *Arabidopsis*. *Plant Physiol.* **2003**, *131*, 632–642. [CrossRef] [PubMed]

21. Sattler, S.E.; Gilliland, L.U.; Magallanes-Lundback, M.; Pollard, M.; DellaPenna, D. Vitamin E is essential for seed longevity and for preventing lipid peroxidation during germination. *Plant Cell* **2004**, *16*, 1419–1432. [CrossRef] [PubMed]

22. Savidge, B.; Weiss, J.D.; Wong, Y.H.H.; Lassner, M.W.; Mitsky, T.A.; Shewmaker, C.K.; Post-Beittenmiller, D.; Valentin, H.E. Isolation and characterization of homogentisate phytyltransferase genes from *Synechocystis* sp. PCC 6803 and *Arabidopsis*. *Plant Physiol.* **2002**, *129*, 321–332. [CrossRef] [PubMed]

23. Venkatesh, T.V.; Karunanandaa, B.; Free, D.L.; Rottnek, J.M.; Baszis, S.R.; Valentin, H.E. Identification and characterization of an *Arabidopsis* homogentisate phytyltransferase paralog. *Planta* **2006**, *223*, 1–11. [CrossRef] [PubMed]

24. Motohashi, R.; Ito, T.; Kobayashi, M.; Taji, T.; Nagata, N.; Asami, T.; Yoshida, S.; Yamaguchi-Shinozaki, K.; Shinozaki, K. Functional analysis of the 37 kDa inner envelope membrane polypeptide in chloroplast biogenesis using a Ds-tagged *Arabidopsis* pale-green mutant. *Plant J.* **2003**, *34*, 719–731. [CrossRef] [PubMed]

25. Cheng, Z.; Sattler, S.; Maeda, H.; Sakuragi, Y.; Bryant, D.A.; DellaPenna, D. Highly divergent methyltransferases catalyze a conserved reaction in tocopherol and plastoquinone synthesis in cyanobacteria and photosynthetic eukaryotes. *Plant Cell* **2003**, *15*, 2343–2356. [CrossRef] [PubMed]
26. Van Eenennaam, A.L.; Lincoln, K.; Durrett, T.P.; Valentin, H.E.; Shewmaker, C.K.; Thorne, G.M.; Jiang, J.; Baszis, S.R.; Levering, C.K.; Aasen, E.D.; et al. Engineering vitamin E content: From *Arabidopsis* mutant to soy oil. *Plant Cell* **2003**, *15*, 3007–3019. [CrossRef] [PubMed]
27. Porfirova, S.; Bergmüller, E.; Tropf, S.; Lemke, R.; Dörmann, P. Isolation of an *Arabidopsis* mutant lacking vitamin E and identification of a cyclase essential for all tocopherol biosynthesis. *Proc. Natl. Acad. Sci. USA* **2002**, *99*, 12495–12500. [CrossRef] [PubMed]
28. Kanwischer, M.; Porfirova, S.; Bergmuller, E.; Dormann, P. Alterations in tocopherol cyclase activity in transgenic and mutant plants of *Arabidopsis* affect tocopherol content, tocopherol composition, and oxidative stress. *Plant Physiol.* **2005**, *137*, 713–723. [CrossRef] [PubMed]
29. Sattler, S.E.; Cahoon, E.B.; Coughlan, S.J.; DellaPenna, D. Characterization of tocopherol cyclases from higher plants and cyanobacteria. Evolutionary implications for tocopherol synthesis and function. *Plant Physiol.* **2003**, *132*, 2184–2195. [CrossRef] [PubMed]
30. Semchuk, N.M.; Lushchak, O.V.; Falk, J.; Krupinska, K.; Lushchak, V.I. Inactivation of genes, encoding tocopherol biosynthetic pathway enzymes, results in oxidative stress in outdoor grown *Arabidopsis thaliana*. *Plant Physiol. Biochem.* **2009**, *47*, 384–390. [CrossRef] [PubMed]
31. Bergmüller, E.; Porfirova, S.; Dörmann, P. Characterization of an *Arabidopsis* mutant deficient in γ-tocopherolmethyltransferase. *Plant Mol. Biol.* **2003**, *52*, 1181–1190. [CrossRef] [PubMed]
32. Maeda, H.; Song, W.; Sage, T.L.; DellaPenna, D. Tocopherols play a crucial role in low-temperature adaptation and Phloem loading in *Arabidopsis*. *Plant Cell* **2006**, *18*, 2710–2732. [CrossRef] [PubMed]
33. Shintani, D.; DellaPenna, D. Elevating the vitamin E content of plants through metabolic engineering. *Science* **1998**, *282*, 2098–2100. [CrossRef] [PubMed]
34. Brigelius-Flohe, R.; Traber, M.G. Vitamin E: Function and metabolism. *FASEB J.* **1999**, *13*, 1145–1155. [PubMed]
35. Krieger-Liszkay, A.; Fufezan, C.; Trebst, A. Singlet oxygen production in photosystem II and related protection mechanism. *Photosynth. Res.* **2008**, *98*, 551–564. [CrossRef] [PubMed]
36. Kamal-Eldin, A.; Appelqvist, L.A. The chemistry and antioxidant properties of tocopherols and tocotrienols. *Lipids* **1996**, *31*, 671–701. [CrossRef] [PubMed]
37. Liebler, D.C. The role of metabolism in the antioxidant function of vitamin E. *Crit. Rev. Toxicol.* **1993**, *23*, 147–169. [CrossRef] [PubMed]
38. Fukuzawa, K.; Tokumura, A.; Ouchi, S.; Tsukatani, H. Antioxidant activities of tocopherols on Fe^{2+}-ascorbate-induced lipid peroxidation in lecithin liposomes. *Lipids* **1982**, *17*, 511–513. [CrossRef] [PubMed]
39. Halliwell, B.; Gutteridge, J.M. *Free Radicals in Biology and Medicine*; Oxford University Press: New York, NY, USA, 2015.
40. Straight, R.C.; Spikes, J.D. Photosensitized oxidation of biomolecules. In *Singlet O_2*; Frimer, A.A., Ed.; CRC Press: Boca Raton, FL, USA, 1985; Volume 4, pp. 91–143.
41. Lass, A.; Sohal, R.S. Electron transport-linked ubiquinone-dependent recycling of alpha-tocopherol inhibits autooxidation of mitochondrial membranes. *Arch. Biochem. Biophys.* **1998**, *352*, 229–236. [CrossRef] [PubMed]
42. Siegel, D.; Bolton, E.M.; Burr, J.A.; Liebler, D.C.; Ross, D. The reduction of α-tocopherolquinone by human NAD(P)H: Quinone oxidoreductase: The role of α-tocopherolhydroquinone as a cellular antioxidant. *Mol. Pharmacol.* **1997**, *52*, 300–305. [PubMed]
43. Wu, J.H.; Croft, K.D. Vitamin E metabolism. *Mol. Aspects Med.* **2007**, *28*, 437–452. [CrossRef] [PubMed]
44. Horvath, G.; Wessjohann, L.; Bigirimana, J.; Jansen, M.; Guisez, Y.; Caubergs, R.; Horemans, N. Differential distribution of tocopherols and tocotrienols in photosynthetic and non-photosynthetic tissues. *Phytochemistry* **2006**, *67*, 1185–1195. [CrossRef] [PubMed]
45. Velasco, L.; Fernández-Martínez, J.; Garcia-Ruiz, R.; Domínguez, J. Genetic and environmental variation for tocopherol content and composition in sunflower commercial hybrids. *J. Agric. Sci.* **2002**, *139*, 425–429. [CrossRef]
46. Bruni, R.; Muzzoli, M.; Ballero, M.; Loi, M.C.; Fantin, G.; Poli, F.; Sacchetti, G. Tocopherols, fatty acids and sterols in seeds of four Sardinian wild Euphorbia species. *Fitoterapia* **2004**, *75*, 50–61. [CrossRef] [PubMed]

47. Horvath, G.; Wessjohann, L.; Bigirimana, J.; Monica, H.; Jansen, M.; Guisez, Y.; Caubergs, R.; Horemans, N. Accumulation of tocopherols and tocotrienols during seed development of grape (*Vitis vinifera* L. cv. Albert Lavallee). *Plant Physiol. Biochem.* **2006**, *44*, 724–731. [CrossRef] [PubMed]
48. Cayuela, J.A.; García, J.F. Sorting olive oil based on alpha-tocopherol and total tocopherol content using near-infra-red spectroscopy (NIRS) analysis. *J. Food Eng.* **2017**, *202*, 79–88. [CrossRef]
49. Gotor, A.A.; Farkas, E.; Berger, M.; Labalette, F.; Centis, S.; Daydé, J.; Calmon, A. Determination of tocopherols and phytosterols in sunflower seeds by NIR spectrometry. *Eur. J. Lipid Sci. Technol.* **2007**, *109*, 525–530. [CrossRef]
50. Abbasi, A.R.; Hajirezaei, M.; Hofius, D.; Sonnewald, U.; Voll, L.M. Specific roles of alpha- and gamma-tocopherol in abiotic stress responses of transgenic tobacco. *Plant Physiol.* **2007**, *143*, 1720–1738. [CrossRef] [PubMed]
51. Arango, Y.; Heise, K.-P. Localization of α-tocopherol synthesis in chromoplast envelope membranes of *Capsicum annuum* L. fruits. *J. Exp. Bot.* **1998**, *49*, 1259–1262. [CrossRef]
52. Abushita, A.A.; Hebshi, E.A.; Daood, H.G.; Biacs, P.A. Determination of antioxidant vitamins in tomatoes. *Food Chem.* **1997**, *60*, 207–212. [CrossRef]
53. Arrom, L.; Munné-Bosch, S. Tocopherol composition in flower organs of *Lilium* and its variations during natural and artificial senescence. *Plant Sci.* **2010**, *179*, 289–295. [CrossRef]
54. Falk, J.; Krauß, N.; Dähnhardt, D.; Krupinska, K. The senescence associated gene of barley encoding 4-hydroxyphenylpyruvate dioxygenase is expressed during oxidative stress. *J. Plant Physiol.* **2002**, *159*, 1245–1253. [CrossRef]
55. Falk, J.; Munne-Bosch, S. Tocochromanol functions in plants: Antioxidation and beyond. *J. Exp. Bot.* **2010**, *61*, 1549–1566. [CrossRef] [PubMed]
56. Evans, H.M.; Bishop, K.S. On the Existence of a Hitherto Unrecognized Dietary Factor Essential for Reproduction. *Science* **1922**, *56*, 650–651. [CrossRef] [PubMed]
57. Azzi, A.; Gysin, R.; Kempna, P.; Munteanu, A.; Negis, Y.; Villacorta, L.; Visarius, T.; Zingg, J.M. Vitamin E mediates cell signaling and regulation of gene expression. *Ann. N. Y. Acad. Sci.* **2004**, *1031*, 86–95. [CrossRef] [PubMed]
58. Azzi, A.; Ricciarelli, R.; Zingg, J.M. Non-antioxidant molecular functions of α-tocopherol (vitamin E). *FEBS Lett.* **2002**, *519*, 8–10. [CrossRef]
59. Zingg, J.M.; Azzi, A. Non-antioxidant activities of vitamin E. *Curr. Med. Chem.* **2004**, *11*, 1113–1133. [CrossRef] [PubMed]
60. Schneider, C. Chemistry and biology of vitamin E. *Mol. Nutr. Food Res.* **2005**, *49*, 7–30. [CrossRef] [PubMed]
61. Kushi, L.H.; Folsom, A.R.; Prineas, R.J.; Mink, P.J.; Wu, Y.; Bostick, R.M. Dietary antioxidant vitamins and death from coronary heart disease in postmenopausal women. *N. Engl. J. Med.* **1996**, *334*, 1156–1162. [CrossRef] [PubMed]
62. Weinstein, S.J.; Wright, M.E.; Lawson, K.A.; Snyder, K.; Mannisto, S.; Taylor, P.R.; Virtamo, J.; Albanes, D. Serum and dietary vitamin E in relation to prostate cancer risk. *Cancer Epidemiol. Biomark. Prev.* **2007**, *16*, 1253–1259. [CrossRef] [PubMed]
63. Bramley, P.M.; Elmadfa, I.; Kafatos, A.; Kelly, F.J.; Manios, Y.; Roxborough, H.E.; Schuch, W.; Sheehy, P.J.A.; Wagner, K.H. Vitamin E. *J. Sci. Food Agric.* **2000**, *80*, 913–938. [CrossRef]
64. Öhrvall, M.; Vessby, B.; Sundlöf, G. Gamma, but not alpha, tocopherol levels in serum are reduced in coronary heart disease patients. *J. Intern. Med.* **1996**, *239*, 111–117. [CrossRef] [PubMed]
65. Schuelke, M.; Mayatepek, E.; Inter, M.; Becker, M.; Pfeiffer, E.; Speer, A.; Hubner, C.; Finckh, B. Treatment of ataxia in isolated vitamin E deficiency caused by alpha-tocopherol transfer protein deficiency. *J. Pediatr.* **1999**, *134*, 240–244. [CrossRef]
66. Witztum, J.L.; Steinberg, D. Role of oxidized low density lipoprotein in atherogenesis. *J. Clin. Investig.* **1991**, *88*, 1785–1792. [CrossRef] [PubMed]
67. Traber, M.G.; Frei, B.; Beckman, J.S. Vitamin E revisited: Do new data validate benefits for chronic disease prevention? *Curr. Opin. Lipidol.* **2008**, *19*, 30–38. [CrossRef] [PubMed]
68. Niki, E. Do free radicals play causal role in atherosclerosis? Low density lipoprotein oxidation and vitamin E revisited. *J. Clin. Biochem. Nutr.* **2010**, *48*, 3–7. [CrossRef] [PubMed]
69. Colombo, M.L. An update on vitamin E, tocopherol and tocotrienol-perspectives. *Molecules* **2010**, *15*, 2103–2113. [CrossRef] [PubMed]

70. Azzi, A. Many tocopherols, one vitamin E. *Mol. Asp. Med.* **2017**. [CrossRef] [PubMed]
71. Azzi, A.; Meydani, S.N.; Meydani, M.; Zingg, J.M. The rise, the fall and the renaissance of vitamin E. *Arch. Biochem. Biophys.* **2016**, *595*, 100–108. [CrossRef] [PubMed]
72. Jiang, Q. Natural forms of vitamin E: Metabolism, antioxidant, and anti-inflammatory activities and their role in disease prevention and therapy. *Free Radic. Biol. Med.* **2014**, *72*, 76–90. [CrossRef] [PubMed]
73. Dietrich, M.; Traber, M.G.; Jacques, P.F.; Cross, C.E.; Hu, Y.; Block, G. Does γ-tocopherol play a role in the primary prevention of heart disease and cancer? A review. *J. Am. Coll. Nutr.* **2006**, *25*, 292–299. [CrossRef] [PubMed]
74. Kloz, M.; Pillai, S.; Kodis, G.; Gust, D.; Moore, T.A.; Moore, A.L.; van Grondelle, R.; Kennis, J.T. Carotenoid photoprotection in artificial photosynthetic antennas. *J. Am. Chem. Soc.* **2011**, *133*, 7007–7015. [CrossRef] [PubMed]
75. Li, Y.; Zhou, Y.; Wang, Z.A.; Sun, X.F.; Tang, K.X. Engineering tocopherol biosynthetic pathway in *Arabidopsis* leaves and its effect on antioxidant metabolism. *Plant Sci.* **2010**, *178*, 312–320. [CrossRef]
76. Asensi-Fabado, M.A.; Munne-Bosch, S. Vitamins in plants: Occurrence, biosynthesis and antioxidant function. *Trends Plant Sci.* **2010**, *15*, 582–592. [CrossRef] [PubMed]
77. Azzi, A. Molecular mechanism of α-tocopherol action. *Free Radic. Biol. Med.* **2007**, *43*, 16–21. [CrossRef] [PubMed]
78. Sattler, S.E.; Mene-Saffrane, L.; Farmer, E.E.; Krischke, M.; Mueller, M.J.; DellaPenna, D. Nonenzymatic lipid peroxidation reprograms gene expression and activates defense markers in *Arabidopsis* tocopherol-deficient mutants. *Plant Cell* **2006**, *18*, 3706–3720. [CrossRef] [PubMed]
79. Hyun, T.K.; Kumar, K.; Rao, K.P.; Sinha, A.K.; Roitsch, T. Role of α-tocopherol in cellular signaling: α-tocopherol inhibits stress-induced mitogen-activated protein kinase activation. *Plant Biotechnol. Rep.* **2011**, *5*, 19–25. [CrossRef]
80. Denoya, C.D.; Skinner, D.D.; Morgenstern, M.R. A *Streptomyces avermitilis* gene encoding a 4-hydroxyphenylpyruvic acid dioxygenase-like protein that directs the production of homogentisic acid and an ochronotic pigment in *Escherichia coli*. *J. Bacteriol.* **1994**, *176*, 5312–5319. [CrossRef] [PubMed]
81. Singh, R.K.; Ali, S.A.; Nath, P.; Sane, V.A. Activation of ethylene-responsive *p*-hydroxyphenylpyruvate dioxygenase leads to increased tocopherol levels during ripening in mango. *J. Exp. Bot.* **2011**, *62*, 3375–3385. [CrossRef] [PubMed]
82. Fritsche, S.; Wang, X.; Nichelmann, L.; Suppanz, I.; Hadenfeldt, S.; Endrigkeit, J.; Meng, J.; Jung, C. Genetic and functional analysis of tocopherol biosynthesis pathway genes from rapeseed (*Brassica napus* L.). *Plant Breed.* **2014**, *133*, 470–479. [CrossRef]
83. Falk, J.; Andersen, G.; Kernebeck, B.; Krupinska, K. Constitutive overexpression of barley 4-hydroxy phenylpyruvate dioxygenase in tobacco results in elevation of the vitamin E content in seeds but not in leaves. *FEBS Lett.* **2003**, *540*, 35–40. [CrossRef]
84. Rippert, P.; Scimemi, C.; Dubald, M.; Matringe, M. Engineering plant shikimate pathway for production of tocotrienol and improving herbicide resistance. *Plant Physiol.* **2004**, *134*, 92–100. [CrossRef] [PubMed]
85. Li, Y.; Wang, Z.; Sun, X.; Tang, K. Current opinions on the functions of tocopherol based on the genetic manipulation of tocopherol biosynthesis in plants. *J. Integr. Plant Biol.* **2008**, *50*, 1057–1069. [CrossRef] [PubMed]
86. Karunanandaa, B.; Qi, Q.; Hao, M.; Baszis, S.R.; Jensen, P.K.; Wong, Y.H.; Jiang, J.; Venkatramesh, M.; Gruys, K.J.; Moshiri, F.; et al. Metabolically engineered oilseed crops with enhanced seed tocopherol. *Metab. Eng.* **2005**, *7*, 384–400. [CrossRef] [PubMed]
87. Raclaru, M.; Gruber, J.; Kumar, R.; Sadre, R.; Lühs, W.; Zarhloul, M.; Friedt, W.; Frentzen, M.; Weier, D. Increase of the tocochromanol content in transgenic *Brassica napus* seeds by overexpression of key enzymes involved in prenylquinone biosynthesis. *Mol. Breed.* **2006**, *18*, 93–107. [CrossRef]
88. Naqvi, S.; Farre, G.; Zhu, C.; Sandmann, G.; Capell, T.; Christou, P. Simultaneous expression of *Arabidopsis* rho-hydroxyphenylpyruvate dioxygenase and MPBQ methyltransferase in transgenic corn kernels triples the tocopherol content. *Transgenic Res.* **2011**, *20*, 177–181. [CrossRef] [PubMed]
89. Kleber-Janke, T.; Krupinska, K. Isolation of cDNA clones for genes showing enhanced expression in barley leaves during dark-induced senescence as well as during senescence under field conditions. *Planta* **1997**, *203*, 332–340. [CrossRef] [PubMed]

90. Keller, Y.; Bouvier, F.; D'Harlingue, A.; Camara, B. Metabolic compartmentation of plastid prenyllipid biosynthesis—Evidence for the involvement of a multifunctional geranylgeranyl reductase. *Eur. J. Biochem.* **1998**, *251*, 413–417. [CrossRef] [PubMed]

91. Zhang, C.; Zhang, W.; Ren, G.; Li, D.; Cahoon, R.E.; Chen, M.; Zhou, Y.; Yu, B.; Cahoon, E.B. Chlorophyll synthase under epigenetic surveillance is critical for vitamin E synthesis, and altered expression affects tocopherol levels in *Arabidopsis*. *Plant Physiol.* **2015**, *168*, 1503–1511. [CrossRef] [PubMed]

92. Ischebeck, T.; Zbierzak, A.M.; Kanwischer, M.; Dormann, P. A salvage pathway for phytol metabolism in *Arabidopsis*. *J. Biol. Chem.* **2006**, *281*, 2470–2477. [CrossRef] [PubMed]

93. Furuya, T.; Yoshikawa, T.; Kimura, T.; Kaneko, H. Production of tocopherols by cell culture of safflower. *Phytochemistry* **1987**, *26*, 2741–2747. [CrossRef]

94. Almeida, J.; Azevedo Mda, S.; Spicher, L.; Glauser, G.; vom Dorp, K.; Guyer, L.; del Valle Carranza, A.; Asis, R.; de Souza, A.P.; Buckeridge, M.; et al. Down-regulation of tomato PHYTOL KINASE strongly impairs tocopherol biosynthesis and affects prenyllipid metabolism in an organ-specific manner. *J. Exp. Bot.* **2016**, *67*, 919–934. [CrossRef] [PubMed]

95. Diepenbrock, C.H.; Kandianis, C.B.; Lipka, A.E.; Magallanes-Lundback, M.; Vaillancourt, B.; Gongora-Castillo, E.; Wallace, J.G.; Cepela, J.; Mesberg, A.; Bradbury, P.; et al. Novel Loci Underlie Natural Variation in Vitamin E Levels in Maize Grain. *Plant Cell* **2017**, *29*. [CrossRef] [PubMed]

96. Collakova, E.; DellaPenna, D. Isolation and functional analysis of homogentisate phytyltransferase from *Synechocystis* sp. PCC 6803 and *Arabidopsis*. *Plant Physiol.* **2001**, *127*, 1113–1124. [CrossRef] [PubMed]

97. Schledz, M.; Seidler, A.; Beyer, P.; Neuhaus, G. A novel phytyltransferase from *Synechocystis* sp. PCC 6803 involved in tocopherol biosynthesis. *FEBS Lett.* **2001**, *499*, 15–20. [CrossRef]

98. Sattler, S.E.; Cheng, Z.; DellaPenna, D. From *Arabidopsis* to agriculture: Engineering improved Vitamin E content in soybean. *Trends Plant Sci.* **2004**, *9*, 365–367. [CrossRef] [PubMed]

99. Ren, W.; Zhao, L.; Wang, Y.; Cui, L.; Tang, Y.; Sun, X.; Tang, K. Overexpression of homogentisate phytyltransferase in lettuce results in increased content of vitamin E. *AJB* **2011**, *10*, 14046–14051.

100. Mene-Saffrane, L.; Davoine, C.; Stolz, S.; Majcherczyk, P.; Farmer, E.E. Genetic removal of tri-unsaturated fatty acids suppresses developmental and molecular phenotypes of an *Arabidopsis* tocopherol-deficient mutant. Whole-body mapping of malondialdehyde pools in a complex eukaryote. *J. Biol. Chem.* **2007**, *282*, 35749–35756. [CrossRef] [PubMed]

101. Mene-Saffrane, L.; Jones, A.D.; DellaPenna, D. Plastochromanol-8 and tocopherols are essential lipid-soluble antioxidants during seed desiccation and quiescence in *Arabidopsis*. *Proc. Natl. Acad. Sci. USA* **2010**, *107*, 17815–17820. [CrossRef] [PubMed]

102. Ksas, B.; Becuwe, N.; Chevalier, A.; Havaux, M. Plant tolerance to excess light energy and photooxidative damage relies on plastoquinone biosynthesis. *Sci. Rep.* **2015**, *5*, 10919. [CrossRef] [PubMed]

103. Olejnik, D.; Gogolewski, M.; Nogala-Kałucka, M. Isolation and some properties of plastochromanol-8. *Mol. Nutr. Food Res.* **1997**, *41*, 101–104. [CrossRef]

104. Maeda, H.; Song, W.; Sage, T.; Dellapenna, D. Role of callose synthases in transfer cell wall development in tocopherol deficient *Arabidopsis* mutants. *Front. Plant Sci.* **2014**, *5*, 46. [CrossRef] [PubMed]

105. Kumar, R.; Raclaru, M.; Schusseler, T.; Gruber, J.; Sadre, R.; Lühs, W.; Zarhloul, K.M.; Friedt, W.; Enders, D.; Frentzen, M.; et al. Characterisation of plant tocopherol cyclases and their overexpression in transgenic *Brassica napus* seeds. *FEBS Lett.* **2005**, *579*, 1357–1364. [CrossRef] [PubMed]

106. Zbierzak, A.M.; Kanwischer, M.; Wille, C.; Vidi, P.A.; Giavalisco, P.; Lohmann, A.; Briesen, I.; Porfirova, S.; Brehelin, C.; Kessler, F.; et al. Intersection of the tocopherol and plastoquinol metabolic pathways at the plastoglobule. *Biochem. J.* **2010**, *425*, 389–399. [CrossRef] [PubMed]

107. Rastogi, A.; Yadav, D.K.; Szymanska, R.; Kruk, J.; Sedlarova, M.; Pospisil, P. Singlet oxygen scavenging activity of tocopherol and plastochromanol in *Arabidopsis thaliana*: Relevance to photooxidative stress. *Plant Cell Environ.* **2014**, *37*, 392–401. [CrossRef] [PubMed]

108. Havaux, M.; Eymery, F.; Porfirova, S.; Rey, P.; Dormann, P. Vitamin E protects against photoinhibition and photooxidative stress in *Arabidopsis thaliana*. *Plant Cell* **2005**, *17*, 3451–3469. [CrossRef] [PubMed]

109. Munné-Bosch, S.; Alegre, L. Interplay between ascorbic acid and lipophilic antioxidant defences in chloroplasts of water-stressed *Arabidopsis* plants. *FEBS Lett.* **2002**, *524*, 145–148. [CrossRef]

110. Liu, X.; Hua, X.; Guo, J.; Qi, D.; Wang, L.; Liu, Z.; Jin, Z.; Chen, S.; Liu, G. Enhanced tolerance to drought stress in transgenic tobacco plants overexpressing VTE1 for increased tocopherol production from *Arabidopsis thaliana*. *Biotechnol. Lett.* **2008**, *30*, 1275–1280. [CrossRef] [PubMed]
111. Ouyang, S.; He, S.; Liu, P.; Zhang, W.; Zhang, J.; Chen, S. The role of tocopherol cyclase in salt stress tolerance of rice (*Oryza sativa*). *Sci. China Life Sci.* **2011**, *54*, 181–188. [CrossRef] [PubMed]
112. Munne-Bosch, S. Linking tocopherols with cellular signaling in plants. *New Phytol.* **2005**, *166*, 363–366. [CrossRef] [PubMed]
113. Munné-Bosch, S.; Weiler, E.W.; Alegre, L.; Müller, M.; Düchting, P.; Falk, J. α-Tocopherol may influence cellular signaling by modulating jasmonic acid levels in plants. *Planta* **2007**, *225*, 681–691. [CrossRef] [PubMed]
114. Schaller, F. Enzymes of the biosynthesis of octadecanoid-derived signalling molecules. *J. Exp. Bot.* **2001**, *52*, 11–23. [CrossRef] [PubMed]
115. Creelman, R.A.; Mullet, J.E. Biosynthesis and Action of Jasmonates in Plants. *Annu. Rev. Plant Physiol. Plant Mol. Biol.* **1997**, *48*, 355–381. [CrossRef] [PubMed]
116. Wasternack, C. Jasmonates: An update on biosynthesis, signal transduction and action in plant stress response, growth and development. *Ann. Bot.* **2007**, *100*, 681–697. [CrossRef] [PubMed]
117. Botha, C.; Cross, R.; Van Bel, A.; Peter, C. Phloem loading in the sucrose-export-defective (SXD-1) mutant maize is limited by callose deposition at plasmodesmata in bundle sheath—Vascular parenchyma interface. *Protoplasma* **2000**, *214*, 65–72. [CrossRef]
118. Provencher, L.M.; Miao, L.; Sinha, N.; Lucas, W.J. Sucrose export defective1 encodes a novel protein implicated in chloroplast-to-nucleus signaling. *Plant Cell* **2001**, *13*, 1127–1141. [CrossRef] [PubMed]
119. Russin, W.A.; Evert, R.F.; Vanderveer, P.J.; Sharkey, T.D.; Briggs, S.P. Modification of a Specific Class of Plasmodesmata and Loss of Sucrose Export Ability in the sucrose export defective1 Maize Mutant. *Plant Cell* **1996**, *8*, 645–658. [CrossRef] [PubMed]
120. Hofius, D.; Hajirezaei, M.R.; Geiger, M.; Tschiersch, H.; Melzer, M.; Sonnewald, U. RNAi-mediated tocopherol deficiency impairs photoassimilate export in transgenic potato plants. *Plant Physiol.* **2004**, *135*, 1256–1268. [CrossRef] [PubMed]
121. Cela, J.; Chang, C.; Munné-Bosch, S. Accumulation of γ-rather than α-tocopherol alters ethylene signaling gene expression in the *vte4* mutant of *Arabidopsis thaliana*. *Plant Cell Physiol.* **2011**, *52*, 1389–1400. [CrossRef] [PubMed]
122. Hass, C.G.; Tang, S.; Leonard, S.; Traber, M.G.; Miller, J.F.; Knapp, S.J. Three non-allelic epistatically interacting methyltransferase mutations produce novel tocopherol (vitamin E) profiles in sunflower. *Theor. Appl. Genet.* **2006**, *113*, 767–782. [CrossRef] [PubMed]
123. Collakova, E.; DellaPenna, D. The role of homogentisate phytyltransferase and other tocopherol pathway enzymes in the regulation of tocopherol synthesis during abiotic stress. *Plant Physiol.* **2003**, *133*, 930–940. [CrossRef] [PubMed]
124. Endrigkeit, J.; Wang, X.; Cai, D.; Zhang, C.; Long, Y.; Meng, J.; Jung, C. Genetic mapping, cloning, and functional characterization of the *BnaX.VTE4* gene encoding a gamma-tocopherol methyltransferase from oilseed rape. *Theor. Appl. Genet.* **2009**, *119*, 567–575. [CrossRef] [PubMed]
125. Hunter, S.C.; Cahoon, E.B. Enhancing vitamin E in oilseeds: Unraveling tocopherol and tocotrienol biosynthesis. *Lipids* **2007**, *42*, 97–108. [CrossRef] [PubMed]
126. Fritsche, S.; Wang, X.; Li, J.; Stich, B.; Kopisch-Obuch, F.J.; Endrigkeit, J.; Leckband, G.; Dreyer, F.; Friedt, W.; Meng, J.; et al. A candidate gene-based association study of tocopherol content and composition in rapeseed (*Brassica napus*). *Front Plant Sci.* **2012**, *3*, 129. [CrossRef] [PubMed]
127. Muzhingi, T.; Palacios-Rojas, N.; Miranda, A.; Cabrera, M.L.; Yeum, K.J.; Tang, G. Genetic variation of carotenoids, vitamin E and phenolic compounds in Provitamin A biofortified maize. *J. Sci. Food Agric.* **2017**, *97*, 793–801. [CrossRef] [PubMed]
128. Wang, X.Q.; Yoon, M.Y.; He, Q.; Kim, T.S.; Tong, W.; Choi, B.W.; Lee, Y.S.; Park, Y.J. Natural variations in OsgammaTMT contribute to diversity of the alpha-tocopherol content in rice. *Mol. Genet. Genomics* **2015**, *290*, 2121–2135. [CrossRef] [PubMed]
129. Shaw, E.J.; Rajcan, I.; Morris, B. Molecular mapping of soybean seed tocopherols in the cross 'OAC Bayfield' × 'OAC Shire'. *Plant Breed.* **2017**, *136*, 83–93. [CrossRef]

130. Graebner, R.C.; Wise, M.; Cuesta-Marcos, A.; Geniza, M.; Blake, T.; Blake, V.C.; Butler, J.; Chao, S.; Hole, D.J.; Horsley, R.; et al. Quantitative Trait Loci Associated with the Tocochromanol (Vitamin E) Pathway in Barley. *PLoS ONE* **2015**, *10*, e0133767. [CrossRef] [PubMed]
131. Mauricio, R. Mapping quantitative trait loci in plants: Uses and caveats for evolutionary biology. *Nat. Rev. Genet.* **2001**, *2*, 370–381. [CrossRef] [PubMed]
132. Wang, X.; Zhang, C.; Li, L.; Fritsche, S.; Endrigkeit, J.; Zhang, W.; Long, Y.; Jung, C.; Meng, J. Unraveling the genetic basis of seed tocopherol content and composition in rapeseed (*Brassica napus* L.). *PLoS ONE* **2012**, *7*, e50038. [CrossRef] [PubMed]
133. Lipka, A.E.; Gore, M.A.; Magallanes-Lundback, M.; Mesberg, A.; Lin, H.; Tiede, T.; Chen, C.; Buell, C.R.; Buckler, E.S.; Rocheford, T.; et al. Genome-wide association study and pathway-level analysis of tocochromanol levels in maize grain. *G3 (Bethesda)* **2013**, *3*, 1287–1299. [CrossRef] [PubMed]
134. Luby, C.H.; Maeda, H.A.; Goldman, I.L. Genetic and phenological variation of tocochromanol (vitamin E) content in wild (*Daucus carota* L. var. carota) and domesticated carrot (*D. carota* L. var. sativa). *Hortic. Res.* **2014**, *1*, 14015. [CrossRef] [PubMed]
135. Rani, R.; Sheoran, R.; Sharma, B. Perspectives of breeding for altering sunflower oil quality to obtain novel oils. *Int. J. Curr. Microbiol. App. Sci.* **2017**, *6*, 949–962. [CrossRef]
136. Rauf, S.; Jamil, N.; Tariq, S.A.; Khan, M.; Kausar, M.; Kaya, Y. Progress in modification of sunflower oil to expand its industrial value. *J. Sci. Food Agric.* **2017**, *97*, 1997–2006. [CrossRef] [PubMed]
137. Seyis, F.; Snowdon, R.; Luhs, W.; Friedt, W. Molecular characterization of novel resynthesized rapeseed (*Brassica napus)* lines and analysis of their genetic diversity in comparison with spring rapeseed cultivars. *Plant Breed.* **2003**, *122*, 473–478. [CrossRef]
138. Hasan, M.; Seyis, F.; Badani, A.; Pons-Kühnemann, J.; Friedt, W.; Lühs, W.; Snowdon, R.J. Analysis of genetic diversity in the *Brassica napus* L. gene pool using SSR markers. *Genet. Resour. Crop Evol.* **2006**, *53*, 793–802. [CrossRef]
139. Quadrana, L.; Almeida, J.; Asis, R.; Duffy, T.; Dominguez, P.G.; Bermudez, L.; Conti, G.; Correa da Silva, J.V.; Peralta, I.E.; Colot, V.; et al. Natural occurring epialleles determine vitamin E accumulation in tomato fruits. *Nat. Commun.* **2014**, *5*, 3027. [CrossRef] [PubMed]
140. Farre, G.; Sudhakar, D.; Naqvi, S.; Sandmann, G.; Christou, P.; Capell, T.; Zhu, C. Transgenic rice grains expressing a heterologous rho-hydroxyphenylpyruvate dioxygenase shift tocopherol synthesis from the gamma to the alpha isoform without increasing absolute tocopherol levels. *Transgenic Res.* **2012**, *21*, 1093–1097. [CrossRef] [PubMed]
141. Chaudhary, N.; Khurana, P. Cloning, functional characterisation and transgenic manipulation of vitamin E biosynthesis genes of wheat. *Funct. Plant Biol.* **2013**, *40*, 1129–1136. [CrossRef]
142. Espinoza, A.; San Martin, A.; Lopez-Climent, M.; Ruiz-Lara, S.; Gomez-Cadenas, A.; Casaretto, J.A. Engineered drought-induced biosynthesis of alpha-tocopherol alleviates stress-induced leaf damage in tobacco. *J. Plant Physiol.* **2013**, *170*, 1285–1294. [CrossRef] [PubMed]
143. Chen, D.; Chen, H.; Zhang, L.; Shi, X.; Chen, X. Tocopherol-deficient rice plants display increased sensitivity to photooxidative stress. *Planta* **2014**, *239*, 1351–1362. [CrossRef] [PubMed]
144. Jin, S.; Daniell, H. Expression of gamma-tocopherol methyltransferase in chloroplasts results in massive proliferation of the inner envelope membrane and decreases susceptibility to salt and metal-induced oxidative stresses by reducing reactive oxygen species. *Plant Biotechnol. J.* **2014**, *12*, 1274–1285. [CrossRef] [PubMed]
145. Tanaka, H.; Yabuta, Y.; Tamoi, M.; Tanabe, N.; Shigeoka, S. Generation of transgenic tobacco plants with enhanced tocotrienol levels through the ectopic expression of rice homogentisate geranylgeranyl transferase. *Plant Biotechnol. J.* **2015**, *32*, 233–238. [CrossRef]
146. Che, P.; Zhao, Z.Y.; Glassman, K.; Dolde, D.; Hu, T.X.; Jones, T.J.; Obukosia, S.; Wambugu, F.; Albertsen, M.C. Elevated vitamin E content improves all-trans beta-carotene accumulation and stability in biofortified sorghum. *Proc. Natl. Acad. Sci. USA* **2016**, *113*, 11040–11045. [CrossRef] [PubMed]
147. Levac, D.; Cázares, P.; Yu, F.; De Luca, V. A picrinine N-methyltransferase belongs to a new family of γ-tocopherol-like methyltransferases found in medicinal plants that make biologically active monoterpenoid indole alkaloids. *Plant Physiol.* **2016**, *170*, 1935–1944. [CrossRef] [PubMed]
148. Fleta-Soriano, E.; Munne-Bosch, S. Enhanced plastochromanol-8 accumulation during reiterated drought in maize (*Zea mays* L.). *Plant Physiol. Biochem.* **2017**, *112*, 283–289. [CrossRef] [PubMed]

149. Liao, P.; Chen, X.; Wang, M.; Bach, T.J.; Chye, M.L. Improved fruit α-tocopherol, carotenoid, squalene and phytosterol contents through manipulation of Brassica juncea 3-HYDROXY-3-METHYLGLUTARYL-COA SYNTHASE1 in transgenic tomato. *Plant Biotechnol. J.* **2017**. [CrossRef] [PubMed]
150. Demurin, Y.; Skoric, D.; Karlovic, D. Genetic variability of tocopherol composition in sunflower seeds as a basis of breeding improved oil quality. *Plant Breed.* **1996**, 33–36. [CrossRef]
151. Yusuf, M.A.; Sarin, N.B. Antioxidant value addition in human diets: Genetic transformation of Brassica juncea with gamma-TMT gene for increased alpha-tocopherol content. *Transgenic Res.* **2007**, *16*, 109–113. [CrossRef] [PubMed]
152. Vinutha, T.; Maheswari, C.; Bansal, N.; Prashat, G.R.; Krishnan, V.; Kumari, S.; Dahuja, A.; Sachdev, A.; Rai, R. Expression analysis of γ-tocopherol methyl transferase genes and α-tocopherol content in developing seeds of soybean [*Glycine max* (L.) Merr.]. *IJBB* **2015**, *52*, 267–273.
153. Tavva, V.S.; Kim, Y.H.; Kagan, I.A.; Dinkins, R.D.; Kim, K.H.; Collins, G.B. Increased alpha-tocopherol content in soybean seed overexpressing the *Perilla frutescens* gamma-tocopherol *methyltransferase* gene. *Plant Cell. Rep.* **2007**, *26*, 61–70. [CrossRef] [PubMed]
154. Siles, L.; Cela, J.; Munne-Bosch, S. Vitamin E analyses in seeds reveal a dominant presence of tocotrienols over tocopherols in the Arecaceae family. *Phytochemistry* **2013**, *95*, 207–214. [CrossRef] [PubMed]
155. Matringe, M.; Ksas, B.; Rey, P.; Havaux, M. Tocotrienols, the unsaturated forms of vitamin E, can function as antioxidants and lipid protectors in tobacco leaves. *Plant Physiol.* **2008**, *147*, 764–778. [CrossRef] [PubMed]
156. Gutierrez-Gonzalez, J.J.; Garvin, D.F. Subgenome-specific assembly of vitamin E biosynthesis genes and expression patterns during seed development provide insight into the evolution of oat genome. *Plant Biotechnol. J.* **2016**, *14*, 2147–2157. [CrossRef] [PubMed]
157. Marwede, V.; Gul, M.K.; Becker, H.C.; Ecke, W. Mapping of QTL controlling tocopherol content in winter oilseed rape. *Plant Breed.* **2005**, *124*, 20–26. [CrossRef]
158. Li, H.Y.; Liu, H.C.; Han, Y.P.; Wu, X.X.; Teng, W.L.; Liu, G.F.; Li, W.B. Identification of QTL underlying vitamin E contents in soybean seed among multiple environments. *Theor. Appl. Genet.* **2010**, *120*, 1405–1413. [CrossRef] [PubMed]
159. Liu, H.; Cao, G.; Wu, D.; Jiang, Z.; Han, Y.; Li, W.; Morris, B. Quantitative trait loci underlying soybean seed tocopherol content with main additive, epistatic and QTL $\times$ environment effects. *Plant Breed.* **2017**. [CrossRef]
160. Ding, Y.; Li, H.; Chen, L.L.; Xie, K. Recent Advances in Genome Editing Using CRISPR/Cas9. *Front. Plant Sci.* **2016**, *7*, 703. [CrossRef] [PubMed]
161. Doudna, J.A.; Gersbach, C.A. Genome editing: The end of the beginning. *Genome Biol.* **2015**, *16*, 292. [CrossRef] [PubMed]
162. Feng, Z.; Zhang, B.; Ding, W.; Liu, X.; Yang, D.L.; Wei, P.; Cao, F.; Zhu, S.; Zhang, F.; Mao, Y.; et al. Efficient genome editing in plants using a CRISPR/Cas system. *Cell Res.* **2013**, *23*, 1229–1232. [CrossRef] [PubMed]
163. Gao, W.; Long, L.; Tian, X.; Xu, F.; Liu, J.; Singh, P.K.; Botella, J.R.; Song, C. Genome Editing in Cotton with the CRISPR/Cas9 System. *Front. Plant Sci.* **2017**, *8*, 1364. [CrossRef] [PubMed]
164. Cardi, T.; Neal Stewart, C., Jr. Progress of targeted genome modification approaches in higher plants. *Plant Cell Rep.* **2016**, *35*, 1401–1416. [CrossRef] [PubMed]
165. Jung, C.; Capistrano-Gossmann, G.; Braatz, J.; Sashidhar, N.; Melzer, S. Recent developments in genome editing and applications in plant breeding. *Plant Breed.* **2017**. [CrossRef]

10

High-Dose Menaquinone-7 Supplementation Reduces Cardiovascular Calcification in a Murine Model of Extraosseous Calcification

Daniel Scheiber [1,†], Verena Veulemans [1,†], Patrick Horn [1], Martijn L. Chatrou [2], Sebastian A. Potthoff [3], Malte Kelm [1,4], Leon J. Schurgers [2,†] and Ralf Westenfeld [1,†,*]

[1] Division of Cardiology, Pulmonology, and Vascular Medicine, Medical Faculty, University Duesseldorf, Duesseldorf 40225, Germany; E-Mails: daniel.scheiber@med.uni-duesseldorf.de (D.S.); verena.veulemanns@med.uni-duesseldorf.de (V.V.); patrick.horn@med.uni-duesseldorf.de (P.H.); malte.kelm@med.uni-duesseldorf.de (M.K.)

[2] Department of Biochemistry, Cardiovascular Research Institute Maastricht, Maastricht University, Maastricht 6229 ER, The Netherlands; E-Mails: m.chatrou@maastrichtuniversity.nl (M.L.C.); l.schurgers@maastrichtuniversity.nl (L.J.S.)

[3] Department of Nephrology, University Duesseldorf, Medical Faculty, Duesseldorf 40225, Germany; E-Mail: sebastian.potthoff@med.uni-duesseldorf.de

[4] Cardiovascular Research Institute Duesseldorf, University Duesseldorf, Medical Faculty, Duesseldorf 40225, Germany

* Author to whom correspondence should be addressed; E-Mail: ralf.westenfeld@med.uni-duesseldorf.de

† These authors contributed equally to this work.

Abstract: Cardiovascular calcification is prevalent in the aging population and in patients with chronic kidney disease (CKD) and diabetes mellitus, giving rise to substantial morbidity and mortality. Vitamin K-dependent matrix Gla-protein (MGP) is an important inhibitor of calcification. The aim of this study was to evaluate the impact of high-dose menaquinone-7 (MK-7) supplementation (100 μg/g diet) on the development of extraosseous calcification in a murine model. Calcification was induced by 5/6 nephrectomy combined with high phosphate diet in rats. Sham operated animals served as controls. Animals received high or low MK-7 diets for 12 weeks. We assessed vital parameters, serum chemistry, creatinine clearance, and cardiac function. CKD provoked increased aortic (1.3 fold; $p < 0.05$) and myocardial (2.4 fold; $p < 0.05$) calcification in line with increased alkaline phosphatase levels (2.2 fold; $p < 0.01$). MK-7 supplementation inhibited cardiovascular calcification and decreased aortic alkaline phosphatase tissue concentrations. Furthermore, MK-7 supplementation increased aortic MGP messenger ribonucleic acid (mRNA) expression (10-fold; $p < 0.05$). CKD-induced arterial hypertension with secondary myocardial hypertrophy and increased elastic fiber breaking points in the arterial tunica media did not change with MK-7 supplementation. Our results show that high-dose MK-7 supplementation inhibits the development of cardiovascular calcification. The protective effect of MK-7 may be related to the inhibition of secondary mineralization of damaged vascular structures.

Keywords: menaquinone-7; vitamin K_2; cardiovascular calcification; matrix Gla-protein; chronic kidney disease

---

1. Introduction

Biological aging [1] and diseases like chronic kidney disease (CKD) [2] or diabetes mellitus [3] are associated with an increased incidence of cardiovascular calcification, an independent cardiovascular risk factor accompanied by enhanced morbidity and mortality [4].

For decades vascular calcification (VC) was thought to be the consequence of passive precipitation of calcium (Ca) and phosphate (P) ions resulting from a supersaturated Ca $\times$ P product [5]. Today cardiovascular calcification is appreciated as an actively regulated, cell-mediated process characterized by the interaction of inductive and inhibitory proteins [6]. According to the anatomical localization, VC can be classified as intimal and medial calcification, although a clear-cut distinction is almost impossible in clinical practice [7]. Intimal calcification is linked to atherosclerosis and characterized by inflammatory accumulation of oxidized lipids [8]. Medial calcification develops independently of inflammation and lipid deposition along the elastic fibers. It is a typical consequence of aging and found in patients suffering from chronic kidney disease or diabetes mellitus [9–11]. Despite differences in etiology, the underlying pathophysiological mechanism of intimal and medial calcification is similar [6].

The vitamin K-dependent matrix Gla-protein (MGP) is a potent inhibitor of arterial calcification [12]. MGP was presented first in 1983 by Price and colleagues as a 14kD protein purified from bovine bone matrix [13]. That the function of MGP was mainly vascular became clear from MGP-deficient mice, all of which died within a few months of birth due to blood vessel rupture as a result of VC [14]. Likewise, humans with a hereditary dysfunctional MGP (Keutel syndrome) suffer from widely distributed extraosseous calcifications [15]. There are two posttranslational modifications in MGP: gamma-glutamate carboxylation and serine phosphorylation [16]. While the function of posttranslational MGP phosphorylation is not completely understood, Murshed and colleagues showed that MGP has to be carboxylated to prevent VC [17]. Diminished MGP carboxylation is associated with an increased tendency of calcification of the vasculature [18]. Analogous to vitamin K-dependent blood clotting factors (Factors II, VII, IX, X, and Protein C, S, and Z), the biological activity of MGP depends on the presence of vitamin K as cofactor [19]. Current medical treatment with vitamin K antagonists may, besides providing effective anticoagulation, also increase the risk for VC [20].

Patients with CKD are characterized by widespread extraosseous calcification. We as well as others have shown that CKD patients display vitamin K insufficiency, associated with elevated plasma concentrations of inactive MGP [21–23]. Increased plasma levels of inactive ucMGP are paralleled by enhanced morbidity and mortality in patients suffering from CKD, aortic stenosis, or congestive heart failure [22,24,25]. Supplementation with vitamin K results in a dose- and time-dependent decrease of ucMGP plasma levels [23,26,27]. So far, no trials reported "hard outcomes" such as VC in the context of CKD and vitamin K supplementation.

Fat-soluble vitamin K is an essential micronutrient [28]. There are two forms of vitamin K in nature: phylloquinone (vitamin K_1; VK_1) and the menaquinones (vitamin K_2; VK_2; MK-n). VK_1 is tightly bound to the chloroplast membrane of plants [29]. Menaquinones differ in side chains of varying length. They are described as MK-n, in which n denotes the number of unsaturated isoprenoid residues. MK-7 is produced by bacteria and is present in fermented foods such as cheese or sauerkraut [30]. In this study we used MK-7 because of its long half-life and good bioavailability. Two independent observational studies [31,32] described a protective cardiovascular effect of nutritional intake of menaquinones, whereas no effect was found for phylloquinone. This discrepancy in function was ascribed to the better availability and transport of long-chain menaquinones such as MK-7 as compared to VK_1. However, in animal models of warfarin-induced vascular calcification, the short chain menaquinone MK-4 was tested, which displayed greater potency in the inhibition of vascular calcification [33–35]. The MK-7 supplementation dose of 100 $\mu g/g$ diet used in this present study was based on these MK-4 studies [33–35].

The aim of this study is to evaluate the impact of high-dose MK-7 supplementation on the development of cardiovascular calcification and the impact on cardiovascular function in a murine model of chronic kidney disease characterized by enhanced extraosseous calcification.

2. Materials and Methods

2.1. Animals and Diets

The animal study protocol was authorized by the responsible governmental office called *LANUV* ("Landesamt für Natur, Umwelt und Verbraucherschutz Nordrhein-Westfalen"; file reference 87-51.04.2010.A275). All experiments were executed according to the German animal welfare act in close cooperation with veterinaries of the Heinrich Heine University. We used 42 male Wistar rats aged 12 weeks with a body weight about 300 g at the beginning of the study protocol. Rats were kept in a climate-controlled room (22–24 °C, relative humidity 60%–80%) with a 12-hour light, 12-hour dark cycle. Food and water were given *ad libitum*.

Animals were divided into an interventional group undergoing 5/6 nephrectomy, receiving a high phosphate diet and into a control group undergoing sham operations. Half of each group received a high MK-7 diet, so that we distinguished between four different treatment groups receiving different diets (sniff-Spezialdiäten GmbH) (Table 1).

Pure synthetic MK-7 was provided by NattoPharma ASA (Hovik, Norway).

Table 1. Diets.

Control (Sham-OP)	
Co (n = 10)	Co-K_2 (n = 10)
Standard diet:	MK-7-supplemented standard diet:
0.36% Phosphate	0.36% Phosphate
0.6% Calcium	0.6% Calcium
0.5 μg/g VK_1	0.5 μg/g VK_1
0 MK-7	100 μg/g MK-7
Intervention (5/6-Nephrectomy + high phosphate diet)	
CKD (n = 11)	CKD-K_2 (n = 11)
High phosphate diet:	Phosphate- and MK-7-rich diet:
1.2% Phosphate	1.2% Phosphate
0.6% Calcium	0.6% Calcium
0.5 μg/g VK_1	0.5 μg/g VK_1
0 MK-7	100 μg/g MK-7

Animals were randomly distributed to four study groups, with two diets different in MK-7 and phosphate concentration. Animals in CKD and CKD-K_2 groups were 5/6 nephrectomized. Control animals were sham operated. Co = control group; Co-K_2 = MK-7-supplemented control group; CKD = intervention group; CKD-K_2 = MK-7-supplemented intervention group; MK-7 = menaquinone-7; VK_1 = vitamin K_1.

2.2. Study Design

All animals took part in a three-month study protocol. On the first day we measured blood pressure using a tail-cuff system. Blood samples were taken by retro orbital bleeding. Body weight was taken twice weekly. 5/6 nephrectomy was performed according to a surgical technique initially described by Perez-Ruiz [36]. Briefly, we performed right-sided nephrectomy and one week later following recovery from the initial surgery, rats underwent functional 2/3 nephrectomy of the remaining left kidney by careful ligation of the renal parenchyma. Controls underwent a similar two-step laparotomy exposing the kidneys but without nephrectomy. After three and eight weeks we repeated the measurements from the preoperative day. At the end of the study after three months we collected 24-hour urine samples from six animals in each group in metabolic cages. Animals were sacrificed under anesthesia by puncture of the vena cava inferior. Blood was collected for serum analyses. Heart, aorta, and kidney tissues were collected for further analyses.

2.3. Echocardiography

Echocardiography was performed as described previously [33]. Briefly, rats were anesthetized using Isoflurane and two-dimensional and M-mode measurements were accomplished using Vivid i, GE Healthcare (GE Healthcare, Buckinghamshire, England) with a 12 MHz probe. Animals were placed in the supine-lateral position with ECGs were obtained throughout the procedure. Parasternal long-axis and short-axis views of the left ventricle (LV) were obtained, ensuring that the mitral and aortic valves and apex were well visualized. Area fraction and wall area were determined by planimetry of end-diastolic and systolic volumes in parasternal short axis. Measurements of LV end-diastolic and end-systolic dimensions were obtained in M-mode at mid-papillary level from more than three beats and fractional shortening (FS) was calculated as FS (%) = ((LVIDd − LVIDs)/LVIDd) × 100, where LVID is LV internal diameter, s is systole, and d is diastole. Diastole is defined as the maximum measurable area; systole is defined as the minimum measurable area. Doppler flow spectrum of the ascending aorta was recorded from the suprasternal view. Peak velocity was measured, and the waveform was also traced to obtain a velocity time-integral calculation and peak gradient.

2.4. Blood/Urine Analyses

Blood and urine analyses were performed by Animal Blood Counter (Scil Animal Care Company GmbH, Viernheim, Germany) and in the Institute of Clinical Chemistry of University Hospital Düsseldorf.

2.5. Histology

Tissues were perfused with cold phosphate-buffered saline (PBS) solution by cannulation of left ventricle. Afterwards tissues were embedded in TissueTek (Sakura Finetek Europe B.V., Alphen aan den Rijn, the Netherlands) on dry ice for cryofixation, paraffin embedded, or placed in frozen nitrogen. Different histological and immunohistological stainings were performed and analyzed with a Leica DM4000 M RL microscope mounted with a Leica DFC 425C camera (Leica Mikrosysteme GmbH, Wetzlar, Germany). Quantitative measurements were performed with ImageJ software (National Institutes of Health, Bethesda, MD, USA).

2.6. qRT-PCR

Real-Time PCR mRNA was extracted using the commercial kits RNAlater and RNeasy (Qiagen, Hilden, Germany) with proteinase K digestion before RNA extraction to maximize mRNA yield. Integrity and amount of mRNA were analyzed by capillary electrophoresis (Agilent Bioanalyzer 2100; Agilent Technologies, Böblingen, Germany). Reverse transcription and real-time PCR were performed with Applied Biosystems 7500 Fast Real Time PCR System (Applied Biosystems, Foster City, CA, USA) according to the manufacturer's instructions. The expression level in untreated mice was arbitrarily assigned the value 1.0, and all other expression values were expressed as fold changes thereof. Values were analyzed using REST software tool (Quiagen, Hilden, Germany).

2.7. Statistics

We performed ANOVA with Bonferroni's *post hoc* analysis using GraphPad Prism 5 software (GraphPad, San Diego, CA, USA) to estimate the overall differences between experimental groups. Confidence intervals over 95% were regarded as significant.

3. Results

3.1. Experimental CKD

Combination of surgical 5/6 nephrectomy with supplementation of a high phosphate diet succeeded in mimicking key metabolic features of CKD. Serum creatinine levels were elevated by more than 50% in CKD and CKD-K_2 animals compared to controls (Table 2) (CKD *vs.* Co after 12 weeks, $p < 0.001$). Likewise, blood urea nitrogen (BUN) concentrations were significantly elevated in the CKD groups (CKD *vs.* Co after 12 weeks, $p < 0.001$). 5/6 nephrectomy and phosphate supplementation affected phosphate concentrations in serum and urine: urine phosphate excretion was more than tripled in CKD animals compared to controls (CKD *vs.* Co after 12 weeks, $p < 0.001$) (Table 2) with an apparent hyperphosphatemia only in CKD but not in CKD-K_2 rats. There was no difference in hemoglobin or hematocrit concentration between the experimental groups (Table 2). Since severe renal impairment is associated with cachexia, we repetitively assessed body weight. All animals that were not fully grown at the start of the study gained weight during the 12 weeks of the experimental period. Control animals increased significantly more weight compared to CKD and CKD-K_2 animals (Figure 1) (CKD *vs.* Co after 12 weeks, $p < 0.01$).

Table 2. Serum and urine parameters after 12 weeks of study protocol.

Parameters	Co	Co-K_2	CKD	CKD-K_2
Serum creatinine (mg/dl)				
Week 12	0.3 ± 0	0.3 ± 0	0.5 ± 0	0.5 ± 0
BUN (mg/dl)				
Week 12	40 ± 2.2	42 ± 1.3	51 ± 2.9	50 ± 1.9
Serum phosphate (mmol/l)				
Week 12	1.8 ± 0.1	1.6 ± 0.1	2.2 ± 0.2	1.8 ± 0.1
Hb (g/dl)				
Week 12	15.0 ± 0.5	15.5 ± 0.2	15.5 ± 0.2	15.5 ± 0.1
Hkt (%)				
Week 12	45.8 ± 1.3	47.9 ± 0.9	44.0 ± 1.5	45.0 ± 0.3
Creatinine clearance (ml/min)				
Week 12	3.2 ± 0.6	2.5 ± 0.2	1.7 ± 0.2	1.8 ± 0.1
Urine phosphate excretion (mg/24 h)	33.1 ± 1	23.6 ± 3.6	82.8 ± 29.9	59.8 ± 7.5

BUN = blood urea nitrogen; K_2 = MK-7.

3.2. Cardiovascular Calcification

We directly assessed cardiovascular calcification by histology (von Kossa) and chemical analysis (AAS = atomic absorption spectroscopy) in the aorta, myocardium, and kidneys in the various treatment groups. AAS is a sensitive method for detecting total tissue calcium amount [37]. In the aortas we performed additional immunohistochemistry for alkaline phosphatase to evaluate the downstream effects of mineralization in terms of VSMC dedifferentiation.

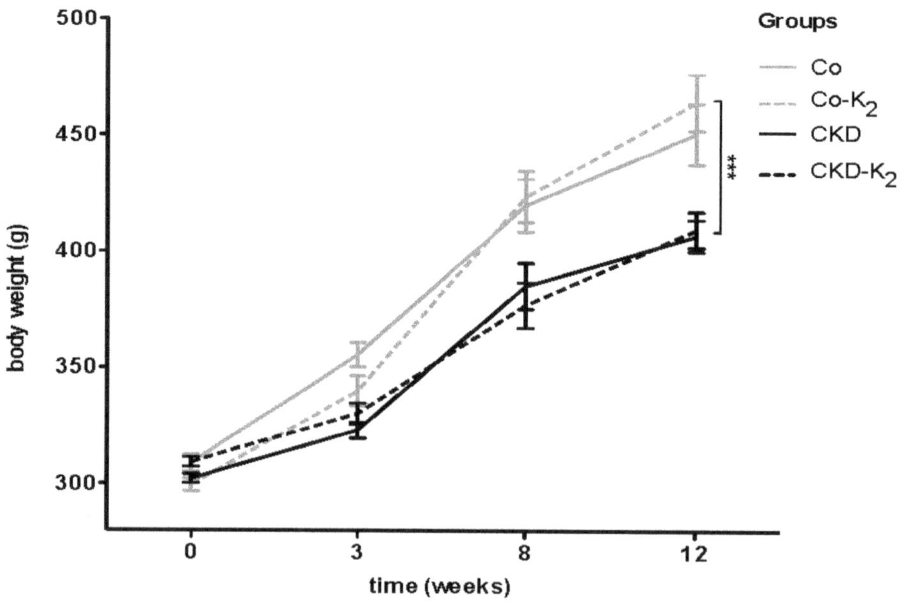

Figure 1. Body weight in grams (g). Body weight of animals was measured repetitively during 12 weeks of study protocol. Experimental animals were not fully grown at start of the experiment; however, all animals gained weight significantly. During the experiment, control animals (Co; Co-K_2) gained significantly more weight compared to CKD and CKD-K_2 animals. Co = control group; Co-K_2 = MK-7 supplemented control group; CKD = 5/6 nephrectomized group; CKD-K_2 = MK-7 supplemented 5/6 nephrectomized group; g = grams. Significant differences: *** $p < 0.001$.

Aorta: While von Kossa staining did not encounter calcification in any treatment group, we detected significant differences in the chemical calcium analysis applying AAS. Animals from the CKD group displayed an induction of aortic calcium content compared to controls by about 30% ($p < 0.05$). MK-7 supplementation abolished aortic calcification, thus CKD-K_2 rats displayed aortic calcium content indistinguishable from controls (Figure 2). In line with the calcium accumulation in the CKD group, we detected an intensified ALP staining in aortic tissue samples of CKD animals compared to control groups (CKD *vs.* Co, $p < 0.01$) and CKD-K_2 animals (Figure 3).

Myocardium: Similar to our observations in aortic tissue, we did not detect overt myocardial calcification by von Kossa staining in any treatment group. Applying chemical analysis by AAS, myocardial tissues of the CKD group displayed a 2.4-fold increased calcium concentration compared to controls (CKD *vs.* Co, $p < 0.05$). Again, MK-7 supplementation inhibited calcium accumulation in the CKD-K_2 rats with calcium tissue concentrations in the range of control rats (Figure 4).

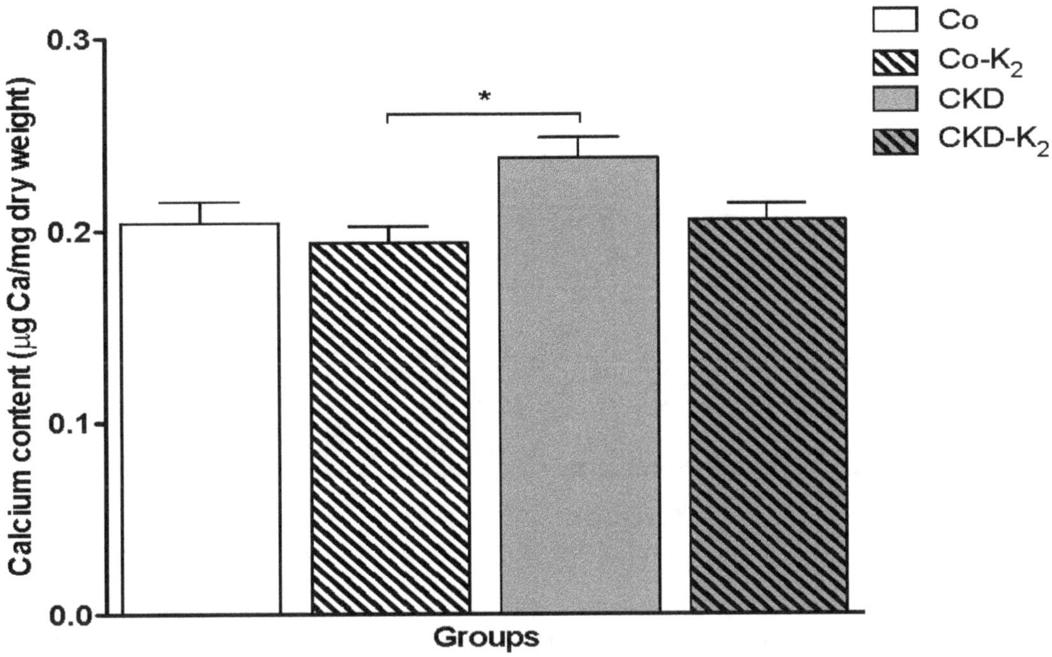

Figure 2. Aortic calcium content. Measurement of aortic calcium content was performed by atomic absorption spectrometry and expressed as μg Ca/mg dry weight tissue. CKD animals display a significant increase in aortic calcium content compared to Co-K_2 animals. Co = control group; Co-K_2 = MK-7 supplemented control group; CKD = 5/6 nephrectomized group; CKD-K_2 = MK-7 supplemented 5/6 nephrectomized group; mg = milligrams; μg = micrograms. Significant differences: * $p < 0.05$.

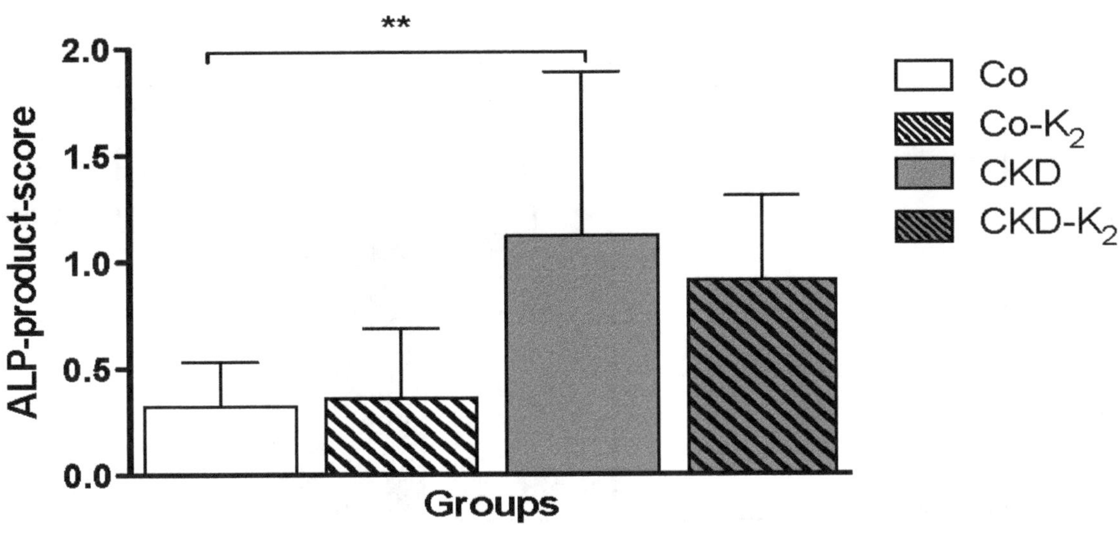

Figure 3. Alkaline phosphatase (ALP) in aortic tissues. ALP was measured to detect local vascular osteochondrogenic activity. Positive staining for ALP is expressed as product score: ALP-positive staining areal × intensity. ALP-product-score is significantly increased in CKD animals as compared to Co animals. Co = control group; Co-K_2 = MK-7 supplemented control group; CKD = 5/6 nephrectomized group; CKD-K_2 = MK-7 supplemented 5/6 nephrectomized group. Significant differences: ** $p < 0.01$.

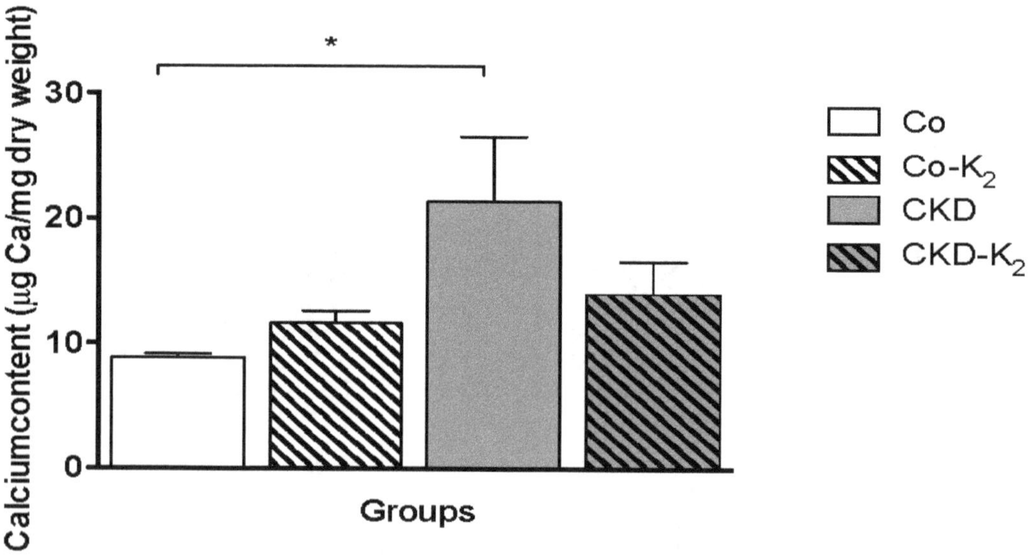

Figure 4. Myocardial calcium content. Measurement of myocardial calcium content using atomic absorption spectrometry in µg Ca/mg dry weight tissue. CKD animals display a significantly increased myocardial calcium content compared to Co animals. Co = control group; Co-K_2 = MK-7 supplemented control group; CKD = 5/6 nephrectomized group; CKD-K_2 = MK-7 supplemented 5/6 nephrectomized group; mg = milligrams; µg = micrograms. Significant differences: * $p < 0.05$.

Kidney: In renal tissues of CKD and CKD-K_2 animals we detected tubular calcification easily visible on von Kossa histology (Figures 5 and 6). Quantitative analysis detected no effect of MK-7 supplementation on renal calcification.

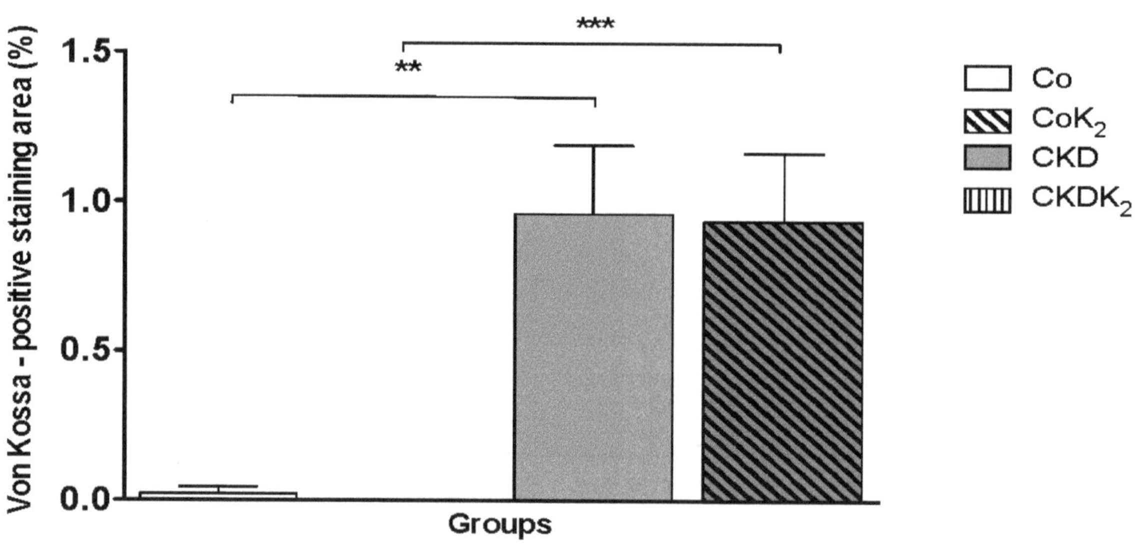

Figure 5. Renal calcification. Von Kossa positive staining area expressed as percentage of tissue area. In 5/6 nephrectomized animals significantly more von Kossa positivity was measured as compared to the control groups. No differences were seen between CKD and CKD-K_2 treated groups. Co = control group; Co-K_2 = MK-7 supplemented control group; CKD = 5/6 nephrectomized group; CKD-K_2 = MK-7 supplemented 5/6 nephrectomized group. Significant differences: ** $p < 0.01$, *** $p < 0.001$.

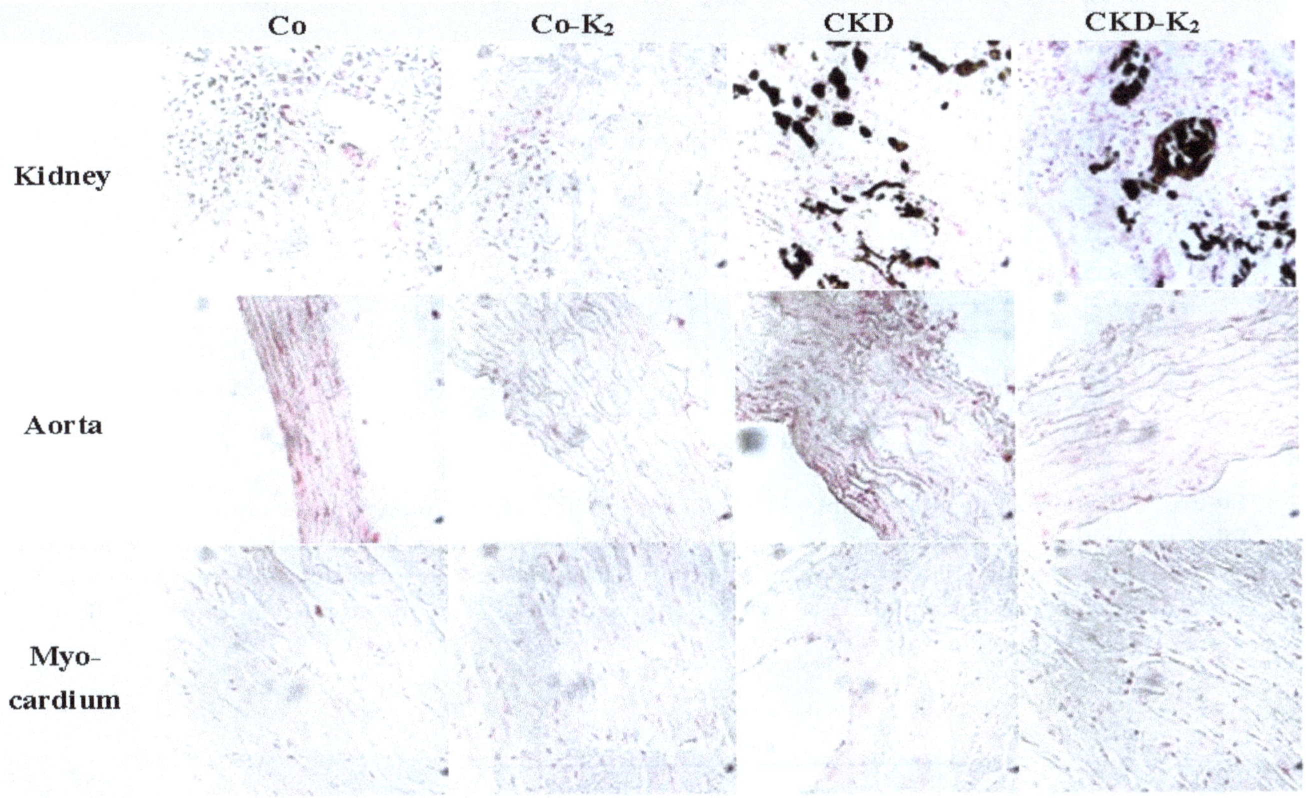

Figure 6. Representative sections of von Kossa stained tissue samples. Microscopically visible von Kossa positive staining was only detected in kidney tissue samples of CKD and CDK-K_2 animals. Magnification 40×; Counterstain: nuclear fast red; Co = control group; Co-K_2 = MK-7 supplemented control group; CKD = 5/6 nephrectomized group; CKD-K_2 = MK-7 supplemented 5/6 nephrectomized group.

3.3. Structural Alterations in Experimental CKD

Fiber breaking points: In order to evaluate the structural alterations induced by 5/6 nephrectomy and a high phosphate diet, we performed Elastica van Gieson staining of the aorta to illustrate elastic fiber breaking points. Both interventional groups (CKD, CKD-K_2) displayed significantly more elastic fiber breaking points compared to the control groups (CKD *vs.* Co, $p < 0.001$) (Figure 7). MK-7 supplementation had no effect on fiber breaking points in controls or CKD rats, respectively.

Proliferative response: Immunofluorescence staining of Ki67/DAPI revealed markedly increased cell proliferation in CKD and CKD-K_2 animals compared to controls (CKD *vs.* Co, $p < 0.001$). MK-7 supplementation did not alter the proliferative response to the CKD stimulus (Figure 8).

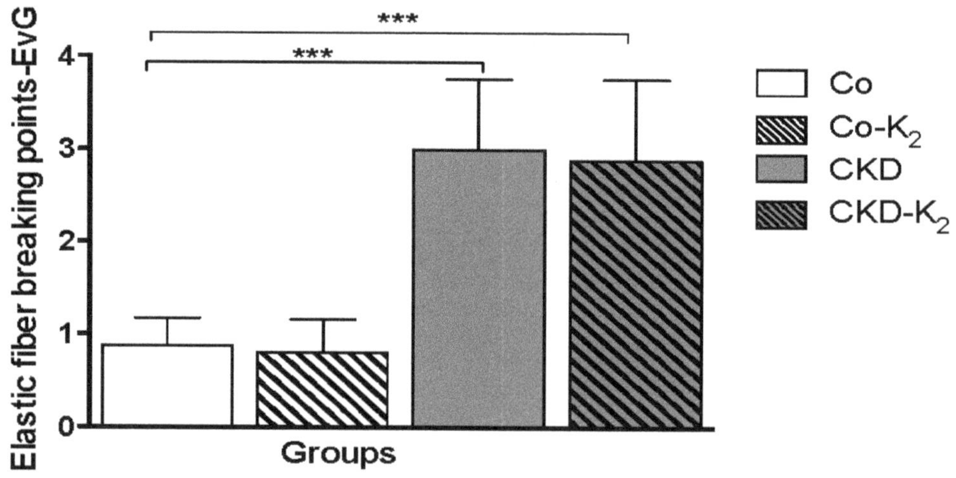

Figure 7. Elastic fiber breaking points. Elastica van Gieson (EvG) staining of aortic tissue samples with focus on elastic fiber breaking points. CKD animals display significantly more elastic fiber breaking points compared to Co animals. Co = control group; Co-K_2 = MK-7 supplemented control group; CKD = 5/6 nephrectomized group; CKD-K_2 = MK-7 supplemented 5/6 nephrectomized group. Significant differences: *** $p < 0.001$.

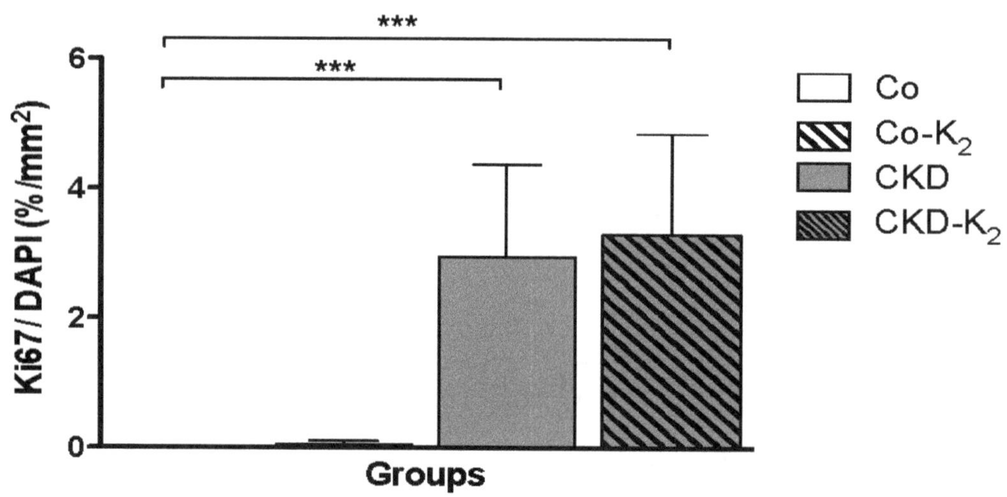

Figure 8. Proliferative response. Ratio of positive staining area for Ki67 per DAPI positive staining area in % per mm^2. DAPI values do not differ significantly between groups. CKD animals display significantly more Ki67 positive staining area per DAPI positive staining area compared to Co animals. Co = control group; Co-K_2 = MK-7 supplemented control group; CKD = 5/6 nephrectomized group; CKD-K_2 = MK-7 supplemented 5/6 nephrectomized group; mm = millimeters. Significant differences: *** $p < 0.001$.

3.4. Cardiovascular Function

Blood pressure: CKD and CKD-K_2 animals developed arterial hypertension (Figure 9). After 12 weeks, systolic as well as diastolic blood pressure values were elevated by 15–20 mmHg in CKD rats compared to controls (CKD-K_2 *vs.* Co-K_2, $p < 0.01$). MK-7 supplementation did not affect blood pressure (Figure 9).

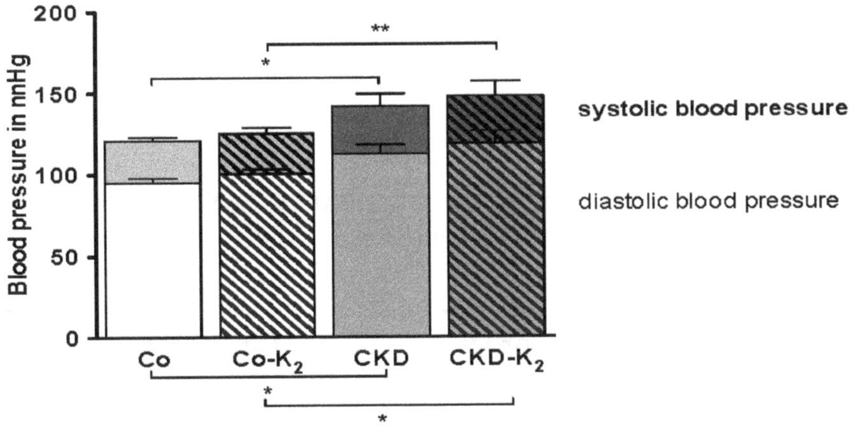

Figure 9. Systolic and diastolic blood pressure. Systolic and diastolic blood pressure after 12 weeks of treatment. CKD animals developed significantly increased systolic and diastolic blood pressure values compared to controls. Co = control group; Co-K_2 = MK-7 supplemented control group; CKD = 5/6 nephrectomized group; CKD-K_2 = MK-7 supplemented 5/6 nephrectomized group; mmHg = millimeters of mercury. Significant differences: * $p < 0.05$, ** $p < 0.01$.

Echocardiography: To quantify the impact of CKD and arterial hypertension on cardiovascular function we analyzed hypertrophy, contractility, and valvular function in the various treatment groups. CKD and CKD-K_2 animals exhibited significant myocardial hypertrophy, as depicted by increased diameters of the interventricular septum (by about 50%; CKD *vs.* Co, $p < 0.01$) (Figure 10). Myocardial contractility, as detected by fractional shortening, remained normal in all the animals studied. No relevant valvular disease or overt signs of valvular calcification were detected throughout the experiments (data not shown).

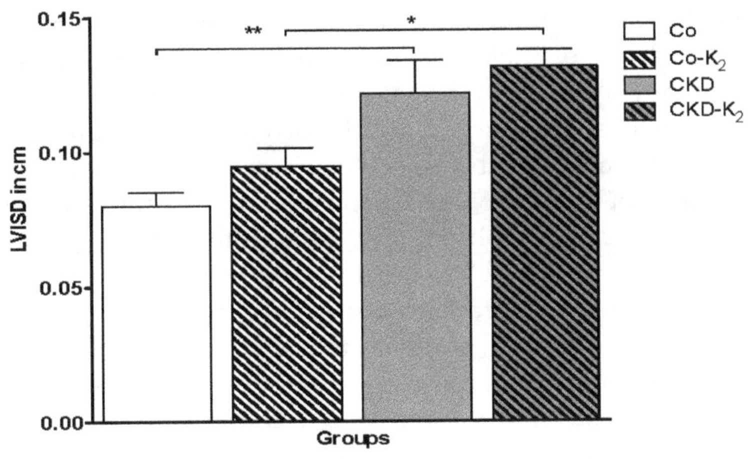

Figure 10. Echocardiography of diastolic interventricular septum diameter (LVISD) in cm. Echocardiography was performed in all animals after 12 weeks of study protocol. CKD animals developed significantly increased LVISD compared to controls. Co = control group; Co-K_2 = MK-7 supplemented control group; CKD = 5/6 nephrectomized group; CKD-K_2 = MK-7 supplemented 5/6 nephrectomized group; cm = centimeters. Significant differences: * $p < 0.05$, ** $p < 0.01$.

3.5. Aortic mRNA Expression

We analyzed regulation of relevant activators and inhibitors of VC in aortic tissue samples by quantitative real-time PCR. In a stepwise analysis, we investigated separately the effect of CKD (Figure 11a), MK-7 supplementation (Figure 11b), and finally the effect of MK-7 supplementation in CKD rats (Figure 11c), each compared to controls. For more clarity, pro-calcific changes are depicted by red columns while alterations associated with potential calcification inhibition are assigned with blue columns.

CKD compared to controls: The induction of CKD was associated with pro-calcific mRNA alterations within the aortas of the animals. MGP and SM22α gene expression was markedly decreased in CKD animals, while periostin and BMP-2 gene expression was increased compared to controls (Figure 11a).

MK-7 supplementation compared to controls: MK-7 supplementation revealed a significant induction of aortic MGP mRNA while procalcifing periostin mRNA levels were found to be significantly reduced (Figure 11b).

MK-7 supplementation and CKD compared to controls: MK-7 supplementation in CKD was associated with a calcification inhibitory effect in the aortic mRNA repertoire. Of note, we detected a significant induction of MGP mRNA levels. Moreover, the CKD-mediated reduction of SM22α mRNA was abolished, as depicted by a trend towards increased SM22α mRNA (Figure 11c).

4. Discussion

In this study we demonstrate that high-dose MK-7 supplementation inhibits calcification in a murine model of CKD-induced cardiovascular calcification. The effect of MK-7 is—at least in part—mediated via MGP and subsequent inhibition of ectopic calcification.

4.1. CKD and High Phosphate Diet

In our study we used a murine model of 5/6 nephrectomy and high phosphate diet to induce CKD-related cardiovascular damage. Shobeiri *et al.* compared different experimental CKD models for the induction of VC [38]. They observed a 2.2-fold increased serum creatinine concentration in 5/6 nephrectomized rats eight weeks after surgery, with corresponding values for BUN and creatinine clearance [38]. Our findings are similar with respect to serum creatinine and BUN levels and creatinine clearance but differ in severity of kidney injury. We observed moderate kidney injury, whereas others report severe kidney injury after 5/6 nephrectomy. This difference might arise from the technique we used to perform the 5/6 nephrectomy. We used unilateral nephrectomy, followed by ligation of the poles of the remaining kidney, whereas most studies describe surgical resection of the kidney poles or embolization of the pole-supplying arteries to induce renal impairment [38,39]. As expected, animals from CKD and CKD-K_2 groups gained less weight as compared to control animals, which is in accordance with previous studies [39]. Moreover, CKD and CKD-K_2 animals did not developed anemia. This finding is consistent with moderate kidney injury, since anemia is most frequently seen in patients with severe renal impairment [40].

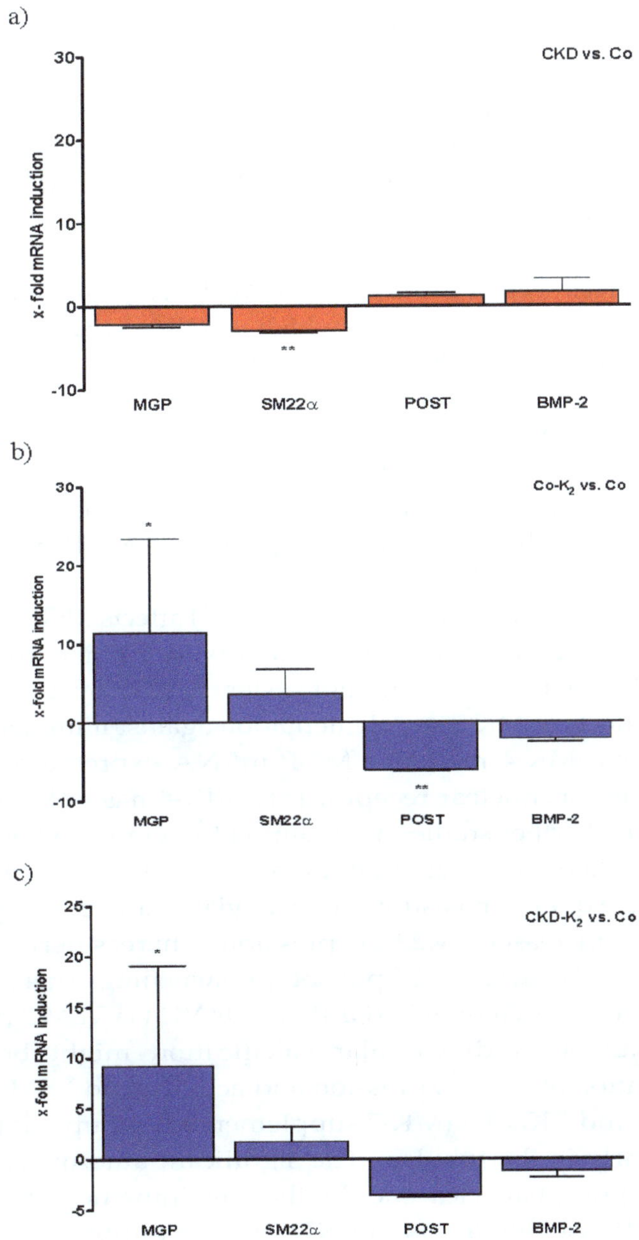

Figure 11. Aortic gene expression. The effect of CKD and MK-7 supplementation on aortic gene expression of calcification modifiers as x-fold induction compared to control group. Red columns depict pro-calcific changes, while alterations associated with potential calcification inhibition are assigned with blue columns. (**a**) In CKD animals SM22α expression is significantly decreased, whereas MGP expression is non-significantly decreased as compared to Co animals. (**b**) In Co-K_2 animals MGP mRNA concentration is significantly increased, whereas POST mRNA concentration is significantly decreased compared to Co animals. (**c**) In CKD-K_2 animals MGP mRNA concentration is significantly and SM22α mRNA concentration is tendentially increased compared to Co animals. Co = control group; Co-K_2 = MK-7 supplemented control group; CKD = 5/6 nephrectomized group; CKD-K_2 = MK-7 supplemented 5/6 nephrectomized group; MGP = matrix Gla-protein; POST = periostin; BMP-2 = bone morphogenetic protein 2. Significant differences: * $p < 0.05$, ** $p < 0.01$.

4.2. Cardiovascular Calcification

Animals in the CKD groups exhibited modest VCs with concomitant alkaline phosphatase presence. ALP may serve as a marker for osteoblastic activity [41]. However, increased deposits of ALP in the vasculature of animals in the CKD groups are also associated with the transdifferentiation of VSMCs towards osteochondrogenic-like cells [42]. These data are supported by the significantly decreased expression of SM22α, a protein specific for VSMCs. Our data are in line with previous observations that SM22α mRNA levels are decreased in a murine model of VC [43,44]. Moreover, we detected increased expression levels of periostin and BMP-2. Periostin is associated with increased extracellular matrix turnover, as seen in diseases like CKD [45,46]. Additionally, periostin is inversely correlated with decreased kidney function [47], which is in line with our results. BMP-2 expression is increased in atherosclerotic plaques [48] and in *in vitro* models of VC [49], supporting our data of CKD-induced VC.

MGP is a vitamin K-dependent protein known to inhibit VC. Functionality of MGP is dependent on vitamin K. We demonstrate that MGP expression is decreased in CKD animals as compared to controls. It has been described that MGP synthesis increases in response to VC [18,49]. Diabetes and CKD have an inhibitory effect on the protective upregulation of MGP expression, which is a possible pathomechanism for CKD-induced VC [50].

For the first time, we demonstrate that vitamin K (MK-7) affects MGP mRNA expression (>10-fold induction in controls and CKD rats) within the vascular wall. Earlier studies [17] showed that only locally expressed MGP in the arterial wall—and not systemic MGP over-expression—inhibits VC. Our results point to protective effects of MK-7 supplementation against imminent VC at the transcriptional level. There is evidence that MK-4 mediates MGP mRNA expression via activation of the SXR (steroid and xenobiotic receptor) nuclear receptor [51]. MK-4 has been shown to activate SXR in a dose-dependent manner [51]. Further studies are required to examine whether this observation can be replicated by MK-7. It is well known that vitamin K is a cofactor for the posttranslational carboxylation of MGP [16]. In our study we did not measure uncarboxylated and carboxylated MGP status.

MK-7 supplementation increased SM22α expression, whereas periostin and BMP-2 expression decreased, indicating that MK-7 affects VSMC phenotypic switching. This corroborates recent findings that the vitamin K-dependent Gla-rich protein (GRP) affects VC via VSMC phenotype modulation [52]. Thus, the impact of CKD on cardiovascular calcification might be counteracted by MK-7 supplementation via regulation of MGP expression and activity, and VSMC phenotypic switching.

Animals in both CKD and CKD-K_2 (MK-7 supplemented) groups significantly developed renal calcium deposits, particularly in the tubules. The significant amount of calcium deposits may be explained by the increased phosphate clearance by the remaining nephrons in combination with the high phosphate diet [53]. Phosphate levels in CKD play an important role in the development of cardiovascular calcification [54,55].

Interestingly, MK-7 supplementation normalized CKD-induced increased serum phosphate concentrations. More importantly, MK-7 supplementation inhibited both vascular and myocardial calcification in CKD animals on a high phosphate diet. Our results demonstrate a protective effect of MK-7 supplementation on early stages of cardiovascular calcification. Our results support previous data from our group, showing that both VK_1 and MK-4 supplementation reverses vitamin K antagonist-induced VC in rats [34]. To our best knowledge, this is the first study demonstrating a protective effect of MK-7 supplementation in a murine model of 5/6 nephrectomy-induced CKD. Compared to commonly applied models to induce VC (adenine diet, gene knockout animals, high-dose warfarin treatment), the VC calcification model applied in the current manuscript with mild CKD and phosphate loading more closely resembles the clinical situation of early CKD. As a matter of fact, cardiovascular mortality is already profoundly increased at early stages of CKD (e.g., below 60 mL/min GFR), rendering this model an attractive option to study the pathophysiological processes of imminent calcification and potential treatment options related to early CKD. Our results support the rationale for prophylactic supplementation of MK-7 in patients at risk for development of cardiovascular calcification. It has been shown that MK-7 supplementation is safe and has no side effects, both in experimental animals and humans [31,32,56]. Patients with CKD have been shown to be subclinically vitamin K deficient [21,22,57]. In an observational study in hemodialysis patients it was reported that a low circulating concentration of MK-4 was a predictor of aortic calcification [58], but this claim remains to be confirmed or refuted. Our group showed that MK-7 supplementation reduces levels of inactive MGP, osteocalcin, and PIVKA-II in hemodialysis patients [27]. It is tempting to speculate whether these results can be transferred to patients, a hypothesis that is currently being investigated in several studies [59].

4.3. Structural and Functional Alterations

In our model, CKD and a high phosphate diet induced increased systolic and diastolic blood pressure with cardiac hypertrophy. It is known that CKD and VC are associated with arterial hypertension [54] and reduced vascular compliance, with subsequent increased systolic and decreased diastolic blood pressure values [60]. Hypertension is most likely a consequence of kidney disease since blood pressure values were similarly elevated in both CKD and CKD-K_2 animals. CKD and hypertension are associated with vascular remodeling and increased cell proliferation [61,62]. VSMC proliferation increased in CKD and CKD-K_2 groups but was not affected by MK-7 treatment. Additionally, we detected increased elastic fiber breaking points in the tunica media, indicative of loss of vascular integrity in animals of the CKD and CKD-K_2 groups [63].

Importantly, we observed an inhibition of calcification of damaged tissues by MK-7 supplementation, whereas MK-7 was not able to continuously block the overwhelming harmful milieu of CKD and a high phosphate diet.

5. Conclusions

Our data provide evidence for a protective effect of high-dose MK-7 supplementation on cardiovascular calcification. MK-7 supplementation could not prevent CKD-associated hypertension and hypertrophy but prevented calcification of affected tissues. Since vitamin K has no reported side effects, it seems a promising therapeutic agent [59]. The effect of MK-7 is likely to act via vitamin K-dependent proteins such as MGP and it is tempting to speculate whether these results can be transferred to CKD patients.

Acknowledgments: This work was supported by: The Forschungskommission of the Medical Faculty, University Düsseldorf, Germany and the Susanne-Brunnenberg-Stiftung at Duesseldorf Heart Center.

Author Contributions: Ralf Westenfeld and Leon J. Schurgers conceived and designed the experiments. Verena Veulemans and Daniel Scheiber performed the experiments. Ralf Westenfeld, Verena Veulemans, and Daniel Scheiber analyzed the data. Patrick Horn, Marijn L. Chatrou, Sebastian Potthoff, and Malte Kelm contributed reagents, materials, and analysis tools. Ralf Westenfeld, Leon J. Schurgers, and Daniel Scheiber wrote the paper.

References

1. Allison, M.A.; Criqui, M.H.; Wright, C.M. Patterns and risk factors for systemic calcified atherosclerosis. *Arterioscler. Thromb. Vasc. Biol.* **2004**, *24*, 331–336. [CrossRef] [PubMed]
2. Giachelli, C.M. The emerging role of phosphate in vascular calcification. *Kidney Int.* **2009**, *75*, 890–897. [CrossRef] [PubMed]
3. Schurgin, S.; Rich, S.; Mazzone, T. Increased prevalence of significant coronary artery calcification in patients with diabetes. *Diabetes Care* **2001**, *24*, 335–338. [CrossRef] [PubMed]
4. Vliegenthart, R.; Oudkerk, M.; Hofman, A.; Oei, H.H.; van Dijck, W.; van Rooij, F.J.; Witteman, J.C. Coronary calcification improves cardiovascular risk prediction in the elderly. *Circulation* **2005**, *112*, 572–577. [CrossRef] [PubMed]

5. Ketteler, M.; Schlieper, G.; Floege, J. Calcification and cardiovascular health—New insights into an old phenomenon. *Hypertension* **2006**, *47*, 1027–1034. [CrossRef] [PubMed]
6. Wu, M.; Rementer, C.; Giachelli, C.M. Vascular calcification: An update on mechanisms and challenges in treatment. *Calcif. Tissue Int.* **2013**, *93*, 365–373. [CrossRef] [PubMed]
7. Moe, S.M.; O'Neill, K.D.; Duan, D.; Ahmed, S.; Chen, N.X.; Leapman, S.B.; Fineberg, N.; Kopecky, K. Medial artery calcification in esrd patients is associated with deposition of bone matrix proteins. *Kidney Int.* **2002**, *61*, 638–647. [CrossRef] [PubMed]
8. Demer, L.L.; Tintut, Y. Vascular calcification: Pathobiology of a multifaceted disease. *Circulation* **2008**, *117*, 2938–2948. [CrossRef] [PubMed]
9. Chatrou, M.L.; Winckers, K.; Hackeng, T.M.; Reutelingsperger, C.P.; Schurgers, L.J. Vascular calcification: The price to pay for anticoagulation therapy with vitamin K-antagonists. *Blood Rev.* **2012**, *26*, 155–166. [CrossRef] [PubMed]
10. Reaven, P.D.; Sacks, J. Coronary artery and abdominal aortic calcification are associated with cardiovascular disease in type 2 diabetes. *Diabetologia* **2005**, *48*, 379–385. [CrossRef] [PubMed]
11. Okuno, S.; Ishimura, E.; Kitatani, K.; Fujino, Y.; Kohno, K.; Maeno, Y.; Maekawa, K.; Yamakawa, T.; Imanishi, Y.; Inaba, M.; *et al.* Presence of abdominal aortic calcification is significantly associated with all-cause and cardiovascular mortality in maintenance hemodialysis. *Am. J. Kidney Dis.* **2007**, *49*, 417–425. [CrossRef] [PubMed]
12. Schurgers, L.J.; Cranenburg, E.C.M.; Vermeer, C. Matrix gla-protein: The calcification inhibitor in need of vitamin k. *Thromb. Haemost.* **2008**. [CrossRef]
13. Price, P.A.; Urist, M.R.; Otawara, Y. Matrix gla protein, a new gamma-carboxyglutamic acid-containing protein which is associated with the organic matrix of bone. *Biochem. Biophys. Res. Commun.* **1983**, *117*, 765–771. [CrossRef]
14. Luo, G.; Ducy, P.; McKee, M.D.; Pinero, G.J.; Loyer, E.; Behringer, R.R.; Karsenty, G. Spontaneous calcification of arteries and cartilage in mice lacking matrix gla protein. *Nature* **1997**, *386*, 78–81. [CrossRef] [PubMed]
15. Munroe, P.B.; Olgunturk, R.O.; Fryns, J.P.; van Maldergem, L.; Ziereisen, F.; Yuksel, B.; Gardiner, R.M.; Chung, E. Mutations in the gene encoding the human matrix gla protein cause keutel syndrome. *Nat. Genet.* **1999**, *21*, 142–144. [CrossRef] [PubMed]
16. Schurgers, L.J.; Uitto, J.; Reutelingsperger, C.P. Vitamin k-dependent carboxylation of matrix gla-protein: A crucial switch to control ectopic mineralization. *Trends Mol. Med.* **2013**, *19*, 217–226. [CrossRef] [PubMed]
17. Murshed, M.; Schinke, T.; McKee, M.D.; Karsenty, G. Extracellular matrix mineralization is regulated locally; different roles of two gla-containing proteins. *J. Cell Biol.* **2004**, *165*, 625–630. [CrossRef] [PubMed]
18. Schurgers, L.J.; Teunissen, K.J.; Knapen, M.H.; Kwaijtaal, M.; van Diest, R.; Appels, A.; Reutelingsperger, C.P.; Cleutjens, J.P.; Vermeer, C. Novel conformation-specific antibodies against matrix gamma-carboxyglutamic acid (gla) protein: Undercarboxylated matrix gla protein as marker for vascular calcification. *Arterioscler. Thromb. Vasc. Biol.* **2005**, *25*, 1629–1633. [CrossRef] [PubMed]
19. Berkner, K.L.; Runge, K.W. The physiology of vitamin k nutriture and vitamin k-dependent protein function in atherosclerosis. *J. Thromb. Haemost.* **2004**, *2*, 2118–2132. [CrossRef] [PubMed]
20. Rennenberg, R.J.M.W.; van Varik, B.J.; Schurgers, L.J.; Hamulyak, K.; ten Cate, H.; Leiner, T.; Vermeer, C.; de Leeuw, P.W.; Kroon, A.A. Chronic coumarin treatment is associated with increased extracoronary arterial calcification in humans. *Blood* **2010**, *115*, 5121–5123. [CrossRef] [PubMed]
21. Pilkey, R.M.; Morton, A.R.; Boffa, M.B.; Noordhof, C.; Day, A.G.; Su, Y.H.; Miller, L.M.; Koschinsky, M.L.; Booth, S.L. Subclinical vitamin k deficiency in hemodialysis patients. *Am. J. Kidney Dis.* **2007**, *49*, 432–439. [CrossRef] [PubMed]
22. Schurgers, L.J.; Barreto, D.V.; Barreto, F.C.; Liabeuf, S.; Renard, C.; Magdeleyns, E.J.; Vermeer, C.; Choukroun, G.; Massy, Z.A. The circulating inactive form of matrix gla protein is a surrogate marker for vascular calcification in chronic kidney disease: A preliminary report. *Clin. J. Am. Soc. Nephrol.* **2010**, *5*, 568–575. [CrossRef] [PubMed]
23. Shea, M.K.; O'Donnell, C.J.; Vermeer, C.; Magdeleyns, E.J.P.; Crosier, M.D.; Gundberg, C.M.; Ordovas, J.M.; Kritchevsky, S.B.; Booth, S.L. Circulating uncarboxylated matrix gla protein is associated with vitamin k nutritional status, but not coronary artery calcium, in older adults. *J. Nutr.* **2011**, *141*, 1529–1534. [CrossRef] [PubMed]

24. Ueland, T.; Gullestad, L.; Dahl, C.P.; Aukrust, P.; Aakhus, S.; Solberg, O.G.; Vermeer, C.; Schurgers, L.J. Undercarboxylated matrix gla protein is associated with indices of heart failure and mortality in symptomatic aortic stenosis. *J. Intern. Med.* **2010**, *268*, 483–492. [CrossRef] [PubMed]
25. Ueland, T.; Dahl, C.P.; Gullestad, L.; Aakhus, S.; Broch, K.; Skardal, R.; Vermeer, C.; Aukrust, P.; Schurgers, L.J. Circulating levels of non-phosphorylated undercarboxylated matrix gla protein are associated with disease severity in patients with chronic heart failure. *Clin. Sci.* **2011**, *121*, 119–127. [CrossRef] [PubMed]
26. Cranenburg, E.C.; Koos, R.; Schurgers, L.J.; Magdeleyns, E.J.; Schoonbrood, T.H.; Landewe, R.B.; Brandenburg, V.M.; Bekers, O.; Vermeer, C. Characterisation and potential diagnostic value of circulating matrix gla protein (mgp) species. *Thromb. Haemost.* **2010**, *104*, 811–822. [PubMed]
27. Westenfeld, R.; Krueger, T.; Schlieper, G.; Cranenburg, E.C.; Magdeleyns, E.J.; Heidenreich, S.; Holzmann, S.; Vermeer, C.; Jahnen-Dechent, W.; Ketteler, M.; *et al.* Effect of vitamin k2 supplementation on functional vitamin k deficiency in hemodialysis patients: A randomized trial. *Am. J. Kidney Dis.* **2012**, *59*, 186–195. [CrossRef] [PubMed]
28. Gonnet, M.; Lethuaut, L.; Boury, F. New trends in encapsulation of liposoluble vitamins. *J. Control. Release* **2010**, *146*, 276–290. [CrossRef] [PubMed]
29. Gijsbers, B.L.; Jie, K.S.; Vermeer, C. Effect of food composition on vitamin k absorption in human volunteers. *Br. J. Nutr.* **1996**, *76*, 223–229. [CrossRef] [PubMed]
30. Schurgers, L.J.; Vermeer, C. Determination of phylloquinone and menaquinones in food. Effect of food matrix on circulating vitamin k concentrations. *Haemostasis* **2000**, *30*, 298–307. [PubMed]
31. Beulens, J.W.J.; Bots, M.L.; Atsma, F.; Bartelink, M.L.E.L.; Prokop, M.; Geleijnse, J.M.; Witteman, J.C.M.; Grobbee, D.E.; van der Schouw, Y.T. High dietary menaquinone intake is associated with reduced coronary calcification. *Atherosclerosis* **2009**, *203*, 489–493. [CrossRef] [PubMed]
32. Geleijnse, J.M.; Vermeer, C.; Grobbee, D.E.; Schurgers, L.J.; Knapen, M.H.; van der Meer, I.M.; Hofman, A.; Witteman, J.C. Dietary intake of menaquinone is associated with a reduced risk of coronary heart disease: The rotterdam study. *J. Nutr.* **2004**, *134*, 3100–3105. [PubMed]
33. Kruger, T.; Oelenberg, S.; Kaesler, N.; Schurgers, L.J.; van de Sandt, A.M.; Boor, P.; Schlieper, G.; Brandenburg, V.M.; Fekete, B.C.; Veulemans, V.; *et al.* Warfarin induces cardiovascular damage in mice. *Arterioscler. Thromb. Vasc. Biol.* **2013**, *33*, 2618–2624. [CrossRef] [PubMed]
34. Schurgers, L.J.; Spronk, H.M.; Soute, B.A.; Schiffers, P.M.; DeMey, J.G.; Vermeer, C. Regression of warfarin-induced medial elastocalcinosis by high intake of vitamin k in rats. *Blood* **2007**, *109*, 2823–2831. [CrossRef] [PubMed]
35. Spronk, H.M.; Soute, B.A.; Schurgers, L.J.; Thijssen, H.H.; de Mey, J.G.; Vermeer, C. Tissue-specific utilization of menaquinone-4 results in the prevention of arterial calcification in warfarin-treated rats. *J. Vasc. Res.* **2003**, *40*, 531–537. [CrossRef] [PubMed]
36. Perez-Ruiz, L.; Ros-Lopez, S.; Cardus, A.; Fernandez, E.; Valdivielso, J.M. A forgotten method to induce experimental chronic renal failure in the rat by ligation of the renal parenchyma. *Nephron. Exp. Nephrol.* **2006**, *103*, e126–e130. [CrossRef] [PubMed]
37. Ng, K.; Hildreth, C.M.; Phillips, J.K.; Avolio, A.P. Aortic stiffness is associated with vascular calcification and remodeling in a chronic kidney disease rat model. *Am. J. Physiol. Renal Physiol.* **2011**, *300*, F1431–F1436. [CrossRef] [PubMed]
38. Shobeiri, N.; Adams, M.A.; Holden, R.M. Vascular calcification in animal models of ckd: A review. *Am. J. Nephrol.* **2010**, *31*, 471–481. [CrossRef] [PubMed]
39. Fleck, C.; Appenroth, D.; Jonas, P.; Koch, M.; Kundt, G.; Nizze, H.; Stein, G. Suitability of 5/6 nephrectomy (5/6nx) for the induction of interstitial renal fibrosis in rats—Influence of sex, strain, and surgical procedure. *Exp. Toxicol. Pathol.* **2006**, *57*, 195–205. [CrossRef] [PubMed]
40. El-Achkar, T.M.; Ohmit, S.E.; McCullough, P.A.; Crook, E.D.; Brown, W.W.; Grimm, R.; Bakris, G.L.; Keane, W.F.; Flack, J.M. Higher prevalence of anemia with diabetes mellitus in moderate kidney insufficiency: The kidney early evaluation program. *Kidney Int.* **2005**, *67*, 1483–1488. [CrossRef] [PubMed]
41. Shioi, A.; Katagi, M.; Okuno, Y.; Mori, K.; Jono, S.; Koyama, H.; Nishizawa, Y. Induction of bone-type alkaline phosphatase in human vascular smooth muscle cells: Roles of tumor necrosis factor-alpha and oncostatin m derived from macrophages. *Circ. Res.* **2002**, *91*, 9–16. [CrossRef]
42. Kendrick, J.; Chonchol, M. The role of phosphorus in the development and progression of vascular calcification. *Am. J. Kidney Dis.* **2011**, *58*, 826–834. [CrossRef] [PubMed]

43. El-Abbadi, M.M.; Pai, A.S.; Leaf, E.M.; Yang, H.Y.; Bartley, B.A.; Quan, K.K.; Ingalls, C.M.; Liao, H.W.; Giachelli, C.M. Phosphate feeding induces arterial medial calcification in uremic mice: Role of serum phosphorus, fibroblast growth factor-23, and osteopontin. *Kidney Int.* **2009**, *75*, 1297–1307. [CrossRef] [PubMed]
44. Steitz, S.A.; Speer, M.Y.; Curinga, G.; Yang, H.Y.; Haynes, P.; Aebersold, R.; Schinke, T.; Karsenty, G.; Giachelli, C.M. Smooth muscle cell phenotypic transition associated with calcification: Upregulation of cbfa1 and downregulation of smooth muscle lineage markers. *Circ. Res.* **2001**, *89*, 1147–1154. [CrossRef] [PubMed]
45. Hakuno, D.; Kimura, N.; Yoshioka, M.; Mukai, M.; Kimura, T.; Okada, Y.; Yozu, R.; Shukunami, C.; Hiraki, Y.; Kudo, A.; *et al.* Periostin advances atherosclerotic and rheumatic cardiac valve degeneration by inducing angiogenesis and mmp production in humans and rodents. *J. Clin. Invest.* **2010**, *120*, 2292–2306. [CrossRef] [PubMed]
46. Hixson, J.E.; Shimmin, L.C.; Montasser, M.E.; Kim, D.K.; Zhong, Y.; Ibarguen, H.; Follis, J.; Malcom, G.; Strong, J.; Howard, T.; *et al.* Common variants in the periostin gene influence development of atherosclerosis in young persons. *Arterioscler. Thromb. Vasc. Biol.* **2011**, *31*, 1661–1667. [CrossRef] [PubMed]
47. Sen, K.; Lindenmeyer, M.T.; Gaspert, A.; Eichinger, F.; Neusser, M.A.; Kretzler, M.; Segerer, S.; Cohen, C.D. Periostin is induced in glomerular injury and expressed de novo in interstitial renal fibrosis. *Am. J. Pathol.* **2011**, *179*, 1756–1767. [CrossRef] [PubMed]
48. Bostrom, K.; Watson, K.E.; Horn, S.; Wortham, C.; Herman, I.M.; Demer, L.L. Bone morphogenetic protein expression in human atherosclerotic lesions. *J. Clin. Invest.* **1993**, *91*, 1800–1809. [CrossRef] [PubMed]
49. Ciceri, P.; Elli, F.; Brenna, I.; Volpi, E.; Romagnoli, S.; Tosi, D.; Braidotti, P.; Brancaccio, D.; Cozzolino, M. Lanthanum prevents high phosphate-induced vascular calcification by preserving vascular smooth muscle lineage markers. *Calcif. Tissue Int.* **2013**, *92*, 521–530. [CrossRef] [PubMed]
50. Kaesler, N.; Magdeleyns, E.; Herfs, M.; Schettgen, T.; Brandenburg, V.; Fliser, D.; Vermeer, C.; Floege, J.; Schlieper, G.; Kruger, T. Impaired vitamin k recycling in uremia is rescued by vitamin k supplementation. *Kidney Int.* **2014**, *86*, 286–293. [CrossRef] [PubMed]
51. Tabb, M.M.; Sun, A.; Zhou, C.; Grun, F.; Errandi, J.; Romero, K.; Pham, H.; Inoue, S.; Mallick, S.; Lin, M.; *et al.* Vitamin k2 regulation of bone homeostasis is mediated by the steroid and xenobiotic receptor sxr. *J. Biol. Chem.* **2003**, *278*, 43919–43927. [CrossRef] [PubMed]
52. Viegas, C.S.; Rafael, M.S.; Enriquez, J.L.; Teixeira, A.; Vitorino, R.; Luis, I.M.; Costa, R.M.; Santos, S.; Cavaco, S.; Neves, J.; *et al.* Gla-rich protein acts as a calcification inhibitor in the human cardiovascular system. *Arterioscler. Thromb. Vasc. Biol.* **2015**, *35*, 399–408. [CrossRef]
53. Tsuchiya, N.; Matsushima, S.; Takasu, N.; Kyokawa, Y.; Torii, M. Glomerular calcification induced by bolus injection with dibasic sodium phosphate solution in sprague-dawley rats. *Toxicol. Pathol.* **2004**, *32*, 408–412. [CrossRef] [PubMed]
54. Eknoyan, G.; Levin, N.W. K/doqi clinical practice guidelines for chronic kidney disease: Evaluation, classification, and stratification. *Am. J. Kidney Dis.* **2002**, *39*, S14–S266.
55. McCarty, M.F.; DiNicolantonio, J.J. Bioavailable dietary phosphate, a mediator of cardiovascular disease, may be decreased with plant-based diets, phosphate binders, niacin, and avoidance of phosphate additives. *Nutrition* **2014**, *30*, 739–747. [CrossRef] [PubMed]
56. Pucaj, K.; Rasmussen, H.; Moller, M.; Preston, T. Safety and toxicological evaluation of a synthetic vitamin k2, menaquinone-7. *Toxicol. Mech. Methods* **2011**, *21*, 520–532. [CrossRef] [PubMed]
57. Holden, R.M.; Morton, A.R.; Garland, J.S.; Pavlov, A.; Day, A.G.; Booth, S.L. Vitamins k and d status in stages 3–5 chronic kidney disease. *Clin. J. Am. Soc. Nephrol.* **2010**, *5*, 590–597. [CrossRef] [PubMed]
58. Fusaro, M.; Noale, M.; Viola, V.; Galli, F.; Tripepi, G.; Vajente, N.; Plebani, M.; Zaninotto, M.; Guglielmi, G.; Miotto, D.; *et al.* Vitamin k, vertebral fractures, vascular calcifications, and mortality: Vitamin k italian (viki) dialysis study. *J. Bone Miner. Res.* **2012**, *27*, 2271–2278. [CrossRef] [PubMed]
59. Brandenburg, V.M.; Schurgers, L.J.; Kaesler, N.; Pusche, K.; van Gorp, R.H.; Leftheriotis, G.; Reinartz, S.; Koos, R.; Kruger, T. Prevention of vasculopathy by vitamin k supplementation: Can we turn fiction into fact? *Atherosclerosis* **2015**, *240*, 10–16. [CrossRef] [PubMed]
60. Taddei, S.; Nami, R.; Bruno, R.M.; Quatrini, I.; Nuti, R. Hypertension, left ventricular hypertrophy and chronic kidney disease. *Heart Fail. Rev.* **2011**, *16*, 615–620. [CrossRef] [PubMed]
61. Feihl, F.; Liaudet, L.; Levy, B.I.; Waeber, B. Hypertension and microvascular remodelling. *Cardiovasc. Res.* **2008**, *78*, 274–285. [CrossRef] [PubMed]

62. Li, S.; Wang, X.; Li, Y.; Kost, C.K., Jr.; Martin, D.S. Bortezomib, a proteasome inhibitor, attenuates angiotensin ii-induced hypertension and aortic remodeling in rats. *PLoS One* **2013**, *8*, e78564. [CrossRef] [PubMed]
63. Ro, A.; Kageyama, N. Pathomorphometry of ruptured intracranial vertebral arterial dissection: Adventitial rupture, dilated lesion, intimal tear, and medial defect. *J. Neurosurg.* **2013**, *119*, 221–227. [CrossRef] [PubMed]

11

Genotypic and Environmental Effects on Tocopherol Content in Almond

Ossama Kodad [1], Rafel Socias i Company [2,*] and José M. Alonso [2]

[1] Département Arboriculture-Viticulture, École Nationale d'Agriculture de Meknès, Meknès BP S/40, Morocco; osama.kodad@yahoo.es

[2] Unidad de Hortofruticutura, Centro de Investigación y Tecnología Agroalimentaria de Aragón (CITA), Av. Montañana 930, 50059 Zaragoza, Spain; jmalonsos@aragon.es

* Correspondence: rsocias@cita-aragon.es

Abstract: Almond is the most important nut species worldwide and almond kernels show the highest levels of tocopherols among all nuts. In almond, tocopherols not only play a substantial role as a healthy food for human consumption, but also in protecting lipids against oxidation and, thus, lengthening the storage time of almond kernels. The main tocopherol homologues detected in almond in decreasing content and biological importance are α-, γ-, δ-, and β-tocopherol. Tocopherol concentration in almond depends on the genotype and the environment, such as the climatic conditions of the year and the growing management of the orchard. The range of variability for the different tocopherol homologues is of 335–657 mg/kg of almond oil for α-, 2–50 for γ-, and 0.1–22 for β-tocopherol. Drought and heat have been the most important stresses affecting tocopherol content in almond, with increased levels at higher temperatures and in water deficit conditions. The right cultivar and the most appropriate growing conditions may be selected to obtain crops with effective kernel storage and for the most beneficial effects of almond consumption for human nutrition and health.

Keywords: almond; *Prunus amygdalus*; tocopherols; genotype; climate

---

1. Introduction

Almond is the most important tree nut crop in terms of commercial production [1]. An adaptation to harsh climates combined with an ability to develop a deep and extensive root system has allowed almond to exploit a wide range of ecological niches. Almond is well-adapted to the Mediterranean climate, characterized by mild winters and dry, hot summers. This adaptation has led to early bloom and rapid early shoot growth because of the low chilling requirements of almond. Almond also shows high tolerance to summer drought and heat. Almond has traditionally been the earliest temperate fruit tree crop to bloom, which limited growing to areas relatively free from spring frosts before the release of late-blooming cultivars by different breeding programs, since frosts at bloom or early fruit development can reduce, and even completely nullify, the crop. Since almond is naturally self-incompatible, it often requires cross-pollination, which further acts to promote genetic variability and adaptability to diverse environments [2].

The edible part of the almond nut is the kernel, considered an important food crop with a high nutritional and medicinal value. The oldest and most extensive medical system that first recorded the health uses for almonds derives from ancient Greeks and then the Persians, and later in traditional Chinese medicine and Indian Ayurvedic medicine [3]. From medieval times to the 18th century, almond nuts were a source of substitute "milk" [4], and also it was used as thickener before starch was "discovered" [3]. Almond consumption has almost doubled in the last 20 years [5], a fact that highlights how this consumption has evolved from a convenient snack food and component of a high number of confectioneries, to an important food which is increasingly recognized as essential for maintaining and increasing human health. Recent nutritional and medical studies have associated the regular consumption of almonds with a wide range of health benefits, including protection from cancer [6,7], obesity [8–10], diabetes [11,12], and heart diseases [13–17]. Almond kernels may be consumed in many different ways, blanched or unblanched, raw or combined, and/or mixed with other nuts. They can also be transformed to produce marzipan, nougat, almond milk, and almond flour, incorporated in many pastries and ice creams. Almonds may also be combined in other products and gastronomic specialties [18]. The high nutritive value of almond kernels is mainly due to their high lipid content. This lipid fraction, even constituting an important source of calories, does not contribute to cholesterol formation because of their high level of unsaturated fatty acids, mainly mono-unsaturated fatty acids [19]. Although almond kernels are high in energy, humans compensate their effect with their high satiety value [20]. The absorption of energy from almond kernels is rather inefficient, having been suggested that their chronic consumption may raise resting energy expenditure [21]. Acute and longer-term almond ingestion may help in regulating body weight [17], modulating fluctuations of blood glucose [22], total low density/high density lipoprotein cholesterol ratio, and triglycerides [23].

Almond kernel quality must be high in order to fulfill not only the industry requirements, but also to be attractive for the consumers [24]. Until recently only the kernel physical traits were considered when trying to establish almond quality [18], but the kernel chemical composition appears to be essential when establishing the best raw material for the different industrial applications and the high diversity of almond confectioneries [24]. In view of the high lipid fraction in the almond kernel, the quality of the almond oil is considered as the most important feature in the evaluation of almond quality. Different parameters related to the lipid fraction have been suggested for quality evaluation of the almond kernels, such as the amount of oil content in the kernel (fat percentage over the kernel dry weight), the percentage of oleic acid of the total fatty acids, the ratio of the percentages of oleic/linoleic acids (O/L), and, especially, the tocopherol concentration in the almond oil [24,25].

Early reviews on the composition of the almond nuts [18,26] did not include tocopherols as an important component of almond kernels. More recently tocopherols were already included in several reviews [27,28], but most of them were primarily descriptive without attempts to assess quality, particularly as it relates not only to industrial requirements, but also to breeding goals and approaches. Extensive variability in the chemical composition has been demonstrated among cultivars; additionally the importance of differences in geographical origins, as well as climatic and growing conditions have also been demonstrated. Despite this extensive information, little is known concerning the genetic control and inheritance of biochemical components of almond quality. For all these reasons, this review summarizes the current knowledge of the almond kernel tocopherol composition and factors affecting its variability.

2. Tocopherol Variability in Almond

Almost all studies carried out on vitamin content in almond are limited to those having an antioxidant effect, mainly tocopherols. The main tocopherol homologues detected in almond in decreasing importance are α-, γ-, δ-, and β-tocopherol. The main biochemical function of tocopherols is considered to be the protection of polyunsaturated fatty acids against peroxidation [29]. They also have protective roles in human health since recent data indicate that they have hypo-cholesterolemic, anti-cancer, and neuroprotective properties [30]. Tocopherol concentrations have been determined in many vegetable oils, having been correlated with their antioxidant activity, since this activity may depend on the ratio of % total tocopherols/% polyunsaturated fatty acids [31]. Tocopherol concentration plays an important role in protecting almond lipids against oxidation, thus increasing the possibilities of lengthening kernel storage [31–33].

The range of variability of the different tocopherol homologues has been reported for different almond cultivars and genotypes from different countries [27,34–44], being summarized in Table 1. The most biologically active form of vitamin E is α-tocopherol, being preferentially utilized in the human body over the other homologues [45], ranging from 200 mg/kg oil in some Australian cultivars [44] to 656.7 mg/kg oil in some local accessions from Morocco [37]. At high temperatures γ-tocopherol has been reported to be much more effective as an inhibitor of polymerization and protection against oxidation than α-tocopherol [46,47]. The range of variability of this homologue was from 2.4 mg/kg oil in some local Moroccan almond seedlings [37] to 50.2 mg/kg oil in some almond selections from the CITA breeding program [35,48]. For δ-tocopherol, the range of variability is reduced as compared to the other homologues and ranged from 0.1 mg/kg oil in some local Moroccan almond seedlings [37] to 22.0 mg/kg oil in some Spanish almond cultivars [39].

Table 1. Tocopherol homologue concentration in almond kernel and kernel oil.

Tocopherol Homologue	Range of Variability		Origin	Reference
	mg/kg Kernel	mg/kg Oil		
α-tocopherol	85–190		Spain	[42]
		335.3–551.7	Spain	[39]
		309–656.7	Morocco	[37]
	180–320		California	[38]
	250–840		Italy	[32]
		350–471	Italy	[43]
		370–571	Argentina	[40]
		200	Australia	[44]
β-tocopherol	50–80		Italy	[32]
	1.2		Australia	[44]
γ-tocopherol		6.1–50.2	Spain	[34,39]
	1.4–8.4		Spain	[42]
		75	Italy	[31]
		2.4–13.5	Morocco	[37]
	5.7		Australia	[44]
δ-tocopherol	0.2–1.6		Spain	[42]
		0.2–22	Spain	[34,39]
		0.1–0.3	Morocco	[37]

3. Environmental Effects

Tocopherol levels increase in response to a variety of abiotic stresses, considered as evidence of its protective role [49]. Tocopherol concentration in almond oil depends on the genotype and the climatic conditions of the year [36,38–40,42], as well as on the environmental conditions of the growing region [36,38]. Drought and heat have been the most important stresses studied until now on the expression of the chemical compounds in fruit trees, including almond. The climatic conditions of the year, mainly temperature, affect the concentration of the different tocopherol homologues in several nut crops [50], indicating that these components depend on the temperature and the occurrence of drought during fruit or nut growth.

The effect of drought stress on the oil percentage in almond kernels and on its composition is not clear since the results of different studies undertaken in this field are ambiguous. However, studies in other species reported that water stress appears to promote tocopherol synthesis [51–53]. In almond there was no obvious relationship between almond tocopherol content and the degree of water deficiency [54], since little variation in kernel oil tocopherols was observed under moderate water stress, except for the more severe deficit of 70% SDI (sustained deficit irrigation) which for all components, except γ-tocopherol, had higher values than the control. In this study, the minor tocopherol homologues appeared to be slightly more responsive to deficit irrigation than the main homologue, α-tocopherol, but their small proportion had little impact on the amount of the total tocopherol content [54]. In the "Nonpareil" almond cultivar, the highest accumulation rate of α-tocopherol takes place during the period from 74 to 94 days after anthesis [44], indicating that the critical period to add nutrient and water to ensure normal accumulation of these chemical compounds is during this period. Tocopherol concentration has been reported to be affected by drought stress in olive oil [55], but not in *Brassica napus* [56], by temperature in soybean [57], and by a combination of both in shea butter (*Vitellaria paradoxa* C.F. Gaertn.) [50]. In olive oil, the total tocopherols and α-tocopherol were highly influenced by the crop-year rainfalls, with the highest concentration from olives harvested during the driest year [58]. The increase in tocopherol content might contribute to the prevention of plant oxidative damage in drought conditions [59,60].

Higher tocopherol concentrations were found in almond kernels harvested in years with higher temperatures suggesting that this environmental factor could affect tocopherol synthesis during kernel development [34]. A study on the effect of two contrasting environments, with drought and heat conditions in Morocco, and irrigated and cold conditions in Spain, concluded that the tocopherol content, mainly of α-tocopherol, increased under the warmer climate conditions of Morocco [37]. More recently, higher α-tocopherol concentrations (~646 μg/g in average) were found when the almond kernel development mostly coincided with spring and summer months with warmer mean temperature in a study in arid Northwestern Argentina [40]. Similar results were reported for α-tocopherol in some almond genotypes grown under hot and dry conditions in Afghanistan [61]. Temperature during seed development in sunflower has shown to affect oil yield and tocopherol concentration since high temperatures may have a negative effect in oil synthesis, but not in tocopherol concentration [62,63]. In soybean seed, it has been reported that the increasing temperature from 23 °C to 28 °C can significantly increase tocopherol levels [64]. Thus, the temperature could be considered an important parameter playing a great role in tocopherol accumulation in different species, including almond.

Concerning the effect of solar radiation, in "Nonpareil" almond kernels the concentration of α-tocopherol was increased after a mild solar UV radiation supplement using the white weed mat, which may have altered metabolic pathways and stimulated α-tocopherol accumulation in almond lipids [44]. In sunflower, it has been reported that an increase in intercepted solar radiation per plant increased the amount of tocopherol per grain [65].

4. Genetic Effects

The evaluation of tocopherol concentration in the oil of different almond cultivars and genotypes showed high variability of the different tocopherol homologues, with a great effect of the environment [28]. However, it has been reported that the cultivars "Atocha", "Desmayo Rojo", "Desmayo Largueta" from Spain, and "Ferraduel" from France showed stable and similar year to year values for α-tocopherol; whereas "Atocha", "Ferraduel", and "Fournat de Brézenaud", and "Yaltinskij" from Ukraine were also stable for γ-tocopherol content in almond kernels produced under contrasting climatic conditions, with drought and heat conditions in Morocco, and irrigated and cold conditions in Spain [36]. These results confirmed that the stability of each tocopherol homologue depends on the specific characteristics of the genotype [34,35]. The estimation of the heritability of the different tocopherols isomers were estimated for the first time in almond [35], reporting that the content of γ-tocopherol showed high heritability estimates, with $h^2 = 60.0\%$, whereas α-tocopherol showed lower heritability ($h^2 = 20.5\%$). These results confirm that the tocopherol content in almond oil kernel is under polygenic control, as previously suggested [28].

The biosynthetic pathway of vitamin E in plants was biochemically elucidated several years ago, and all enzymes in this pathway were localized to the inner chloroplast envelope [66–68]. Today, the availability of complete genome sequences, in particular from *Arabidopsis* and *Synechocystis* sp. PCC6803, all biosynthetic genes in tocopherol biosynthesis have been identified and cloned to date [69,70]. A mutation in the gene VTE5 (PCT) of *Arabidopsis* lead to the discovery of its function, since it is encoding a protein with phytol kinase activity, directly involved in the biosynthetic pathway of tocopherol [70,71]. Tocopherol QTL analysis found that up to 65% of the markers were co-located in certain genomic regions of maize, including the candidate genes PDS1 (p-hydroxyphenylpyruvate dioxygenase; HPPD) and VTE4 (γ-tocopherol methyltransferase; γ-TMT), thus showing that a single QTL may affect more than one tocopherol homologue [71]. After exploring mutant inbred lines in sunflower, three loci (m = *Tph*1, g = *Tph*2, and d) were shown to disrupt synthesis in α-tocopherol production; additionally, the loci losing function in these mutations enhanced synthesis of other tocopherols [72]. In almond no studies have been conducted to elucidate the pathway biosynthesis of tocopherol isomers and the genes involved in this process, but, recently, five different QTLs believed to control the tocopherol concentration in the almond kernel oil have been identified [73]. More studies are required to understand the biosynthetic pathway of these biochemicals components to elucidate the gene involved in these pathways. This information will be of great interest for the breeders to improve tocopherol content in the future, since the almond kernel is used more and more in different industrial processes using high temperatures in their application [24].

5. Conclusions

The present information on the different effects on tocopherol content in almond is scarce. Only descriptive results have been published, not allowing a critical comparison among them, since some results are given as tocopherol content in the almond kernel and others in the kernel oil, not always stating the oil concentration of the almond kernel. Although genetic and environmental effects affecting tocopherol content in almond have been described, no interaction between them has ever been established. The present scenario of climatic change and of the shift of almond growing to warmer regions [1] may have a positive effect on the tocopherol content in almond kernels due to the effect of higher temperatures increasing this content. Consequently, the right cultivar and the most appropriate growing conditions may be selected in order to have almond crops not only allowing a better effective kernel storage, but also holding the most beneficial effects for human nutrition and health with their consumption. The objective of selecting for high tocopherol content in a breeding progeny is easily attainable because of its high heritability, whenever the adequate parents are chosen. As a consequence, these components could be considered as selection criteria in almond breeding programs as already suggested [24]. At present the possibilities of selecting cultivars, growing regions, and orchard practices offer an optimistic outlook for increasing tocopherol content in almond.

Acknowledgments: This work was supported by the grant RTA2014-00062-00-00 of the Spanish INIA, and the activity of the Consolidated Research Group A12 of Aragon.

References

1. Gradziel, T.M.; Curtis, R.; Socias i Company, R. Production and growing regions. In *Almonds: Botany, Production and Uses*; Socias i Company, R., Gradizel, T.M., Eds.; CABI: Wallingford, UK, 2017; pp. 70–86.
2. Socias i Company, R.; Felipe, A.J. Almond: A diverse germplasm. *HortScience* **1992**, *27*, 717–718.
3. Albala, K. Almonds along the Silk Road: The exchange and adaptation of ideas from West to East. *Petits Propos Culin.* **2009**, *88*, 17–32.
4. Mori, A.M.; Considine, R.V.; Mattes, R.D. Acute and second-meal effects of almond form in impaired glucose tolerant adults: A randomized crossover trial. *Nutr. Metab.* **2011**, *8*, 6. [CrossRef] [PubMed]
5. Ryan, N.T. World almond market. In *Almonds: Botany, Production and Uses*; Socias i Company, R., Gradizel, T.M., Eds.; CABI: Wallingford, UK, 2017; pp. 449–459.
6. Davis, P.A.; Iwasashi, C.K. Whole almonds and almond fractions reduce aberrant crypt foci in a rat model of colon carcinogenesis. *Cancer Lett.* **2001**, *165*, 27–33. [CrossRef]
7. Davis, P.A.; Law, S.; Wong, J. Colonic interposition after esophagectomy for cancer. *Arch. Surg.* **2003**, *138*, 303–308. [CrossRef] [PubMed]

8. Ren, Y.; Waldron, K.W.; Pacy, J.F.; Ellis, P.R. Chemical and histochemical characterization of cell wall polysaccharides in almond seeds in relation to lipid bioavailability. In *Biologically Active Phytochemicals in Food*; Pfannhauser, W., Fenwick, G.R., Khokhar, S., Eds.; Royal Society of Chemistry: Cambridge, UK, 2001; pp. 448–452.
9. Fraser, G.E.; Bennett, H.W.; Jaceldo, K.B.; Sabaté, J. Effect on body weight of a free 76 kilojoule (320 calorie) daily supplement of almonds for six months. *J. Am. Coll. Nutr.* **2002**, *21*, 275–283. [CrossRef] [PubMed]
10. Kendall, C.W.; Jenkins, D.J.; Marchie, A.; Ren, Y.; Ellis, P.R.; Lapsley, K.G. Energy availability from almonds: Implications for weight loss and cardiovascular health. A randomized controlled dose-response trial. *FASEB J.* **2003**, *17*, A339.
11. Lovejoy, J.C.; Most, M.M.; Lefevre, M.; Greenway, F.L.; Rood, J.C. Effect of diets enriched in almonds on insulin action and serum lipids in adults with normal glucose tolerance or type 2 diabetes. *Am. J. Clin. Nutr.* **2002**, *76*, 1000–1006. [PubMed]
12. Scott, L.W.; Balasubramanyam, A.; Kimball, K.T.; Ahrens, A.K.; Fordis, C.M.; Ballantyne, C.M. Long-term, randomonized clinical trial of two diets in the metabolic syndrome and type 2 diabetes. *Diabetes Care* **2003**, *26*, 2481–2482. [CrossRef] [PubMed]
13. Spiller, G.A.; Jenkins, D.J.A.; Cragen, L.N.; Gates, J.E.; Bosello, O.; Berra, K.; Rudd, C.; Stevenson, M.; Superko, R. Effect of a diet high in monounsaturated fat from almonds on plasma-cholesterol and lipoproteins. *J. Am. Coll. Nutr.* **1992**, *11*, 126–130. [PubMed]
14. Fulgoni, V.L.; Abbey, M.; Davis, P.; Jenkins, D.; Lovejoy, J.; Most, M.; Sabaté, J.; Spiller, G. Almonds lower blood cholesterol and LDL-cholesterol but not HDL-cholesterol in human subjects: Results of a meta-analysis. *FASEB J.* **2002**, *16*, A981–A982.
15. Hyson, D.A.; Schneeman, B.O.; Davis, P.A. Almonds and almond oil have similar effects on plasma lipids and LDL oxidation in healthy men and women. *J. Nutr.* **2002**, *132*, 703–707. [PubMed]
16. Jenkins, D.J.A.; Kendall, C.W.C.; Marchie, A.; Parker, T.L.; Connelly, P.W.; Qian, W.; Haight, J.S.; Faulkner, D.; Vidgen, E.; Lapsley, K.G.; et al. Dose response of almonds on coronary heart disease risk factors—Blood lipids, oxidized LDL, lipoprotein(a), homocysteine and pulmonary nitric oxide: A randomized controlled cross-over trial. *Circulation* **2002**, *106*, 1327–1332. [CrossRef] [PubMed]
17. Sabaté, J.; Haddad, E.; Tanzman, J.S.; Jambazian, P.; Rajaram, S. Serum lipid response to the graduated enrichment of a Step I diet with almonds: A randomized feeding trial. *Am. J. Clin. Nutr.* **2003**, *77*, 1379–1384. [PubMed]
18. Schirra, M. Postharvest technology and utilization of almonds. *Hortic. Rev.* **1997**, *20*, 267–292.
19. Sabaté, J.; Hook, D.G. Almonds, walnuts, and serum lipids. In *Lipids in Human Nutrition*; Spiller, G.A., Ed.; CRC Press: Boca Raton, FL, USA, 1996; pp. 137–144.
20. Hollis, J.; Mattes, R. Effect of chronic consumption of almonds on body weight in healthy humans. *Br. J. Nutr.* **2007**, *98*, 651–656. [CrossRef] [PubMed]
21. Cassady, B.A.; Hollis, J.H.; Fulford, A.D.; Considine, R.V.; Mattes, R.D. Mastication of almonds: Effects of lipid bioaccessibility, appetite, and hormone response. *Am. J. Clin. Nutr.* **2009**, *89*, 794–800. [CrossRef] [PubMed]
22. Jenkins, D.J.; Kendall, C.W.; Josse, A.R.; Salvatore, S.; Brighenti, F.; Augustin, L.S.; Ellis, P.R.; Vidgen, E.; Rao, A.V. Almonds decrease postprandial glycemia, insulinemia, and oxidative damage in healthy individuals. *J. Nutr.* **2006**, *136*, 2987–2992. [PubMed]
23. Foster, G.D.; Shantz, K.L.; Vander Veur, S.S.; Oliver, T.L.; Lent, M.R.; Virus, A.; Szapary, P.; Rader, D.J.; Zemel, B.S.; Gilden-Tsai, A. A randomized trial of the effects of an almond-enriched, hypocaloric diet in the treatment of obesity. *Am. J. Clin. Nutr.* **2012**, *96*, 249–254. [CrossRef] [PubMed]
24. Socias i Company, R.; Kodad, O.; Alonso, J.M.; Gradziel, T.M. Almond quality: A breeding perspective. *Hortic. Rev.* **2008**, *34*, 197–238.
25. Kodad, O.; Socias i Company, R. Variability of oil content and of major fatty acid composition in almond (*Prunus amygdalus* Batsch) and its relationshipwith kernel quality. *J. Agric. Food Chem.* **2008**, *56*, 4096–4101. [CrossRef] [PubMed]
26. Saura Calixto, F.; Cañellas, J.; Soler, L. *La Almendra: Composición, Variedades, Desarrollo y Maduración*; INIA: Madrid, Spain, 1988.
27. Yada, S.; Lapsley, K.; Huang, G. A review of composition studies of cultivated almonds: Macronutrients and micronutrients. *J. Food Compos. Anal.* **2011**, *24*, 469–480. [CrossRef]

28. Kodad, O. Chemical composition of almond nuts. In *Almonds: Botany, Production and Uses*; Socias i Company, R., Gradizel, T.M., Eds.; CABI: Wallingford, UK, 2017; pp. 428–449.
29. Kamal-Eldin, A.; Appelqvist, L.A. The chemistry and antioxidant properties of tocopherols and tocotrienols. *Lipids* **1996**, *31*, 671–701. [CrossRef] [PubMed]
30. Sen, C.K.; Khanna, S.; Roy, S. Tocotrienols in health and disease: The other half of the natural vitamin E family. *Mol. Asp. Med.* **2007**, *28*, 692–728. [CrossRef] [PubMed]
31. Senesi, E.; Rizzolo, A.; Colombo, C.; Testoni, A. Influence of pre-processing storage conditions on peeled almond quality. *Ital. J. Food Sci.* **1996**, *2*, 115–125.
32. Zacheo, G.; Cappello, M.S.; Gallo, A.; Santino, A.; Cappello, A.R. Changes associated with postharvest ageing in almond seeds. *Lebensm. Wiss. Technol.* **2000**, *33*, 415–423. [CrossRef]
33. García-Pascual, P.; Mateos, M.; Carbonell, V.; Salazar, D.M. Influence of storage conditions on the quality of shelled and roasted almonds. *Biosyst. Eng.* **2003**, *84*, 201–209. [CrossRef]
34. Kodad, O.; Socias i Company, R.; Prats, M.S.; López Ortiz, M.C. Variability in tocopherol concentrations in almond oil and its use as a selection criterion in almond breeding. *J. Hortic. Sci. Biotechnol.* **2006**, *81*, 501–507. [CrossRef]
35. Font i Forcada, C.; Kodad, O.; Juan, T.; Estopañán, G.; Socias i Company, R. Genetic variability and pollen effect on the transmission of the chemical components of the almond kernel. *Span. J. Agric. Res.* **2011**, *9*, 781–789. [CrossRef]
36. Kodad, O.; Estopañán, G.; Juan, T.; Mamouni, A.; Socias i Company, R. Tocopherol concentration in almond oil: Genetic variation and environmental effect under warm conditions. *J. Agric. Food Chem.* **2011**, *59*, 6137–6141. [CrossRef] [PubMed]
37. Kodad, O.; Estopañán, G.; Juan, T.; Socias i Company, R. Protein content and oil composition of almond from Moroccan seedlings: Genetic diversity, oil quality and geographical origin. *J. Am. Oil Chem. Soc.* **2013**, *90*, 243–252. [CrossRef]
38. Yada, S.; Huang, G.; Lapsley, K. Natural variability in the nutrient composition of California-grown almonds. *J. Food Compos. Anal.* **2013**, *30*, 80–85. [CrossRef]
39. Kodad, O.; Estopañán, G.; Juan, T.; Socias i Company, R. Tocopherol concentration in almond oil from Moroccan seedlings: Geographical origin and post-harvest implications. *J. Food Compos. Anal.* **2014**, *33*, 161–165. [CrossRef]
40. Maestri, D.; Martínez, M.; Bodoira, R.; Rossi, Y.; Oviedo, A.; Pierantozzi, P.; Torres, M. Variability in almond oil chemical traits from traditional cultivars and native genetic resources from Argentina. *Food Chem.* **2015**, *170*, 55–61. [CrossRef] [PubMed]
41. Kodad, O.; Alonso, J.M.; Espiau, M.T.; Estopañán, G.; Juan, T.; Socias i Company, R. Chemometric characterization of almond germplasm: Compositional aspects involved in quality and breeding. *J. Am. Soc. Hortic. Sci.* **2011**, *136*, 273–281.
42. López-Ortiz, C.M.; Prats-Moya, S.; Beltrán Sanahuja, A.; Maestre-Pérez, S.E.; Grané-Teruel, N.; Martín-Carratalá, M.L. Comparative study of tocopherol homologue content in four almond oil cultivars during two consecutive years. *J. Food Compos. Anal.* **2008**, *21*, 144–151. [CrossRef]
43. Rizzolo, A.; Baldo, C.; Polesello, A. Application of high-performance liquid chromatography to the analysis of niacin and biotin in Italian almond cultivars. *J. Chromatogr.* **1991**, *553*, 187–192. [CrossRef]
44. Zhu, Y. Almond (*Prunus dulcis* (Mill.) D.A. Webb) Fatty Acids and Tocopherols under Different Conditions. Ph.D. Thesis, University of Adelaide, Adelaide, Australia, March 2014.
45. Brigelius-Flohé, R.; Kelly, F.J.; Salonen, J.T.; Neuzil, J.; Zingg, J.M.; Azzi, A. The European perspective on vitamin E: Current knowledge and future research. *Am. J. Clin. Nutr.* **2002**, *76*, 703–716. [PubMed]
46. Lampi, A.M.; Kamal-Eldin, A. Effect of α-and γ-tocopherols on thermal polymerization of purified high-oleic sunflower triacylglycerols. *J. Am. Oil Chem. Soc.* **1998**, *75*, 1699–1703. [CrossRef]
47. Warner, K.; Neff, W.E.; Eller, E.J. Enhancing quality and oxidative stability of aged fried food with gamma-tocopherol. *J. Agric. Food Chem.* **2003**, *51*, 623–627. [CrossRef] [PubMed]
48. Kodad, O. Criterios de Selección y de Evaluación de Nuevas Obtenciones Autocompatibles en un Programa de Mejora Genética del Almendro. Ph.D. Thesis, University of Lleida, Lleida, Spain, 2006.
49. Munné-Bosch, S.; Alegre, L. The function of tocopherols and tocotrienols in plants. *Crit. Rev. Plant Sci.* **2002**, *21*, 31–57. [CrossRef]

50. Maranz, S.; Wiesman, Z. Influence of climate on the tocopherol content of sheabutter. *J. Agric. Food Chem.* **2004**, *52*, 2934–2937. [CrossRef] [PubMed]

51. Ali, Q.; Ashraf, M.; Anwar, F. Physico-chemical attributes of seed oil from drought stressed sunflower (*Helianthus annus* L.) plants. *Grasas Aceites* **2009**, *60*, 475–481.

52. Ali, Q.; Ashraf, M.; Anwar, F. Seed composition and seed oil antioxidant activity of maize under water stress. *J. Am. Oil Chem. Soc.* **2010**, *87*, 1179–1187. [CrossRef]

53. Britz, S.J.; Kremer, D.F. Warm temperatures or drought during seed maturation increase free α-tocopherol in seed of soybean (*Glycine max* [L.] Merr.). *J. Agric. Food Chem.* **2002**, *50*, 6058–6063. [CrossRef] [PubMed]

54. Zhu, Y.; Taylor, C.; Sommer, K.; Wilkinson, K.; Wirthensohn, M. Influence of deficit irrigation strategies on fatty acid and tocopherol concentration of almond (*Prunus dulcis*). *Food Chem.* **2015**, *173*, 821–826. [CrossRef] [PubMed]

55. Romero, M.P.; Tovar, M.J.; Ramos, T.; Motilva, M.J. Effect of crop season on the composition of virgin olive oil with protected designation of "Les Garrigues". *J. Am. Oil Chem. Soc.* **2003**, *80*, 423–430. [CrossRef]

56. Richards, A.; Wijesundera, C.; Salisbury, P. Genotype and growing environment effects on the tocopherols and fatty acids of *Brassica napus* and *B. juncea*. *J. Am. Oil Chem. Soc.* **2008**, *87*, 469–481. [CrossRef]

57. Almonor, G.O.; Fenner, G.P.; Wilson, R.F. Temperature effects on tocopherols composition in soybeans with genetically improved oil quality. *J. Am. Oil Chem. Soc.* **1998**, *75*, 591–596. [CrossRef]

58. Beltrán, G.; Jiménez, A.; del Rio, C.; Sánchez, S.; Martínez, L.; Uceda, M.; Aguilera, M.P. Variability of vitamin E in virgin olive oil by agronomical and genetic factors. *J. Food Compos. Anal.* **2010**, *23*, 633–639. [CrossRef]

59. Munné-Bosch, S.; Schwarz, K.; Alegre, L. Enhanced formation of alpha-tocopherol and highly oxidized abietane diterpenes in water-stressed rosemary plants. *Plant Physiol.* **1999**, *121*, 1047–1052. [CrossRef] [PubMed]

60. Munné-Bosch, S.; Peñuelas, J. Drought-induced oxidative stress in strawberry tree (*Arbutus unedo* L.) growing in Mediterranean field conditions. *Plant Sci.* **2004**, *166*, 1105–1110. [CrossRef]

61. Zamany, A.J.; Samadi, G.R.; Kim, D.H.; Keum, Y.S.; Saini, R.K. Comparative study of tocopherol contents and fatty acids composition in twenty almond cultivars of Afghanistan. *J. Am. Oil Chem. Soc.* **2017**, *6*, 805–817. [CrossRef]

62. Baydar, H.; Erbaf, S. Influence of seed development and seed position on oil, fatty acids and total tocopherol contents in sunflower (*Helianthus annuus* L.). *Turk. J. Agric. For.* **2005**, *29*, 179–186.

63. Ayerdi-Gotor, A.; Berger, M.; Labalette, F.; Centis, S.; Daydé, J.; Calmon, A. Variabilité des teneurs et compositions des composés mineurs dans l'huile de tournesol au cours du développement du capitule. Partie I—Tocophérols. *OCL* **2006**, *13*, 206–212. [CrossRef]

64. Britz, S.J.; Kremer, D.F.; Kenworthy, W.J. Tocopherols in soybean seeds: Genetic variation and environmental effects in field-grown crops. *J. Am. Oil Chem. Soc.* **2008**, *85*, 931–936. [CrossRef]

65. Izquierdo, N.G.; Nolasco, S.; Mateo, C.; Santos, D.; Aguirrezábal, L.A.N. Relationship between oil tocopherol concentration and oil weight per grain in several crop species. *Crop Pasture Sci.* **2011**, *62*, 1088–1097. [CrossRef]

66. Soll, J.; Schultz, G. Comparison of geranylgenariol and phytyl substituted methyl-quinols in the tocopherol synthesis of spinach chloroplasts. *Biochem. Biophys. Res. Commun.* **1979**, *91*, 715–720. [CrossRef]

67. Soll, J.; Kemmerling, M.; Schultz, G. Tocopherol and plastoquinone synthesis in spinach chloroplast subfractions. *Arch. Biochem. Biophys.* **1980**, *204*, 544–550. [CrossRef]

68. Soll, J.; Schultz, G. Phytol synthesis from geranylgeraniol in spinach chloroplasts. *Biochem. Biophys. Res. Commun.* **1981**, *99*, 907–912. [CrossRef]

69. Herbers, K. Vitamin production in transgenic plants. *J. Plant Physiol.* **2003**, *160*, 821–829. [CrossRef] [PubMed]

70. Gilliland, L.U.; Magallanes-Lundback, M.; Hemming, C.; Supplee, A.; Koornneef, M.; Leo, B.; Della Penna, D. Genetic basis for natural variation in seed vitamin E levels in *Arabidopsis thaliana*. *Proc. Natl. Acad. Sci. USA* **2006**, *49*, 18834–18841. [CrossRef] [PubMed]

71. Chander, S.; Guo, Y.G.; Yang, X.H.; Yan, J.B.; Zhang, Y.R.; Song, T.M.; Li, J.S. Genetic dissection of tocopherol concentration and composition in maize grain using quantitative trait loci analysis and the candidate gene approach. *Mol. Breed.* **2008**, *22*, 353–365. [CrossRef]

72. Tang, S.; Hass, C.G.; Knapp, S.J. *Ty3/gypsy*-like retrotransposon knockout of a 2-methyl-6-phytyl-1, 4-benzoquinone methyltransferase is non-lethal, uncovers a cryptic paralogous mutation, and produces novel tocopherol (vitamin E) profiles in sunflower. *Theor. Appl. Genet.* **2006**, *113*, 783–799. [CrossRef] [PubMed]
73. Font i Forcada, C.; Fernández i Martí, A.; Socias i Company, R. Mapping quantitative trait loci for kernel composition in almond. *BMC Genet.* **2012**, *13*, 47. [CrossRef] [PubMed]

12

Total and Differential Phylloquinone (Vitamin K1) Intakes of Preterm Infants from All Sources during the Neonatal Period

Paul Clarke [1,*], Simon J. Mitchell [2] and Martin J. Shearer [3]

1 Neonatal Unit, Norfolk and Norwich University Hospitals NHS Foundation Trust, Colney Lane, Norwich, Norfolk NR4 7UY, UK
2 Newborn Intensive Care, St Mary's Hospital, Oxford Road, Manchester M13 9WL, UK; simon.mitchell@cmft.nhs.uk
3 The Centre for Haemostasis and Thrombosis, St. Thomas' Hospital, Westminster Bridge Road, London SE1 7EH, UK; martin.shearer@gstt.nhs.uk
* Correspondence: paul.clarke@nnuh.nhs.uk

Abstract: All newborns require phylloquinone after birth to prevent vitamin K deficiency bleeding. Babies born prematurely may be at particular risk of deficiency without adequate supplementation during infancy. The main sources of phylloquinone in preterm babies during the neonatal period are the prophylactic dose of phylloquinone given at birth, and that derived from parenteral and/or enteral feeding. This observational study formed part of a prospective, multicentre, randomised, controlled trial that examined the vitamin K status of preterm infants after random allocation to one of three phylloquinone prophylactic regimens at birth (0.5 or 0.2 mg intramuscularly or 0.2 mg intravenously). In this nutritional sub-study we quantified the proportional and total phylloquinone intakes of preterm infants within the neonatal period from all sources. Almost all infants had average daily phylloquinone intakes that were in excess of the currently recommended amounts. In infants who did not receive parenteral nutrition, the bolus dose of phylloquinone given at birth was the major source of phylloquinone intake, whereas in infants who received parenteral nutrition, the intake from the parenteral preparation exceeded that from the bolus dose by a ratio of approximately 3:1. Our study supports the concern of others that preterm infants who receive current parenteral nutrition formulations may be receiving excessive vitamin K.

Keywords: phylloquinone; prophylaxis; prematurity; deficiency; bleeding; dietary; micronutrients; supplement; nutrition

---

1. Introduction

Vitamin K-dependent coagulation factors are synthesised exclusively in the liver and so the maintenance of adequate hepatic vitamin K reserves is essential for normal haemostasis. Preterm as well as term babies are born with extremely low hepatic stores of vitamin K [1,2]. Unlike in adults, the major hepatic form of vitamin K in neonates is phylloquinone (vitamin K_1) which is also the major form of the vitamin in human breast milk. After birth, the combination of low hepatic reserves and relatively low concentrations of phylloquinone in breast milk (compared to formula milks) places the breast-fed infant at increased risk of developing vitamin K deficiency. They are consequently dependent upon adequate intakes of vitamin K postnatally and during early infancy to keep them healthy. Supplementary vitamin K prophylaxis is offered at birth to protect against vitamin K deficiency bleeding (VKDB), a now rare but still potentially lethal disorder which may cause devastating brain injury and lifelong impairment in survivors [3–5]. Preterm infants may be at higher risk of developing VKDB without adequate ongoing phylloquinone intakes following birth [6], so a baseline understanding of their current typical intakes from various sources during the neonatal period is clearly important.

In both term and preterm infants the very large bolus dose of phylloquinone given prophylactically at birth is considered to be the major source of phylloquinone in early infancy [7,8], and, therefore, to provide the mainstay of protection provided against VKDB during early infancy. Preterm neonates receive an on-going supply of phylloquinone from dietary sources, including from enteral and often parenteral feeding. No previous study has reported in detail the total phylloquinone intakes of preterm infants from all the various sources during their first weeks of life. The aims of this study were: (i) to quantify phylloquinone intake by preterm infants from all sources during the first postnatal weeks of life; and (ii) to assess the relative contribution of the various sources to the total phylloquinone intake of preterm infants during the neonatal period.

2. Experimental Section

2.1. Study Design

This observational study was done as part of a prospective, multicentre, randomised controlled trial that examined the vitamin K status of preterm infants after random allocation to one of three phylloquinone prophylactic regimens at birth [9]. The setting was three neonatal intensive care units (NICUs) in the United Kingdom (UK). The present study reports the detailed phylloquinone intakes of these infants during the first weeks after birth. Data on the functional outcome measures of phylloquinone status and metabolism in this cohort, including undercarboxylated prothrombin (PIVKA-II), prothrombin time, and factor II concentrations, were reported previously [9]. Assessment of other vitamin-K dependent proteins (such as osteocalcin and matrix Gla protein) was beyond the scope of the study.

2.2. Subjects

Infants eligible for inclusion were born at a gestational age of <32 completed weeks and admitted to one of the three participating NICUs. Exclusion criteria included fetal intracranial haemorrhage suspected antenatally, history of maternal antiplatelet antibodies or alloimmune thrombocytopenia, maternal drug treatment with known vitamin K antagonists, life-threatening congenital abnormality, and marked bruising present from birth. Infants with bowel diseases (such as necrotising enterocolitis) or other expected complications of prematurity were not excluded or discontinued from the study. Written parental consent was obtained for inclusion, and the period of recruitment was between November 2001 and February 2003.

2.3. Sources of Vitamin K Intake

There are only three prospective sources of phylloquinone intake by preterm infants during the neonatal period: (i) the prophylactic bolus dose received soon after birth and any extra bolus doses given while in the NICU; (ii) enteral milk feeds and human milk fortifiers (HMFs); and (iii) parenteral nutrition (PN).

2.3.1. Prophylactic Phylloquinone Formulation and Dose

The phylloquinone preparation provided for prophylaxis and for any subsequent bolus dose for infants in this study was Konakion® Neonatal Ampoules (Roche Ltd, Basel, Switzerland). This formulation contained phytomenadione 2 mg/mL and had Cremophor EL (BASF AG, Ludwigshafen, Germany) as the solubilising excipient. Although unlicensed for use in preterm infants, this vitamin K formulation was at the time the commonest preparation used for prophylaxis in the UK [10].

For the main study [2,9], infants were randomly allocated to receive one of three vitamin K prophylaxis regimens within a few hours of birth: phylloquinone 0.5 mg intramuscularly (IM), 0.2 mg IM, or 0.2 mg intravenously (IV). As a safety provision, the study protocol provided that a 0.2 mg IM additional bolus dose of phylloquinone would be given during the study period to any infant with abnormal coagulation values or clinical bleeding in case these findings represented vitamin K deficiency.

2.3.2. Enteral Feeding and Human Milk Fortifiers

The introduction and grading of enteral feeds proceeded in line with standard practices. In general, small "trophic" volumes (totalling ~20 mL/kg/day) of colostrum/human milk and/or a preterm milk formula were commenced within the first few days postnatal. Maternal expression of breast milk was actively encouraged, and expressed breast milk (EBM) was the preferred milk feed for preterm infants at all participating neonatal units. Bolus aliquots of milk were given via a nasogastric tube, initially on an hourly basis. Any increment in the feed volume was a decision of the clinical ward round and would depend upon an infant's stability and any recent history of feed tolerance. Infants were considered to have established full enteral feeds when they were tolerating a volume of at least 150 mL/kg/day of milk and no longer on PN. An infant who tolerated the gradual feed increase without event or setback would potentially establish full feeds by 7–10 days postnatal.

It was standard clinical practice at all three participating NICUs to add HMF routinely to breast milk once the full enteral feed volume of 150 mL/kg/day was attained. Three commercially-available HMFs were available in the UK during the study period. Infants at the participating units all received Eoprotin HMF (Nutricia Ltd., Trowbridge, UK). Coincidentally, a new formulation of Eoprotin with a higher phylloquinone content was introduced nationally in the UK during the study period. Initially one scoop was given per 100 mL of breast milk, and this was graded up to three scoops (old Eoprotin formulation) or four scoops (new Eoprotin formulation) on successive days as tolerated. Infants discharged to neonatal centres outside of the three trial centres prior to study completion who subsequently received a different HMF had their phylloquinone intake calculated according to the actual fortifier received.

2.3.3. Parenteral Nutrition

Administration of PN solution was routine for the sickest neonates in the participating NICUs. It was generally reserved for all very preterm infants (less than ~29 weeks' gestation), extremely low birth weight infants (ELBW; <1000 g), and also any other neonate that was considered unlikely to achieve full enteral feeding by 7–10 days postnatal. It was expected that many of the more mature and heavier preterm infants in the study group would not require PN.

PN was usually commenced within the first three days of life. The daily volume of lipid infused was routinely graded up over the first three days to minimise fat intolerance and hyperlipidaemia. The phylloquinone-containing components of the PN solution were 20% Intralipid®, an intravenous fat emulsion, and Vitlipid N Infant®, a fat-soluble vitamin emulsion (Fresenius Kabi Ltd, Runcorn, Cheshire, UK). Nursing charts recorded the dates when PN began and ended, and also the exact daily volumes of the respective PN solutions delivered to each infant.

2.4. Assessment of Phylloquinone Intake

Phylloquinone intakes from all sources were calculated between birth and the date that the infant had tolerated full enteral feeds (*i.e.*, ⩾150 mL/kg/day of milk) for a continuous full 2-week period, the latter date being considered the date of "study completion". The total vitamin intake was thus calculated for each enrolled infant between birth and the date that full enteral feeds had been tolerated for two weeks.

Each infant's absolute phylloquinone intake between birth and study completion was calculated from the sum amounts received from: (i) allocated prophylactic phylloquinone dose and any extra bolus phylloquinone doses given during the study period, obtained from review of the prescription charts; (ii) daily enteral feed volumes and HMF, obtained from the daily nursing charts; and (iii) PN intake, with daily volumes of Intralipid and Vitlipid received being obtained from the PN prescription charts and the nursing infusion administration charts.

An average daily phylloquinone intake was calculated for each infant from its total phylloquinone intake (expressed in μg/kg, using the infant's weight at completion of the study) divided by the number of days from birth to study completion. The phylloquinone intake from enteral feeds was calculated from the actual milk types and volumes fed to each infant between birth and study completion, as recorded on the neonatal nursing charts.

2.4.1. Phylloquinone Content of Milk Feeds and Fortifier

Table 1 shows the phylloquinone content of human preterm breast milk, and of the preterm artificial milk formulae that were available in the UK during the study period. The values for phylloquinone content of term infant human breast milk and term infant milk formulae are also provided for comparison purposes. Milk formulae phylloquinone contents are compiled from the various manufacturers' contemporaneous data sheets. Values for the phylloquinone content of HMF-fortified preterm breast milk are also provided; these are based upon the manufacturer-published phylloquinone content of the various HMFs that were commercially-available during the study period, and upon the mean phylloquinone concentration value reported for preterm EBM. The value for mean phylloquinone concentration of human preterm EBM (3.0 μg/L) derives from a study of human milk obtained on postnatal one day from mothers of preterm infants prior to maternal phylloquinone supplementation [11]. To date this study of Bolisetty *et al.* [11] remains the only known study in which breast milk phylloquinone concentrations have been measured in mothers of preterm infants. Nevertheless, this mean value compares well to the mean concentration of phylloquinone in mature human breast milk (2.1 μg/L) from mothers of term infants reported by Haroon *et al.* [12], and to the mean value (2.5 μg/L) that was used in the calculation of the Adequate Intake (AI) by the Food and Nutrition Board [7]. Addition of HMF to EBM provided a total phylloquinone concentration of 5–66 μg/L depending on brand used (Table 1). Artificial preterm milk formulae provided 40–66 μg/L of phylloquinone depending on brand. These values were used to calculate exact phylloquinone intakes from the enteral feeds for all study individuals up to completion of the study.

Table 1. Phylloquinone content of human milk, commercial milk formulae, and fortifiers.

Nutrient	Phylloquinone Content (μg/100 mL)	Phylloquinone Content (μg/L)
Human Milk		
Term colostrum [a]	0.23	2.3
Term mature EBM [a]	0.21	2.1
Preterm colostrum/EBM [b]	0.30	3.0
Formula Milks		
PreAptamil	6.6	66
Aptamil	4.0	40
Nutriprem 1	6.6	66
Nutriprem 2	5.9	59
SMA Low Birth Weight	8.0	80
SMA Gold	6.7	67
C + G Premium	5.1	51
C + G Plus	5.0	50

Table 1. *Cont.*

Nutrient	Phylloquinone Content (μg/100 mL)	Phylloquinone Content (μg/L)
Human Milk Fortifiers		
Eoprotin (old formulation)	0.2 per 3 scoops (3 g powder) [c]	2
Eoprotin (new formulation)	6.3 per 4 scoops (4.2 g powder) [c]	63
Nutriprem HMF	6.2 per 2 sachets (4.2 g powder) [c]	62
SMA Breast Milk Fortifier	11.0 per 2 sachets (4 g powder) [c]	110
Fortified EBM [d]		
Eoprotin old formulation	0.5	5
Eoprotin new formulation	6.6	66
Nutriprem HMF	6.5	65
SMA HMF	11.3	113

EBM, expressed breast milk; HMF, human milk fortifier. [a] Analysis of colostrum and breast milk obtained within five days *post-partum*, from Haroon *et al.* [12]; [b] Mean preterm EBM concentration on the first postnatal day in unsupplemented mothers, from Bolisetty *et al.* [11]; [c] Quantities recommended by manufacturers for addition to each 100 mL of human milk; [d] Values listed refer to content of fortified human milk after adding the recommended amount of HMF according to manufacturers' instructions

2.4.2. Phylloquinone Content of Parenteral Nutrition Solution

The phylloquinone content of Vitlipid N Infant (fat soluble vitamin emulsion) was 20 mg/L. That of 20% Intralipid IV fat emulsion varied between batches, and ranged from 0.50 to 0.77 mg/L [13]; for calculation purposes a figure of 0.6 mg/L was used. Infants on PN received 4 mL/kg of Vitlipid and 5–15 mL/kg of 20% Intralipid per day, providing daily phylloquinone supplementation of 80 μg/kg and 3–9 μg/kg respectively.

2.4.3. Calculation of Total and Proportional Phylloquinone Intake from All Sources

The average daily phylloquinone intake was calculated for each infant from the total phylloquinone intake (expressed as μg/kg body weight at study completion) divided by number of days between birth and study completion. The proportional intake of phylloquinone from each route was also assessed: for each infant the contribution to overall total intake from each phylloquinone source was expressed as a percentage of total intake. In addition to calculating the proportional intake for all infants who completed the study (because not all preterm infants required or received PN feeding) the proportional intake was calculated separately for infants who received PN and for infants who did not receive any PN.

2.4.4. Statistical Analysis

Infants who died before study completion were excluded from analysis. Data for all randomised infants who completed the study were analysed using StatsDirect statistical software (www.statsdirect.com) version 2.4.5. The Mann-Whitney U test was used to compare phylloquinone intakes between the three randomisation cohorts, and a p-value of <0.05 was considered statistically significant.

2.5. Ethics Approvals

The study received prior ethical review board approval from Salford and Trafford Local Research Ethics Committee on 5 November 2001 (Project No. 01198). Further Research Ethics Committee approvals were given on 10 July 2002 and on 10 December 2002 for extension of the study to two additional sites.

3. Results

3.1. Baseline Characteristics

Of 98 infants randomised to the main trial [2,9], 15 died before study completion and three infants with incomplete data were excluded from the analysis. All deaths were related to the common complications of prematurity and no infant in the study had vitamin K deficiency bleeding [9]. A total of 80 infants completed the study. Table 2 shows their baseline characteristics, including feeding characteristics, overall and subgrouped according to initial allocated dose of phylloquinone prophylaxis. There were no significant differences between subgroups for any of these baseline characteristics. As already reported, all infants had satisfactory vitamin K status at study completion and there were no significant differences in any functional outcome measures of phylloquinone status and metabolism between the subgroups in this cohort [9]. No infant suffered any suspected adverse event or reaction in relation to phylloquinone dosage or its route of administration. There were no differences between sub-groups in incidence of significant intraventricular haemorrhage ($n = 6$ infants overall, $p = 0.9$), other significant bleeding, such as gastro-intestinal or pulmonary ($n = 7$ infants overall, $p = 0.2$), or numbers transfused with fresh frozen plasma during the study ($n = 7$ infants overall, $p = 0.7$).

Table 2. Baseline characteristics of the $n = 80$ infants who completed the study and subgroups according to initial phylloquinone prophylaxis regimen.

Characteristic	All Infants ($n = 80$)	0.5 mg IM ($n = 28$)	0.2 mg IM ($n = 26$)	0.2 mg IV ($n = 26$)
Gestational Age, weeks	29.4 (22.4–31.9)	29.0 (24.1–31.9)	29.9 (24.0–31.7)	29.6 (22.4–31.4)
Birth Weight, g	1092 (454–1910)	1033 (454–1910)	1143 (534–1910)	1203 (575–1892)
Male gender, n	36 (45%)	10 (36%)	13 (50%)	13 (50%)
Received any PN, n	56 (70%)	18 (64%)	17 (65%)	21 (81%)
Duration of PN [a], days median (range) (IQR)	10 (3–78) (7–17)	9 (4–78) (7–13)	10 (5–29) (9–21)	9 (3–48) (5–18)
Postnatal age reached full enteral feeds, days	10 (4–80)	9 (4–80)	12 (4–43)	11 (4–49)
Postnatal age at study completion, days	25 (17–90)	24 (19–90)	26 (19–58)	26 (17–64)
Weight at study completion, g	1495 (600–2710)	1281 (605–2650)	1595 (600–2270)	1572 (612–2710)

Data are median (range) unless indicated. IM, intramuscular; IV, intravenous; PN, parenteral nutrition; IQR, inter-quartile range. [a] Data shown here include only babies who received any period of PN. There were no statistically significant differences between any subgroups for any of the baseline characteristics shown.

3.2. Total Phylloquinone Intakes

Table 3 shows total phylloquinone intakes from all sources between birth and study completion overall and for the subgroups. There were no significant differences in absolute phylloquinone intakes from all sources between the three study groups at study completion. However, after correcting for birth weight and days to study completion, the average daily intake of phylloquinone adjusted for birth weight was significantly lower for infants who had received 0.2 mg boluses at birth ($p < 0.05$).

Table 3. Phylloquinone intakes from all sources between birth and study completion (adapted from Clarke *et al.* [9], with permission).

Phylloquinone Intake (μg)	All infants ($n = 80$)	0.5 mg IM ($n = 28$)	0.2 mg IM ($n = 26$)	0.2 mg IV ($n = 26$)
Via bolus doses				
Mean (SD)	378 (256)	629 (264)	238 (80) *	246 (130) *
Median (range)	200 (200–1500)	500 (500–1500)	200 (200–400) *	200 (200–800)
From PN †				
Mean (SD)	784 (939)	610 (972)	754 (768)	1001 (1045)
Median (range)	542 (0–5071)	440 (0–5071)	674 (0–2441)	713 (0–3895)
Via enteral feeds				
Mean (SD)	124 (90)	118 (85)	125 (97)	131 (91)
Median (range)	133 (2–340)	116 (2–340)	122 (6–304)	145 (8–300)
Total phylloquinone intake μg				
Mean (SD)	1286 (1025)	1357 (1133)	1118 (775)	1378 (1136)
Median (range)	1011 (214–6574)	1038 (507–6574)	958 (332–2730)	1020 (214–4822)
μg/kg				
Mean (SD)	914 (597)	1070 (633)	808 (591)	853 (548)
Median (range)	775 (141–2594)	1048 (408–2594)	699 (173–2057)	704 (141–2343)
μg/kg/day				
Mean (SD)	30 (15)	37 (15)	26 (15) ‡	27 (11) ‡
Median (range)	28 (7–75)	39 (18–75)	27 (8–55) ‡	27 (7–65) ‡

SD, standard deviation. † Includes infants who received any period of PN as well as those who did not receive PN; * *Versus* 0.5 mg IM group, $p < 0.001$; ‡ *Versus* 0.5 mg IM group, $p < 0.05$.

3.2.1. Phylloquinone Intakes According to Parenteral Nutrition Administration

Table 4 shows the total phylloquinone intake from all sources in study infants who received any period of PN and completed the study ($n = 56$). PN-derived phylloquinone intake in these 56 infants was comparable in the 0.5 mg IM ($n = 18$) and 0.2 mg IV ($n = 21$) groups, and slightly higher in the 0.2 mg IM group ($n = 17$).

Table 5 shows total phylloquinone intakes by route confined to study infants who did not receive any PN ($n = 24$).

Table 4. Relative intakes of phylloquinone from all sources together with total intakes at study completion in infants who received parenteral nutrition.

Phylloquinone Intake (μg)	All Infants Given PN (*n* = 56)	0.5 mg IM (*n* = 18)	0.2 mg IM (*n* = 17)	0.2 mg IV (*n* = 21)
Via bolus doses				
Mean (SD)	391 (277)	672 (303)	259 (94) *	275 (143) *
Median (range)	200 (200–1500)	500 (500–1500)	200 (200–400) *	200 (200–800) *
From PN				
Mean (SD)	1120 (940)	950 (1077)	1153 (658) †	1240 (1027)
Median (range)	759 (305–5071)	589 (350–5071)	767 (515–2441) †	946 (305–3895)
Via enteral feeds				
Mean (SD)	101 (80)	97 (63)	80 (82)	120 (89)
Median (range)	94 (2–304)	105 (2–198)	79 (6–304)	142 (8–300)
Total phylloquinone intake μg				
Mean (SD)	1612 (1066)	1719 (1280)	1492 (714)	1617 (1140)
Median (range)	1234 (596–6574)	1423 (956–6574)	1189 (771–2730)	1240 (596–4822)
μg/kg				
Mean (SD)	1168 (535)	1410 (540)	1119 (498)	1000 (506) ‡
Median (range)	1136 (438–2594)	1269 (721–2594)	971 (529–2057)	813 (438–2343) ‡
μg/kg/day				
Mean (SD)	37 (13)	46 (12)	34 (11) ‡	30 (10) *
Median (range)	33 (18–75)	44 (28–75)	33 (19–55) ‡	29 (18–65) *

Statistically-significant comparisons (using Mann-Whitney U test) are shown thus: * *versus* 0.5 mg IM group, $p < 0.0001$; † *Versus* 0.5 mg IM group, $p < 0.05$; ‡ *Versus* 0.5 mg IM group, $p < 0.01$.

Table 5. Relative intakes of phylloquinone from bolus doses and enteral feeds together with total intakes at study completion for infants who did not receive parenteral nutrition.

Phylloquinone Intake (μg)	All Infants Not Given PN (*n* = 24)	0.5 mg IM (*n* = 10)	0.2 mg IM (*n* = 9)	0.2 mg IV (*n* = 5)
Via bolus doses				
Mean (SD)	346 (202)	550 (158)	200 (NA) *	200 (NA) †
Median (range)	200 (200–1000)	500 (500–1000)	200 (NA) *	200 (NA) †
Via enteral feeds				
Mean (SD)	181 (88)	156 (107)	212 (55)	176 (94)
Median (range)	195 (7–340)	149 (7–340)	214 (132–292)	208 (14–254)
Total phylloquinone intake μg				
Mean (SD)	527 (187)	706 (145)	412 (55) *	376 (94) †
Median (range)	466 (214–1016)	690 (507–1016)	414 (332–492) *	408 (214–454) †
μg/kg				
Mean (SD)	322 (124)	458 (48)	220 (27) *	233 (54) †
Median (range)	251 (141–562)	439 (408–562)	215 (173–249) *	249 (141-284) †
μg/kg/day				
Mean (SD)	15 (6)	22 (3)	10 (1) *	12 (4) †
Median (range)	13 (7–25)	21 (18–25)	10 (8–12) *	13 (7–17) †

NA, not applicable because all infants received 0.2 mg dose. Statistically-significant comparisons (using Mann-Whitney U test) are shown thus: * *versus* 0.5 mg IM group, $p < 0.0001$; † *Versus* 0.5 mg IM group, $p < 0.001$.

3.2.2. Proportional Contribution of Various Sources to Overall Phylloquinone Intakes

Table 6 shows the proportional intake of phylloquinone from each route as a percentage of the total intake, for all infants and for the subgroups. Analysis of the proportional intake of phylloquinone from the various routes shows that for the infants receiving 0.5 mg phylloquinone after delivery and who received PN, the bolus dose comprised ~40% of total phylloquinone intake over the study period, while PN comprised ~50% of intake, and enteral feeding <10% of intake. In contrast for the 0.2 mg groups, only ~20% of the total phylloquinone intake in the study period came from the bolus prophylaxis dose, whereas 70% came from PN, and <10% came from enteral feeding.

Table 6. Proportional intake of phylloquinone from each route from birth until study completion as a percentage of the total intake.

Proportional Phylloquinone Intake	All Infants	0.5 mg IM	0.2 mg IM	0.2 mg IV
All Infants	*n* = 80	*n* = 28	*n* = 26	*n* = 26
% Via bolus doses				
Mean (SD)	38 (23)	56 (21)	30 (16) *	27 (19) *
Median (range)	33 (5–99)	52 (23–99)	22 (7–60) *	20 (5–94) *
% From PN				
Mean (SD)	46 (33)	32 (26)	49 (37) †	57 (31) *
Median (range)	56 (0–92)	37 (0–77)	69 (0–89) †	68 (0–92) *
% Via enteral feeds				
Mean (SD)	17 (18)	12 (11)	21 (23)	16 (17)
Median (range)	8 (0–59)	8 (0–41)	10 (0–59)	8 (0–56)
Infants given PN	*n* = 56	*n* = 18	*n* = 17	*n* = 21
% Via bolus doses				
Mean (SD)	27 (14)	43 (11)	20 (8) *	19 (8) *
Median (range)	23 (5–64)	45 (23–64)	19 (7–42) *	17 (5–34) *
% From PN				
Mean (SD)	65 (16)	50 (13)	75 (10) *	71 (13) *
Median (range)	68 (28–92)	50 (28–77)	78 (54–89) *	74 (43–92) *
% Via enteral feeds				
Mean (SD)	8 (7)	7 (5)	6 (6)	10 (9)
Median (range)	6 (0–28)	7 (0–16)	3 (0–21)	8 (0–28)
Infants not given PN	n = 24	*n* = 10	*n* = 9	*n* = 5
% Via bolus doses				
Mean (SD)	63 (18)	78 (13)	49 (7) *	57 (21) †
Median (range)	58 (41–99)	77 (60–99)	48 (41–60) *	49 (44–94) †
% Via enteral feds				
Mean (SD)	37 (18)	22 (13)	51 (7) *	43 (21) †
Median (range)	42 (1–59)	23 (1–41)	52 (40–59) *	51 (7–56) †

Statistically-significant comparisons (using Mann-Whitney U test) are shown thus: * *versus* 0.5 mg IM group, $p < 0.0001$; † *Versus* 0.5 mg IM group, $p < 0.05$.

Considering infants who had not received any period of PN, the bolus dose for those receiving 0.5 mg phylloquinone after delivery represented ~80% of the total study intake (with enteral feeding ~20% of the total intake), whereas for the 0.2 mg groups the bolus dose and enteral feeding each comprised ~50% of the total phylloquinone intake.

4. Discussion

This is the first study to describe in detail the absolute phylloquinone intake by preterm infants from all sources during their first weeks of postnatal life. We quantified the relative proportional intake of phylloquinone from the various nutritional routes for infants who received PN and for those who did not receive PN. We found no differences in overall intakes between the three study groups that had been randomly allocated different phylloquinone regimens at birth. However after correcting for birth weight and days to study completion, the average daily intake of phylloquinone adjusted for birth weight was significantly lower for infants who had received the lower dose prophylactic bolus dose of 0.2 mg phylloquinone. We had speculated that the initial bolus doses of phylloquinone given for prophylaxis at birth would assume less importance as a source of the vitamin contributing to the overall intake at study completion, due to the increasing respective contributions to overall phylloquinone intake derived from other nutritional (dietary) sources. In infants who did not receive any PN, the bolus dose given at birth represented approximately 50% of the overall phylloquinone intake at study completion, compared to only approximately 20% in infants who had received PN.

Preterm infants represent a neglected group with respect to current knowledge of their phylloquinone intakes and recommendations for their nutritional requirements. As pointed out by Kumar *et al.* [14], published recommendations for vitamin K intakes and/or supplementation are specific for all ages except for preterm infants. As a result, recommendations for preterm infants are arbitrary and historically have ranged from 5 to 10 μg/kg/day in 1993 [15] and as high as 100 μg/kg/day in 1988 [16]. In this context it is important to note that the principles and knowledge base of dietary recommendations have changed over time. For example, the recommendations of 5–10 μg/kg/day for preterm infants in 1993 [15] came out during the lifespan of the 10th Edition of the US Food and Nutrition Board guidelines published in 1989, at which time they took the form of Recommended Daily Allowances (RDA) instead of the current Dietary Reference Intakes (DRI). At that time the RDA for term infants over the first six months was 5 μg/day, which in turn was based on the adult RDA of 1 μg/kg/day [17]. This means that the 5–10 μg/kg/day recommendation for preterm infants by Greer *et al.* [15] was 5–10 fold greater than the intake recommendations for term infants at that time. More recent guidelines published in 2005 recommended a phylloquinone intake of 8–10 μg/kg/day as an AI for preterm infants [18], representing the top end of the 1993 recommendations [15].

There is an inevitable degree of arbitrariness of recommendations even for healthy term infants. In the current United States recommendations published in 2001, the AI for healthy term infants is based on an average daily milk intake of 0.78 L and an average phylloquinone concentration in human milk of 2.5 μg/L [7]. This gave an AI of 2.0 μg/day after rounding [7]. The weak link in this calculation as a precise AI value lies with the fairly wide variations in the reported concentrations of phylloquinone in breast milk which taking the lower and upper values would result in estimated phylloquinone intakes of ~0.5 μg/day and 2.5 μg/day respectively [8].

Another weakness of current recommendations is that they are based solely on the phylloquinone content of breast milk. Although phylloquinone is the major vitamer of vitamin K in breast milk, it also contains a member of the menaquinone series, namely menaquinone-4 (MK-4) at concentrations that are about half that of phylloquinone [19,20]. There is also evidence that this MK-4 in breast milk is derived from dietary phylloquinone [20]. Future neonatal AI recommendations should also consider the contribution to intakes made by MK-4 as well as its potential contribution to neonatal vitamin K status.

Whether the dietary guidelines have been in the form of an RDA or AI, a common underlying assumption is that the infant is also given a prophylactic dose at birth in amounts recommended by the relevant paediatric societies [7,17]. For any individual infant, the optimal daily ongoing phylloquinone required from feeding will depend in part upon what prophylactic dose was given at birth and any postnatal supplementation received from PN. However there is also likely to be inter-individual variation in storage and metabolism.

For the purposes of discussion we have taken the most recent recommendation of 8–10 μg/kg/day [18] as a benchmark against which the phylloquinone intakes in this study can be compared. The median phylloquinone intake for infants who completed this study was approximately three-fold this recommended amount, and up to five to seven-fold more in some infants (Table 3).

For infants who received PN, there was little difference between allocation groups. The median of the average phylloquinone intake was three to four times the recommended amount, and all had an average phylloquinone intake that ranged between ~20–70 μg/kg/day, *i.e.*, two to seven times the daily recommendation (Table 4). For infants who did not receive any PN, the median average daily intake received by 0.5 mg IM group infants was approximately twice that currently recommended, whereas for infants in the 0.2 mg IM and 0.2 mg IV bolus groups the medians and ranges of average daily intakes were remarkably close to the currently recommended intakes of 8–10 μg/kg/day (Table 5).

For infants who did not receive any PN, the bolus dose(s) of phylloquinone constituted the major source of phylloquinone intake in the study period. In contrast, for infants who had received a period of PN by far their major intake source was, somewhat surprisingly, that delivered by the PN solution. For comparison, the ratio of median phylloquinone intake from PN to that from bolus doses was ~3:1.

In infants given PN, the median overall phylloquinone intake from enteral feeds was 6% (range: 0%–28%) of the total intake. In contrast in the infants not given PN the proportional intake from enteral feeds was significantly higher, and comprised 23% of overall intake for infants receiving a 0.5 mg bolus dose of phylloquinone after delivery, and 50% of overall intake for infants who received a 0.2 mg dose. Thus the contribution towards overall phylloquinone intake made by enteral feeding is small, but becomes more important in infants not given PN and particularly so for infants who receive lower bolus prophylactic doses (0.2 mg) and who do not receive PN.

These data show that in almost all infants, the average daily phylloquinone intake was in excess of the currently recommended amounts. The intakes were particularly high at three to four times the recommended amounts in all who received PN (irrespective of prophylactic dose), and were approximately twice the recommended amounts in infants given 0.5 mg prophylactic doses who did not receive PN. Only infants who received the 0.2 mg dose and who did not receive PN had an intake which approximated well to the current recommended daily phylloquinone intake of 8–10 μg/kg/day. Our data provide further evidence that the amounts of phylloquinone currently added to manufactured PN multivitamin solutions are excessive for the needs of preterm infants and should be reviewed.

Although there are no known clinical manifestations of toxicity from phylloquinone prophylaxis in neonates, nor indeed any known toxic effects in adults consuming high amounts of vitamin K [7], we previously found evidence of hepatic overload in a sub-group of preterm infants from our main study who had received the 0.5 mg rather than the 0.2 mg dose for prophylaxis [9]. The larger dose was more likely to be associated with elevated serum phylloquinone 2,3-epoxide concentrations, and suggested overload of the hepatic vitamin K 2,3-epoxide reductase enzyme in some preterm infants [2,9]. Furthermore, in a separate study we previously obtained evidence of metabolic overload in a subgroup of preterm infants who predominately excreted the less extensively metabolised urinary 7C-side chain metabolite of vitamin K instead of the usual 5C-side chain metabolite [21]. This subgroup also had the highest serum concentrations of phylloquinone together with raised blood concentrations of phylloquinone 2,3-epoxide that is normally undetectable. This combination of increased excretion of the 7C-metabolite, high serum phylloquinone and raised phylloquinone 2,3-epoxide is indicative of a metabolic overload of both vitamin K recycling and catabolic pathways [21]. None of the infants in these studies who had biochemical evidence of overload showed any clinical manifestations of an overload status.

Because of their special nutritional requirements preterm babies are often provided with multivitamin supplements—including the fat-soluble vitamins A, D, and E—at the time of discharge home from the neonatal unit; these are usually continued throughout infancy. However post-discharge phylloquinone supplements are rarely provided to this group at present. Yet without adequate ongoing supplementation preterm infants may be at increased risk of developing vitamin K deficiency in early infancy, particularly if they continue to be exclusively breast fed. National surveillance studies of VKDB continue to report sporadic cases in preterm infants [6]. The most recent study in the United Kingdom and the Irish Republic reported a case of probable VKDB in a 24-week gestation infant who had received 0.4 mg/kg IM at birth [22]. This infant was primarily human milk fed and had no liver disease but suffered gastro-intestinal bleeding aged three months postnatal. Further study is required to assess whether phylloquinone supplements should be given routinely to preterm infants on discharge home from the neonatal unit.

5. Conclusions

In conclusion, this study of phylloquinone intake in the first weeks of life shows that all preterm infants received at least the minimum daily recommended intake of phylloquinone, but that most received an excessive intake. These data support the calls for the amount of phylloquinone added to standard PN multivitamin solutions to be reduced [14,23,24], and also support lower initial phylloquinone bolus doses being used for prophylaxis at birth [6]. For all infants studied, a bolus prophylactic phylloquinone dose of 0.2 mg (or ~0.3 mg/kg) was more appropriate than 0.5 mg because it resulted in an average daily intake over the study period closer to the currently recommended intake amounts. Also, average daily intakes were remarkably close to the currently recommended intake values in infants given 0.2 mg prophylaxis who did not receive any PN. In infants who do not receive PN, a 0.2 mg or 0.5 mg bolus dose given at birth represents a significant proportion of overall phylloquinone intake.

Future research in preterm infants should focus on their post-discharge vitamin K status and address the question whether additional supplementation with phylloquinone during infancy should also be routine.

Acknowledgments: This study was supported by the Hope Neonatal Unit Research Endowment Fund. We thank the staff of the Human Nutristasis Unit at Guy's and St Thomas's Hospital, London, and the respective biochemistry and haematology departments of the participating hospitals. We thank the paediatricians who allowed us to gather follow-up data on back-transferred infants. P.C. wishes to sincerely thank Mark Turner and Suresh Victor for very helpful constructive critical review of this and the other studies that comprised his doctoral thesis. Above all we sincerely thank all the parents who kindly allowed their infants to participate.

Author Contributions: The authors thank the American Academy of Pediatrics for kindly granting us permission to use and adapt the data presented in Table 3 from *Pediatrics* vol. 118, page e1663 [9], Copyright © 2006 by the AAP.

Author Contributions: S.J.M. conceived the idea for this study. P.C. collected the data, performed the statistical analyses, and wrote the first manuscript draft. All authors contributed to manuscript revisions, provided intellectual input in data interpretation, and approve of the final version. P.C. is guarantor.

References

1. Shearer, M.J. Vitamin K metabolism and nutriture. *Blood Rev.* **1992**, *6*, 92–104. [CrossRef]
2. Clarke, P. A Comparison of Vitamin K Status in Preterm Infants Following Intravenous or Intramuscular Prophylaxis and the Effects of Feeding with Preterm Formula or Fortified Human Milk. Ph.D. Thesis, University of Manchester, Manchester, UK, 2008.
3. Lane, P.A.; Hathaway, W.E. Vitamin K in infancy. *J. Pediatr.* **1985**, *106*, 351–359. [CrossRef]
4. Sutor, A.H.; von Kries, R.; Cornelissen, E.A.; McNinch, A.W.; Andrew, M. Vitamin K deficiency bleeding (VKDB) in infancy. ISTH Pediatric/Perinatal Subcommittee. International Society on Thrombosis and Haemostasis. *Thromb. Haemost.* **1999**, *81*, 456–461. [PubMed]
5. Shearer, M.J. Vitamin K deficiency bleeding (VKDB) in early infancy. *Blood Rev.* **2009**, *23*, 49–59. [CrossRef] [PubMed]
6. Clarke, P. Vitamin K prophylaxis for preterm infants. *Early Hum. Dev.* **2010**, *86* (Suppl. 1), 17–20. [CrossRef] [PubMed]

7. Food and Nutrition Board, Institute of Medicine. *Dietary Reference Intakes for Vitamin A, Vitamin K, Arsenic, Boron, Chromium, Copper, Iodine, Iron, Manganese, Molybdenum, Nickel, Silicon, Vanadium, and Zinc*; National Academy Press: Washington, DC, USA, 2001.
8. Shearer, M.J.; Fu, X.; Booth, S.L. Vitamin K nutrition, metabolism, and requirements: Current concepts and future research. *Adv. Nutr.* **2012**, *3*, 182–195. [CrossRef] [PubMed]
9. Clarke, P.; Mitchell, S.J.; Wynn, R.; Sundaram, S.; Speed, V.; Gardener, E.; Roeves, D.; Shearer, M.J. Vitamin K prophylaxis for preterm infants: A randomized, controlled trial of 3 regimens. *Pediatrics* **2006**, *118*, e1657–e1666. [CrossRef] [PubMed]
10. Clarke, P.; Mitchell, S. Vitamin K prophylaxis in preterm infants: Current practices. *J. Thromb. Haemost.* **2003**, *1*, 384–386. [CrossRef] [PubMed]
11. Bolisetty, S.; Gupta, J.M.; Graham, G.G.; Salonikas, C.; Naidoo, D. Vitamin K in preterm breastmilk with maternal supplementation. *Acta Paediatr.* **1998**, *87*, 960–962. [CrossRef] [PubMed]
12. Haroon, Y.; Shearer, M.J.; Rahim, S.; Gunn, W.G.; McEnery, G.; Barkhan, P. The content of phylloquinone (vitamin K_1) in human milk, cows' milk and infant formula foods determined by high-performance liquid chromatography. *J. Nutr.* **1982**, *112*, 1105–1117. [PubMed]
13. Smith, R.J. (Fresenius Kabi Ltd, Runcorn, UK). Personal communication, 2004.
14. Kumar, D.; Greer, F.R.; Super, D.M.; Suttie, J.W.; Moore, J.J. Vitamin K status of premature infants: Implications for current recommendations. *Pediatrics* **2001**, *108*, 1117–1122. [CrossRef] [PubMed]
15. Greer, F. Vitamin K. In *Nutritional Needs of the Preterm Infant: Scientific Basis and Practical Guidelines*; Tsang, R.C., Lucas, A., Eds.; Williams & Wilkins: Baltimore, MD, USA, 1993; pp. 111–119.
16. Greene, H.L.; Hambidge, K.M.; Schanler, R.; Tsang, R.C. Guidelines for the use of vitamins, trace elements, calcium, magnesium, and phosphorus in infants and children receiving total parenteral nutrition: Report of the subcommittee on pediatric parenteral nutrient requirements from the committee on clinical practice issues of the American Society for Clinical Nutrition. *Am. J. Clin. Nutr.* **1988**, *48*, 1324–1342. [PubMed]
17. Food and Nutrition Board Commission on Life Sciences; National Research Council. *Recommended Dietary Allowances*, 10th ed.; National Academy Press: Washington, DC, USA, 1989.
18. Tsang, R.C. *Nutrition of the Preterm Infant: Scientific Basis and Practical Guidelines*, 2nd ed.; Digital Educational Publishing: Cincinnati, OH, USA, 2005.
19. Indyk, H.E.; Woollard, D.C. Vitamin K in milk and infant formulas: Determination and distribution of phylloquinone and menaquinone-4. *Analyst* **1997**, *122*, 465–469. [CrossRef] [PubMed]
20. Thijssen, H.H.; Drittij, M.J.; Vermeer, C.; Schoffelen, E. Menaquinone-4 in breast milk is derived from dietary phylloquinone. *Br. J. Nutr.* **2002**, *87*, 219–226. [CrossRef] [PubMed]
21. Harrington, D.J.; Clarke, P.; Card, D.J.; Mitchell, S.J.; Shearer, M.J. Urinary excretion of vitamin K metabolites in term and preterm infants: Relationship to vitamin K status and prophylaxis. *Pediatr. Res.* **2010**, *68*, 508–512. [CrossRef] [PubMed]
22. Busfield, A.; Samuel, R.; McNinch, A.; Tripp, J.H. Vitamin K deficiency bleeding after NICE guidance and withdrawal of Konakion Neonatal: British Paediatric Surveillance Unit study, 2006–2008. *Arch. Dis. Child.* **2013**, *98*, 41–47. [CrossRef] [PubMed]
23. Costakos, D.T.; Greer, F.R.; Love, L.A.; Dahlen, L.R.; Suttie, J.W. Vitamin K prophylaxis for premature infants: 1 mg *versus* 0.5 mg. *Am. J. Perinatol.* **2003**, *20*, 485–490. [PubMed]
24. Costakos, D.T.; Porte, M. Did "controversies concerning vitamin K and the newborn" cover all the controversies? *Pediatrics* **2004**, *113*, 1466–1467. [CrossRef] [PubMed]

Dietary Vitamin K Intake is Associated with Cognition and Behaviour among Geriatric Patients: The CLIP Study

Justine Chouet [1], Guylaine Ferland [2], Catherine Féart [3,4], Yves Rolland [5], Nancy Presse [2], Kariane Boucher [2], Pascale Barberger-Gateau [3,4], Olivier Beauchet [1] and Cedric Annweiler [1,6,*]

[1] Department of Neuroscience, Division of Geriatric Medicine, Angers University Hospital; Angers University Memory Clinic; UPRES EA 4638, University of Angers, UNAM, Angers F-49933, France; E-Mails: justine.chouet@gmail.com (J.C.); OlBeauchet@chu-angers.fr (O.B.)

[2] Centre de recherche, Institut Universitaire de Gériatrie de Montréal, Montréal, QC H3W 1W5, Canada; E-Mails: guylaine.ferland@umontreal.ca (G.F.); nancy.presse@umontreal.ca (N.P.); kariane.boucher@gmail.com (K.B.)

[3] Université Bordeaux, ISPED, Centre INSERM U897-Epidemiologie-Biostatistique, Bordeaux F-33000, France; E-Mails: catherine.feart@isped.u-bordeaux2.fr (C.F.); Pascale.Barberger-Gateau@isped.u-bordeaux2.fr (P.B.-G.)

[4] INSERM, ISPED, INSERM U897-Epidemiologie-Biostatistique, Bordeaux F-33000, France

[5] Department of Geriatric Medicine, Institut du Vieillissement, University Hospital; INSERM U1027, Toulouse F-31400, France; E-Mail: rolland.y@chu-toulouse.fr

[6] Robarts Research Institute, Department of Medical Biophysics, Schulich School of Medicine and Dentistry, the University of Western Ontario, London, ON N6A 5B7, Canada

* Author to whom correspondence should be addressed; E-Mail: CeAnnweiler@chu-angers.fr

Abstract: Our objective was to determine whether dietary vitamin K intake was associated with cognition and behavior among older adults. 192 consecutive participants $\geqslant$65 years recruited in the cross-sectional CLIP (Cognition and LIPophilic vitamins) study, were separated into two groups according to the tertiles of dietary phylloquinone intake (*i.e.*, lowest third below 207 µg/day *versus* the other two thirds combined). Daily dietary phylloquinone intake was estimated from 50-item interviewer-administered food frequency questionnaire. Cognition was assessed with Mini-Mental State Examination (MMSE); behaviour with Frontotemporal Behavioral Rating Scale (FBRS). Age, gender, social problems, education, body mass index (BMI), comorbidities, history of stroke, use vitamin K antagonists, inadequate fatty fish intake, serum thyroid-stimulating hormone (TSH), vitamin B12, albumin, and estimated glomerular filtration rate were used as confounders. Compared to participants in the lowest third of dietary phylloquinone intake ($n = 64$), those with higher intake had higher (*i.e.*, better) mean MMSE score (22.0 $\pm$ 5.7 *versus* 19.9 $\pm$ 6.2, $p = 0.024$) and lower (*i.e.*, better) FBRS score (1.5 $\pm$ 1.2 *versus* 1.9 $\pm$ 1.3 $p = 0.042$). In multivariate linear regressions, log dietary phylloquinone intake was positively associated with MMSE score (adjusted $\beta = 1.66$, $p = 0.013$) and inversely associated with FBRS score (adjusted $\beta = -0.33$, $p = 0.037$). Specifically, log dietary phylloquinone intake correlated negatively with FBRS subscore of physical neglect ($r = -0.24$, $p = 0.001$). Higher dietary phylloquinone intake was associated with better cognition and behavior among older adults.

Keywords: cognition; behavior; diet; older adults; vitamin K

1. Introduction

Vitamin K is a fat-soluble substance found mainly in green vegetables and some vegetable oils. Vitamin K is classically known for its role as a coenzyme in the biological activation of seven proteins involved in blood coagulation [1]. Recently, a role for vitamin K has been demonstrated in target organs, such as the central nervous system (CNS) [2–10]. At the neuronal level, vitamin K is involved in the synthesis of sphingolipids—a major constituent of the myelin sheath and neuronal membranes—and the biological activation of vitamin K-dependent proteins (VKDPs) involved in neuronal physiology and survival [2,3]. Insufficient levels of vitamin K may, instead, cause neuropathological dysfunction [4]. Accordingly, an epidemiological study has reported a significant association between higher serum phylloquinone concentration (*i.e.*, vitamin K_1) and better verbal episodic memory performance in older adults [5]. Similarly, we found that the use of vitamin K antagonists (VKAs), which deplete the active form of vitamin K, was associated with cognitive impairment [6] and a lower volume of gray matter in the hippocampus [7] among geriatric patients. Taken together, these results suggest the importance of adequate (*i.e.*, high enough) vitamin K levels for optimal cognition in older adults [11]. To date, no randomized controlled trial has explored the benefits of vitamin K supplementation to maintain or improve cognition and related behavioral disorders in older adults. Before conducting such an expensive and time-consuming trial, it seems important and contributory to determine whether the intake of vitamin K relates to cognitive and behavioral performance in older adults.

We had the opportunity to examine the association between dietary vitamin K intake and cognitive behavioral performance in a sample of geriatric patients: the CLIP (Cognition and LIPophilic vitamins) cohort. Our objective was to determine whether dietary vitamin K intake was associated with cognitive and behavioral performance among geriatric patients.

2. Materials and Methods

2.1. Participants

We studied in- and outpatients aged 65 and over, consecutively recruited in the CLIP study. The CLIP study is an observational cross-sectional study designed to examine the relationships between neurocognition and lipophilic vitamins among all patients consecutively hospitalized or seen in consultation in the geriatric acute care unit of the University Hospital of Angers, France, from February to April 2014. After giving their informed consent for research, included participants received a full medical examination consisting of structured questionnaires, a standardized clinical examination, and a blood test. The study was conducted in accordance with the ethical standards set forth in the Helsinki Declaration (1983). The entire study protocol was approved by the local ethical committee (No. 2014-33).

2.2. Explanatory Variable: Dietary Intake of Vitamin K

Dietary vitamin K intake was estimated from a semi-quantitative food frequency questionnaire (FFQ) [12]. The 50-item FFQ used here was specifically designed to determine the daily dietary phylloquinone intake during the previous 12 months. It comprises 50 food items identified as important contributors to phylloquinone intake (e.g., spinach, iceberg lettuce, collards, and broccoli) and items with very high phylloquinone content (⩾500 μg/usual portion). The FFQ was interviewer-administered in 30 min by questioning the patients and/or their relatives, when applicable. Estimated phylloquinone intake was calculated for each food item by multiplying the amount of phylloquinone for that food item by the selected frequency and serving size (calculated as 0.5 for smaller than, and 1.5 for larger than the suggested portion), and all values were added to provide an estimate in μg/day of each participant's daily phylloquinone intake. The vitamin K FFQ shows good relative agreement with five-day food records ($\kappa = 0.60$, $p < 0.001$) [12]. In the present analysis, the participants were categorized into two groups based on the first tertile of the dietary phylloquinone intake: those in the lowest third of dietary phylloquinone intake below 207 μg/day, and those in the other two thirds combined of dietary phylloquinone intake above 207 μg/day.

2.3. Dependent Variables: Neuropsychiatric Measures

Cognition was assessed by one neuropsychologist blinded from participants' vitamin K intake using the Mini-Mental State Examination (MMSE) [13], in the absence of delirium identified with the Confusion Assessment Method [14]. The MMSE is a well-established measure of global cognitive performance in older adults composed of five sections (orientation, registration, attention-calculation, recall, and language). Scores range between 30 and 0 (worst). It shows good test-retest and inter-rater reliability and performs satisfactorily against more detailed measures of cognitive function [13].

Behavior was assessed at the same time as the MMSE using the Frontotemporal Behavioral Rating Scale (FBRS) [15]. The FBRS indicates the presence of symptoms of four domains of behavioral disturbances (*i.e.*, self-control disorder, physical neglect, mood disorders and loss of general interest). Each domain is scored 1 if at least 1 symptom is present, and 0 if no symptoms are present. The total FBRS score ranges from 0 (normal) to 4 (worst). The FBRS is easy to perform and has demonstrated good test-retest reliability [15].

2.4. Covariables

Age, gender, social problems, education level, body mass index, comorbidity burden, history of stroke, use of VKAs, regular fatty fish and eggs intakes, serum concentrations of thyroid-stimulating hormone (TSH), vitamin B12, albumin, and estimated glomerular filtration rate (*i.e.*, creatinine clearance, eGFR) are covariates related to diet and cognitive behavioral performance and were used as potential confounders. Evaluation of education level was based on self-report. Participants who passed at least the Elementary School Recognition Certificate were considered to have high education level. Social problems were defined by a geriatrician (yes/no) as the existence of social and/or familial isolation with consequent difficulties to stay in the usual place of life. Comorbidity burden was estimated with the Cumulative Illness Rating Scale-Geriatrics score (CIRS-G) (range 0–60, worst) [16]. History of stroke was sought by questioning the patients, the family physicians, and the patients' files. Stroke was defined according to the World Health Organization criteria as rapidly developed signs of focal or global disturbance of cerebral function lasting longer than 24 h, with no apparent nonvascular cause [17]. In case of clinical suspicion, computed tomography or magnetic resonance imaging scan was necessary to confirm the diagnosis and to distinguish among ischemic stroke and intracranial hemorrhage. The regular use of VKAs was systematically noted from the primary care physicians' prescriptions and sought by questioning the patients and their relatives, whatever the type of VKA used (*i.e.*, warfarin, acenocoumarol, or fluindione), the indication, length of treatment, and history of international normalized ratio (INR). The regular intake of fatty fish and eggs (*i.e.*, dietary sources of vitamin D and omega-3 polyunsaturated fatty acids (*n*-3 PUFAs), both linked to cognition) was sought using a standardized question: "Do you eat fatty fish at least once a week and/or eggs several times per week?" and was coded as low (*i.e.*, answer "No") or adequate (*i.e.*, answer "Yes"), as previously published [18]. Finally, the serum concentrations of TSH, vitamin B12, albumin and creatinine were measured using automated standard laboratory methods at the University Hospital of Angers, France, and eGFR was calculated using the Cockcroft-Gault formula $(((140 - \text{age}_{\text{years}}) \times \text{weight}_{\text{kg}}/\text{creatinine}_{\mu\text{mol/L}}) \times 1.04$ for females, and $\times 1.25$ for males).

2.5. Statistical Analysis

The participants' characteristics were summarized using means and standard deviations or frequencies and percentages, as appropriate. Statistics were performed on logarithmically-transformed values for the dietary phylloquinone intake to improve the symmetry of the non-Gaussian distribution.

Firstly, comparisons of participants' characteristics according to the dietary phylloquinone intake (*i.e.*, the lowest third *versus* the other two thirds combined) were performed using Student's *t*-test or the Chi-square test, as appropriate. Secondly, the mean difference of neuropsychiatric scores was calculated between participants in the lowest third *versus* the other two thirds combined of dietary phylloquinone intake. Thirdly, multiple linear regressions were used to examine the associations of log dietary phylloquinone intake (independent variable) with the MMSE score and the FBRS score (dependent variables), while adjusting for potential confounders. Separate analyses were conducted for each dependent variable. Finally, we examined the correlation between log dietary phylloquinone intake and each subscore of the FBRS. Lastly, we performed a sensitivity analysis after removing the participants who used VKA ($n = 31$). p-Values < 0.05 were considered significant. All statistics were performed using SPSS (v19.0, IBM corporation, Chicago, IL, USA) and RevMan (v5.1, Nordic Cochrane Centre, Copenhagen, Denmark).

3. Results

Among 192 included participants (mean $\pm$ standard deviation, 82.8 $\pm$ 7.1years; 62.5% female; 63.4% inpatient), the mean dietary phylloquinone intake estimated using a validated food frequency questionnaire (FFQ) [12] was 319.9 $\pm$ 196.3 μg/day. Sixty-four participants were in the lowest third of dietary phylloquinone intake, *i.e.*, below 207 μg/day (Table 1). The mean Mini-Mental State Examination score (MMSE) score was 21.4 $\pm$ 5.9 [13], and the mean Frontotemporal Behavioral Rating Scale (FBRS) score was 1.6 $\pm$ 1.2 [15]. Participants in the other two thirds combined of dietary phylloquinone intake had better MMSE and FBRS scores than those in the lowest third (respectively, 22.0 $\pm$ 5.7 *versus* 19.9 $\pm$ 6.2 with $p = 0.024$, and 1.5 $\pm$ 1.2 *versus* 1.9 $\pm$ 1.3 with $p = 0.042$) (Table 1). The between-group mean difference of MMSE score was −2.14 (95% confidence interval (CI): −3.95; −0.33), and that of FBRS score was 0.39 (95% CI: 0.01; 0.77) (Figure 1).

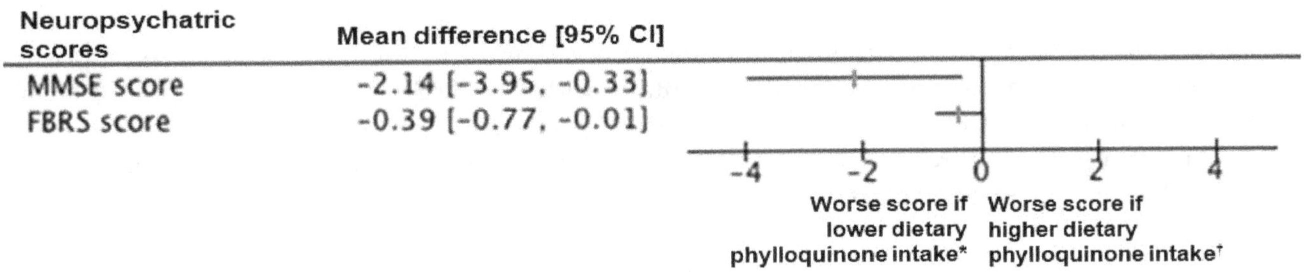

Figure 1. Forest plot for the mean difference of neuropsychiatric scores according to the dietary phylloquinone intake. Horizontal lines correspond to the 95% confidence interval (CI). The vertical line corresponds to a mean difference of 0.00, equivalent to no between-group difference. FBRS: Frontotemporal Behavioral Rating Scale; MMSE: Mini-Mental State Examination; *: lowest third of dietary phylloquinone intake below 206.97 μg/day; †: two other thirds combined of dietary phylloquinone intake.

Table 1. Baseline characteristics of 192 participants by dietary phylloquinone intake.

	Total Cohort (n = 192)	Dietary Phylloquinone Intake *		p-Value
		<207 µg/day (n = 64)	⩾ 207 µg/day (n = 128)	
Demographical measures				
Age, years	82.8 ± 7.1	83.7 ± 5.9	82.4 ± 7.7	0.227
Female gender, n (%)	120 (62.5)	43 (67.2)	77 (60.2)	0.343
Social problems, n (%)	21 (10.9)	10 (15.6)	11 (8.6)	0.141
High education level †, n (%)	152 (79.2)	51 (79.7)	101 (78.9)	0.900
Clinical measures				
Body mass index, kg/m^2	26.2 ± 5.4	25.8 ± 4.9	26.4 ± 5.6	0.492
CIRS-G score, /60	8.3 ± 4.0	9.0 ± 4.4	8.0 ± 3.8	0.118
History of stroke, n (%)	29 (15.2)	10 (15.6)	19 (15.0)	0.904
Use of vitamin K antagonists, n (%)	31 (16.1)	11 (17.2)	20 (15.6)	0.781
Dietary intake of phylloquinone, µg/day	319.9 ± 196.3	125.3 ± 52.1	417.1 ± 167.4	**<0.001**
Low dietary intake of fatty fish and eggs ‡, n (%)	23 (12.2)	9 (14.8)	14 (10.9)	0.453
Neuropsychiatric measures				
MMSE score, /30	21.4 ± 5.9	19.9 ± 6.2	22.0 ± 5.7	**0.024**
FBRS score, /4	1.6 ± 1.2	1.9 ± 1.3	1.5 ± 1.2	**0.042**
Serum measures				
TSH concentration, mIU/L	1.6 ± 1.8	1.5 ± 1.2	1.7 ± 2.0	0.440
Vitamin B12 concentration, ng/L	444.3 ± 266.2	478.5 ± 375.8	427.4 ± 190.6	0.228
Albumin concentration, g/L	34.9 ± 5.5	33.0 ± 5.7	35.9 ± 5.2	**0.001**
Estimated glomerular filtration rate, mL/min	53.7 ± 21.9	50.8 ± 18.2	55.1 ± 23.5	0.217

Data presented as mean ± standard deviation when applicable. CIRS-G: Cumulative Illness Rating Scale for Geriatrics; FBRS: Frontotemporal Behavioral Rating Scale; MMSE: Mini-Mental State Examination; TSH: thyroid stimulating hormone; *: lower dietary phylloquinone intake defined as the lowest third (*i.e.*, below 206.97 µg/day); higher dietary phylloquinone intake defined as the other two thirds combined (*i.e.*, above 206.97 µg/day); †: Elementary School Recognition Certificate passed; ‡: Answer "No" to the question "Do you eat fatty fish at least once a week and/or eggs several times per week?"; p-values < 0.05 indicated in bold.

Results of multiple linear regression models were reported in Table 2. We observed a positive association between log dietary phylloquinone intake and the MMSE score (β = 1.66, p = 0.013), and an inverse association with the FBRS score (β = −0.33, p = 0.037). Higher education level and higher serum concentrations of thyroid-stimulating hormone (TSH) and albumin were also associated with higher (*i.e.*, better) MMSE score, but none was associated with the FBRS score (Table 2).

Finally, Table 3 reports the correlations between the log dietary phylloquinone intake and the subscores of the FBRS. Log dietary intake of phylloquinone correlated negatively with the subscore of physical neglect (r = −0.24, p = 0.001), but not with the subscores of self-control disorders (p = 0.060), mood disorders (p = 0.196) and loss of general interest (p = 0.699).

Table 2. Fully adjusted linear regressions examining the association between the dietary phylloquinone intake (independent variable) and the MMSE and FBRS scores * (dependent variables), adjusted for potential confounders (n = 192).

	Neuropsychiatric Measures					
	MMSE Score			FBRS Score		
	β	(95% CI)	*p*-value	β	(95% CI)	*p*-value
Log dietary phylloquinone intake	1.66	(0.36; 2.95)	0.013	−0.33	(−0.63; −0.02)	0.037
Age	−0.22	(−0.39; −0.06)	0.009	0.02	(−0.03; 0.06)	0.450
Female gender	−0.63	(−2.46; 1.19)	0.492	−0.01	(−0.47; 0.44)	0.953
Social problems	2.75	(−0.31; 5.82)	0.078	0.10	(−0.63; 0.83)	0.792
High education level †	2.52	(0.27; 4.77)	**0.029**	−0.11	(−0.67; 0.45)	0.691
Body mass index	0.02	(−0.18; 0.23)	0.842	0.02	(−0.04; 0.07)	0.561
CIRS-G score	−0.14	(−0.41; 0.13)	0.312	0.03	(−0.04; 0.09)	0.441
History of stroke	−1.56	(−4.26; 1.13)	0.253	0.38	(−0.27; 1.02)	0.248
Use of vitamin K antagonists	−0.07	(−2.69; 2.56)	0.628	−0.10	(−0.75; 0.56)	0.773
Low dietary intake of fatty fish and eggs ‡	−0.09	(−2.83; 2.65)	0.948	0.63	(−0.06; 1.31)	0.072
TSH concentration	0.76	(0.02; 1.49)	**0.044**	0.06	(−0.13; 0.24)	0.556
Vitamin B12 concentration	−0.00	(−0.01; 0.00)	0.513	0.00	(0.00; 0.00)	0.281
Albumin concentration	0.24	(0.04; 0.43)	**0.018**	0.01	(−0.04; 0.06)	0.698
Estimated glomerular filtration rate	−0.02	(−0.07; 0.04)	0.567	−0.01	(−0.02; 0.01)	0.242

β: coefficient of regression corresponding to a change of cognitive score; CI: confidence interval; CIRS-G: Cumulative Illness Rating Scale for Geriatrics; FBRS: Frontotemporal Behavioral Rating Scale; MMSE: Mini-Mental State Examination; TSH: Thyroid Stimulating Hormone; *: Separate models were used for each dependent variable; †: Elementary School Recognition Certificate passed; ‡: Answer "No" to the question "Do you eat fatty fish at least once a week and/or eggs several times per week?"; β significant (*i.e.*, $p < 0.05$) indicated in bold.

Table 3. Correlation matrix of the dietary phylloquinone intake with the subscores of the Frontotemporal Behavioural Rating Scale.

Characteristics	1.	2.	3.	4.	5.
1. Log dietary phylloquinone intake	-	−0.14	−0.24 **	−0.09	−0.03
2. Self-control disorders		-	0.16 *	0.29 ***	0.32 ***
3. Physical neglect			-	0.14	0.25 ***
4. Mood disorders				-	0.35 ***
5. Lower general interest					-

*: $p < 0.05$ (2-tailed); **: $p < 0.01$ (2-tailed); ***: $p < 0.001$ (2-tailed).

Lastly, the sensitivity analysis found unaltered results after removing all participants who used VKA (n = 31). Of the 161 remaining participants, those in the lowest third of dietary phylloquinone intake had worse MMSE score (19.9 ± 6.0 *versus* 22.4 ± 5.8, p = 0.016) and FBRS score (1.9 ± 1.3 *versus* 1.5 ± 1.2, p = 0.035) than those in the other two thirds combined. Log dietary phylloquinone intake was linearly associated with the MMSE score (β = 1.83 (95% CI: 0.46; 3.20), p = 0.009) and with the FBRS score (β = −0.34 (95% CI: −0.66; −0.01), p = 0.041). Log dietary phylloquinone intake correlated negatively with the subscores of physical neglect (r = −0.24, p = 0.003) and self-control disorders (r = −0.17, p = 0.037), but not with mood disorders (p = 0.127) and loss of general interest (p = 0.978).

4. Discussion

The main finding of this cross-sectional study is that, irrespective of all measured potential confounders, increased dietary phylloquinone intake was associated with better cognition and behavior among geriatric patients. Specifically, compared to those in the lowest third of dietary phylloquinone intake, participants with higher dietary phylloquinone intake had 2.1 points more on the MMSE (*i.e.*, better) and 0.4 points less on the FBRS (*i.e.*, better).

These findings are consistent with the emerging epidemiological literature on vitamin K and cognition. Specifically, previous studies have reported that the serum concentration of phylloquinone was lower among patients with Alzheimer's disease (AD) compared to cognitively healthy controls [8], and that higher serum phylloquinone concentration was associated with better verbal episodic memory performance [5]. In line with this, we recently found that the use of VKAs, a drug class that generates a relative state of vitamin K deficiency, was associated among geriatric patients with greater prevalence of cognitive disorders [6], and with lower volume of gray matter in the brain, including in the hippocampus [7]. Here, we found no association between the use of VKAs and the global cognitive performance used as a quantitative variable. Several explanations can be proposed to account for this divergence: first, the potential lack of power of the present study that was not originally designed to assess the covariate VKA; second, the use of the cognitive performance as a continuous variable, unlike the previous study [6], which was focused on the cognitive impairment as a categorical variable; third, the lack of specification on the length of treatment and stability of the INR, which could influence the potential cognitive effect of VKAs. Of note, removing from the analysis the participants who were taking VKAs regularly did not alter our results, which strengthened the possibility of a specific link between dietary vitamin K intake and cognition. To the best of our knowledge, only two case-control studies have specifically examined the intake of phylloquinone in relation to cognition [9,10]. Shatenstein *et al.* found that that the mean dietary phylloquinone intake was persistently two-fold less in 36 community-dwelling patients with early-stage AD followed during 18 months in the Nutrition-Memory Study compared to 58 cognitively healthy control subjects (55.5 $\pm$ 54.3 *versus* 104.5 $\pm$ 83.7 with $p < 0.001$ at baseline) [9]. Consistently, Presse *et al.* found, in an additional analysis of the Nutrition-Memory Study cohort, that 31 cases with mild-to-moderate AD had lower dietary phylloquinone intake compared to 31 age- and gender-matched cognitively-healthy control subjects (37 µg/day *versus* 70 µg/day, $p < 0.0001$), even after adjusting for energy intakes ($p = 0.0003$) [10]. Additional indirect evidence stems from two cohort studies in which the high consumption of green leafy and cruciferous vegetables, rich in vitamin K, was associated with slower rates of age-related cognitive decline [19,20]. Compared to these studies, we did not use diet records to estimate the dietary phylloquinone intake, but a FFQ. Nevertheless, despite this methodological divergence, we observed that the higher the dietary phylloquinone intake, the better the cognitive performance and the lower the behavioural disorders. Specifically, we found a correlation of dietary phylloquinone intake with self-control disorders and physical neglect, but not with mood disorders and loss of interest (Table 3). In other words, the intake of phylloquinone does not appear to be related to emotional and affect regulation, but rather to behavioral disorders in relation with the cognitive sphere, which was confirmed by the finding of a direct association between dietary phylloquinone intake and MMSE score.

The mechanism linking dietary phylloquinone intake with cognition and behavior is not fully elucidated. Causality cannot be inferred from our cross-sectional study. It is possible that worse cognitive performance and greater behavioral disorders precipitate loss of functional autonomy with consequent poorer access to vitamin K-rich food. For instance, lower consumption of green vegetables, a major source of phylloquinone, has been reported in participants with AD compared to cognitively healthy participants [10]. In addition, the association of dietary phylloquinone intake with neuropsychiatric performance could be explained in a more general way by an overall healthy diet, which could also reflect generally healthy lifestyles. However, the latter assumptions should be mitigated here by the fact that the mean BMI of 26.2 kg/m^2 in our study indicated overweight according to the National Heart, Lung, and Blood Institute [21], and because there was no BMI difference between participants in the lowest third of phylloquinone intake and those in the highest thirds ($p = 0.492$, Table 1). Moreover the associations of dietary phylloquinone intake with the MMSE score and the FBRS score were significant even after adjustment for BMI and albumin concentration (Table 2). A scenario of reverse causation is plausible and should be considered. Evidence precisely supports a role for vitamin K in the CNS. Vitamin K modulates the synthesis and metabolism of sphingolipids, which are key players in neuronal proliferation, differentiation, senescence, cell-cell interaction, and transformation [2,3]. Recent research has linked alterations in sphingolipid metabolism to the aging process and neurodegenerative disorders such as AD [3]. In parallel, two VKDPs, Gas6 (growth arrest-specific gene 6) and protein S, are also closely associated with the CNS functioning [2,3]. Gas6 is involved in chemotaxis, mitogenesis, cell growth, and myelination, and has further been shown to rescue cortical neurons from amyloid β-induced apoptosis, a hallmark of AD [22]. Protein S offers neuronal protection during ischemic/hypoxic injury, both *in vivo* and *in vitro* [23]. Vitamin K may also protect neurons from *N*-methyl-D-aspartate-induced toxicity and apoptosis [24]. Finally, other authors have proposed that insufficient vitamin K could contribute to the pathogenesis of AD through a link to the apolipoprotein Eε4 allele, an established risk factor for AD that is also associated with lower vitamin K levels [11]. ApoE genotype was not determined in our cohort, which precludes testing this assumption. All these data suggest that the less available the vitamin K is, the less protected and effective the CNS may be, with subsequently greater risks of brain changes, cognitive decline, and behavioral disorders.

The strengths of our study include the originality of the research question on a highly common condition in older adults, the standardized collection of data from a single research center, the assessment of the dietary phylloquinone intake over preceding 12 months based on a validated tool, the assessment of both cognitive and behavioral outcomes, and the detailed description of the participants' characteristics allowing the use of regression models to measure adjusted associations. Regardless, a number of limitations should be acknowledged. First, due to the limited number of 192 in- and outpatients, our study may lack power and the participants may be not representative of the population of all seniors. Second, our study is cross-sectional at present, which precludes inferring causality. Third, the FFQ was validated on a Canadian population [12], and it is likely that the eating habits of our elderly patients were not strictly the same as those of North Americans. Moreover, it is noticeable that FFQs tend to overestimate intakes [25,26]. Nonetheless, the FFQ used in the present study presents a very good relative agreement with results from 24 h dietary recalls in healthy older adults [12]. It is also possible that the dietary phylloquinone intake may have been poorly estimated by interviewing patients with cognitive disorders. However, to avoid this bias, we double-checked information whenever possible from formal or informal carers. Fourth, although we were able to control for important characteristics that could modify the associations, residual potential confounders such as the determination of energy and homocysteine intakes or the determination of ApoE genotype, might still be present. Fifth, limitations include the use of the MMSE and FBRS tools, which may exhibit ceiling effects and limited sensitivity to subtle abnormalities [27]. In future studies, the screening for cognitive disorders should use other outcomes, e.g., comparing episodic memory or executive functions according to dietary phylloquinone intakes.

5. Conclusions

In conclusion, we report a clinically and statistically significant association between increased dietary phylloquinone intake and better cognition and behavior among geriatric patients. There is a strong need for novel effective preventive and therapeutic strategies for cognitive decline and dementia. The potential role of vitamin K in the development of dementia is therefore of substantial interest. Further prospective nutrition studies and clinical trials are needed to clarify whether older adults with higher dietary vitamin K intake are less likely to experience cognitive and behavioral declines than those with lower intake, and whether enhancing vitamin K intake could improve, or prevent, this process.

Acknowledgments: The authors thank Elena De Neree Tot Babberich, Clemence Gourdeau, Simon Pointel, Bruno Lemarchant, from Medical School, University of Angers, UNAM, Angers F-49933, France, for their help in collecting the participants' data and food records.

Author Contributions: Cedric Annweiler has full access to the data in the study and takes responsibility for the integrity of the data and the accuracy of the data analyses. Study concept and design: Cedric Annweiler;

Acquisition of data: Justine Chouet, Kariane Boucher, Nancy Presse, Guylaine Ferland and Cedric Annweiler; Analysis and interpretation of data: Justine Chouet and Cedric Annweiler; Drafting of the manuscript: Justine Chouet and Cedric Annweiler; Critical revision of the manuscript for important intellectual content: Guylaine Ferland, Catherine Féart, Yves Rolland, Nancy Presse, Kariane Boucher, Pascale Barberger-Gateau, and Olivier Beauchet; Statistical expertise: Cedric Annweiler and Catherine Féart; Administrative, technical, or material support: Cedric Annweiler; Study supervision: Cedric Annweiler.

References

1. Suttie, J.W. *Vitamin K in Health and Disease*; CRC Press: Boca Raton, FL, USA, 2009.
2. Ferland, G. Vitamin K, an emerging nutrient in brain function. *Biofactors* **2012**, *38*, 151–157. [CrossRef] [PubMed]
3. Ferland, G. Vitamin K and the nervous system: An overview of its actions. *Adv. Nutr.* **2012**, *3*, 204–212. [CrossRef] [PubMed]
4. Hall, J.G.; Pauli, R.M.; Wilson, K.M. Maternal and fetal sequelae of anticoagulation during pregnancy. *Am. J. Med.* **1980**, *68*, 122–140. [CrossRef]
5. Presse, N.; Belleville, S.; Gaudreau, P.; Greenwood, C.E.; Kergoat, M.J.; Morais, J.A.; Payette, H.; Shatenstein, B.; Ferland, G. Vitamin K status and cognitive function in healthy older adults. *Neurobiol. Aging* **2013**, *34*, 2777–2783. [CrossRef] [PubMed]
6. Annweiler, C.; Ferland, G.; Barberger-Gateau, P.; Brangier, A.; Rolland, Y.; Beauchet, O. Vitamin K antagonists and cognitive impairment: Results from a cross-sectional pilot study among geriatric patients. *J. Gerontol. A Biol. Sci. Med. Sci.* **2015**, *70*, 97–101. [CrossRef] [PubMed]
7. Annweiler, C.; Denis, S.; Duval, G.; Ferland, G.; Bartha, R.; Beauchet, O. Use of vitamin K antagonists and brain volumetry in seniors: Preliminary results from the GAIT study. *J. Gerontol. A Biol. Sci. Med. Sci.* **2015**. (in press).
8. Sato, Y.; Honda, Y.; Hayashida, N.; Iwamoto, J.; Kanoko, T.; Satoh, K. Vitamin K deficiency and osteopenia in elderly women with Alzheimer's disease. *Arch. Phys. Med. Rehabil.* **2005**, *86*, 576–581. [CrossRef] [PubMed]
9. Shatenstein, B.; Kergoat, M.J.; Reid, I. Poor nutrient intakes during 1-year follow-up with community-dwelling older adults with early stage Alzheimer dementia compared to cognitively intact matched controls. *J. Am. Diet Assoc.* **2007**, *107*, 2091–2099. [CrossRef] [PubMed]
10. Sato, Y.; Honda, Y.; Hayashida, N.; Iwamoto, J.; Kanoko, T.; Satoh, K. Low vitamin K intakes in community-dwelling elders at an early stage of Alzheimer's disease. *J. Am. Diet Assoc.* **2008**, *108*, 2095–2099.
11. Allison, A.C. The possible role of vitamin K deficiency in the pathogenesis of Alzheimer's disease and in augmenting brain damage associated with cardiovascular disease. *Med. Hypotheses* **2001**, *57*, 151–155. [CrossRef] [PubMed]
12. Presse, N.; Shatenstein, B.; Kergoat, M.J.; Ferland, G. Validation of a semi-quantitative food frequency questionnaire measuring dietary vitamin K intake in elderly people. *J. Am. Diet Assoc.* **2009**, *109*, 1251–1255. [CrossRef] [PubMed]
13. Folstein, M.F.; Folstein, S.E.; McHugh, P.R. Mini-mental state: a practical method for grading the cognitive state of patients for the clinician. *J. Psychiatr. Res.* **1975**, *12*, 189–198. [CrossRef]
14. Inouye, S.K.; van Dyck, C.H.; Alessi, C.A.; Balkin, S.; Siegal, A.P.; Horwitz, R.I. Clarifying confusion: The confusion assessment method. A new method for detection of delirium. *Ann. Intern. Med.* **1990**, *113*, 941–948. [CrossRef] [PubMed]
15. Lebert, F.; Pasquier, F.; Souliez, L.; Petit, H. Frontotemporal behavioral scale. *Alzheimer Dis. Assoc. Disord.* **1998**, *12*, 335–339. [CrossRef] [PubMed]
16. Linn, B.S.; Linn, M.W.; Gurel, L. Cumulative illness rating scale. *J. Am. Geriatr. Soc.* **1968**, *16*, 622–626. [CrossRef] [PubMed]
17. Hatano, S. Experience from a multicentre stroke register: A preliminary report. *Bull World Health Organ.* **1976**, *54*, 541–553. [PubMed]
18. Chevallereau, G.; Gleyses, X.; Roussel, L.; Hamdan, S.; Beauchet, O.; Annweiler, C. Proposal and validation of a quick question to rate the influence of diet in geriatric epidemiological studies on vitamin D. *Int. J. Vitam Nutr. Res.* **2013**, *83*, 254–258. [CrossRef] [PubMed]
19. Kang, J.H.; Ascherio, A.; Grodstein, F. Fruit and vegetable consumption and cognitive decline in aging women. *Ann. Neurol.* **2005**, *57*, 713–720. [CrossRef] [PubMed]

20. Morris, M.C.; Evans, D.A.; Tangney, C.C.; Bienias, J.L.; Wilson, R.S. Associations of vegetable and fruit consumption with age-related cognitive change. *Neurology* **2006**, *67*, 1370–1376. [CrossRef] [PubMed]
21. Clinical guideline on the identification, evaluation, and treatment of overweight and obesity in adults: The evidence report. National Heart, Lung, and Blood Institute (online), 1998. Available online: http://www.nhlbi.nih.gov/guidelines/obesity/ob_gdlns.png (accessed on 6 August 2014).
22. Yagami, T.; Ueda, K.; Asakura, K.; Okamura, N.; Sakaeda, T.; Sakaguchi, G.; Itoh, N.; Hashimoto, Y.; Nakano, T.; Fujimoto, M.; *et al.* Effect of Gas6 on secretory phospholipase A(2)-IIA-induced apoptosis in cortical neurons. *Brain Res.* **2003**, *985*, 142–149. [CrossRef]
23. Liu, D.; Guo, H.; Griffin, J.H.; Fernandez, J.A.; Zlokovic, B.V. Protein S confers neuronal protection during ischemic/hypoxic injury in mice. *Circulation* **2003**, *107*, 1791–1796. [CrossRef] [PubMed]
24. Zhong, Z.; Wang, Y.; Guo, H.; Sagare, A.; Fernández, J.A.; Bell, R.D.; Barrett, T.M.; Griffin, J.H.; Freeman, R.S.; Zlokovic, B.V.; *et al.* Protein S protects neurons from excitotoxic injury by activating the TAM receptor Tyro3-phosphatidylinositol 3-kinase-Akt pathway through its sex hormone-binding globulin-like region. *J. Neurosci.* **2010**, *30*, 15521–15534. [CrossRef] [PubMed]
25. Booth, S.L.; Suttie, J.W. Dietary intake and adequacy of vitamin K. *J. Nutr.* **1998**, *128*, 785–788. [PubMed]
26. Holmes, M.V.; Hunt, B.J.; Shearer, M.J. The role of dietary vitamin K in the management of oral vitamin K antagonists. *Blood Rev.* **2012**, *26*, 1–14. [CrossRef] [PubMed]
27. Spencer, R.J.; Wendell, C.R.; Giggey, P.P.; Katzel, L.I.; Lefkowitz, D.M.; Siegel, E.L.; Waldstein, S.R. Psychometric limitations of the mini-mental state examination among nondemented older adults: An evaluation of neurocognitive and magnetic resonance imaging correlates. *Exp. Aging Res.* **2013**, *39*, 382–397. [CrossRef] [PubMed]

Prevalence and Predictors of Functional Vitamin K Insufficiency in Mothers and Newborns in Uganda

Data Santorino [1,*], Mark J. Siedner [2], Juliet Mwanga-Amumpaire [1], Martin J. Shearer [3], Dominic J. Harrington [3] and Unni Wariyar [1]

1 Department of Pediatrics and Child Health, Mbarara University of Science and Technology, Plot 8-18 Mbarara–Kabale Road, P.O. Box 1410, Mbarara, Uganda; jmwanga@must.ac.ug (J.M.-A.); wariyarunniwariyar@gmail.com (U.W.)

2 Department of Medicine and Infectious Diseases, Massachusetts General Hospital and Harvard Medical School, 125 Nashua Street, Boston, MA 02114, USA; MSIEDNER@mgh.harvard.edu

3 Centre for Haemostasis and Thrombosis, St. Thomas' Hospital, Westminster Bridge Road, London SE1 7EH, UK; Martin.Shearer@gstt.nhs.uk (M.J.S.); Dominic.Harrington@viapath.co.uk (D.J.H.)

* Correspondence: boymukedata@gmail.com

Abstract: Vitamin K deficiency bleeding (VKDB) in infancy is a serious but preventable cause of mortality or permanent disability. Lack of epidemiologic data for VKDB in sub-Saharan Africa hinders development and implementation of effective prevention strategies. We used convenience sampling to consecutively enroll mothers delivering in a southwestern Uganda Hospital. We collected socio-demographic and dietary information, and paired samples of maternal venous and neonatal cord blood for the immunoassay of undercarboxylated prothrombin (PIVKA-II), a sensitive marker of functional vitamin K (VK) insufficiency. We used univariable and multivariable logistic regression models to identify predictors of VK insufficiency. We detected PIVKA-II of ⩾0.2 AU (Arbitrary Units per mL)/mL (indicative of VK insufficiency) in 33.3% (47/141) of mothers and 66% (93/141) of newborns. Importantly, 22% of babies had PIVKA-II concentrations ⩾5.0 AU/mL, likely to be associated with abnormal coagulation indices. We found no significant predictors of newborn VK insufficiency, including infant weight (AOR (adjusted odds ratio) 1.85, 95% CI (confidence interval) 0.15–22.49), gender (AOR 0.54, 95% CI 0.26–1.11), term birth (AOR 0.72, 95% CI 0.20–2.62), maternal VK-rich diet (AOR 1.13, 95% CI 0.55–2.35) or maternal VK insufficiency (AOR 0.99, 95% CI 0.47–2.10). VK insufficiency is common among mothers and newborn babies in southwestern Uganda, which in one fifth of babies nears overt deficiency. Lack of identifiable predictors of newborn VK insufficiency support strategies for universal VK prophylaxis to newborns to prevent VKDB.

Keywords: vitamin K; undercarboxylated prothrombin; deficiency; insufficiency; newborn; bleeding; haemorrhage; prophylaxis

1. Introduction

Vitamin K Deficiency Bleeding (VKDB) in infancy is a rare but potentially serious worldwide problem with a high risk of mortality or permanent disability, primarily due to the high incidence of intracranial haemorrhage (ICH) of the later onset syndrome [1–5]. It is a disease of breastfeeding infants [1,6–9] and can be prevented by administration of vitamin K (VK) to newborns shortly after birth [1,9–12]. VKDB is classified according to the age of presentation as early, classical and late [1]. Early VKDB occurs in the first 24 h after birth, it is generally rare and often associated with maternal anticoagulant and or anticonvulsant usage during pregnancy. Classical and late VKDB occur between days 2 to 7, and days 8 to 6 months of life, respectively [9]. In classical VKDB, bleeding typically occurs from the gastrointestinal tract, umbilicus, skin, nose or after circumcision [1,9,10] while in late VKDB, bleeding predominantly occurs within the brain with prevalence rates of ICH as high as 60%–80% [2,3]. Reported incidence rates of classical and late VKDB over the last 50 years in infants who have not been given VK prophylaxis vary widely across different countries.

Apart from reflecting the lack of standardization for case definitions [4,10], there is evidence that the incidence of VKDB reflects economic and nutritional status [6,8,9], social customs such as male circumcision [6,13], and probably genetic variations such as those known to influence the metabolism and intracellular recycling of VK [14]. For classical VKDB, the extremely high incidence rates of 1.7% in Cincinnati, USA in the 1960s [6] and 0.8% in Addis Ababa, Ethiopia from 1982–1991 [8] are noteworthy for the economic deprivation of the populations studied. Incidence rates were strongly influenced by male circumcision in the Cincinnati study [6] but not in the Addis Ababa study where circumcision occurred after 7 days of age and outside the window of classical VKDB [8]. In contrast, the incidence of classical and late VKDB from national surveys in two European countries (Germany and the British Isles) in the late 1980s reveal a markedly lower incidence of 4–7 cases per 10^5 births in infants given no VK prophylaxis [9,10,15]. A much higher prevalence of late VKDB has been reported in countries of South East Asia (e.g., Japan, Thailand, Malaysia, Vietnam and China) with incidence rates ranging from 11 to 116 cases per 10^5 births [3,4,9,16]. There is no data for the prevalence of late VKDB in sub-Saharan Africa. Apart from exclusive breastfeeding [1,6–9], other known risk factors for classical and late VKDB are diarrhea, prolonged antibiotic use and the presence of underlying diseases (e.g., biliary atresia, alpha-1-antitrypsin deficiency, cystic fibrosis) causing malabsorption of VK [1,5,17,18]. Feeding infants with milk formulas (both unsupplemented and supplemented) offers a high protection against VKDB owing to their higher VK content compared to breast milk [19,20] resulting in a greatly superior VK status of formula-fed infants [21].

The lack of data about the epidemiology of VKDB in sub-Saharan Africa has limited the development and implementation of guidelines for prevention of VKDB. As such, VK is not typically listed as a priority drug for children by programmatic organizations such as in the World Health Organization's Model Medicines list for children [13]. To estimate the incidence of neonatal haemorrhage in Uganda, we performed a retrospective chart review from June–August 2010 at Mbarara Regional Referral Hospital (MRRH) in Southwestern Uganda where VK prophylaxis is not routinely administered to newborns at birth. We found a 6.6% incidence of haemorrhage among all neonatal admissions to the Hospital during the observation period (unpublished data). This was higher than the neonatal haemorrhage prevalence previously reported by Lulseged in Ethiopia [8]. Based on this high prevalence of newborn haemorrhage, we conducted a study to determine the epidemiology and predictors of functional VK insufficiency among mothers and their newborns at MRRH. We define "functional VK insufficiency" as a nutritional state in which the hepatic stores of vitamin K are insufficient to ensure full gamma-glutamyl carboxylation of the VK-dependent procoagulant proteins, factors II (prothrombin), VII, IX and X. In states of VK insufficiency, functionally defective undercarboxylated species of factors such as prothrombin are released into the bloodstream where they can be measured [9,22]. Historically the collective name for these undercarboxylated species is PIVKA (Proteins Induced by vitamin K Absence or Antagonism). In the present study functional VK insufficiency was assessed by the measurement of undercarboxylated prothrombin (PIVKA-II) which has been shown to be a highly sensitive and selective functional marker of VK status with respect to its coagulation function [9,22]. Our choice of PIVKA-II has several advantages over traditional biomarkers of VK status. First, global coagulation tests such as the prothrombin time (PT) or activated partial thromboplastin time (APTT) are insufficiently sensitive to detect early VK insufficiency. As reviewed by Suttie [23], a 1–2 second increase in the PT only occurs when the percent of active (carboxylated) prothrombin has dropped to below 50% of normal whereas immunoassays of PIVKA-II can readily detect undercarboxylated species of prothrombin when there are no observable changes in the PT. For example, even when the concentration of active prothrombin is as high as 90% there is a 20-fold increase in the concentrations of PIVKA-II as measured by an immunoassay such as that used in our study [23]. Second, a prolonged PT lacks specificity for VK insufficiency: for example in a VK supplementation trial carried out in 98 preterm infants, 21 infants who had a significantly prolonged PT were shown to have satisfactory VK status as assessed by serum PIVKA-II and phylloquinone measurements [24]. Thus while a prolonged PT (and APTT) are expected findings in advanced vitamin K deficiency, they have important limitations as early biomarkers of VK insufficiency.

2. Experimental Section

2.1. Enrollment and Study Procedures

We consecutively enrolled mothers delivering during daytime hours on the peripartum ward at MRRH. Women in active labour were consented before the onset of second stage of labor and were followed until delivery for blood collection at birth. Women with self-reported liver disease, visible jaundice or taking warfarin were excluded [25,26]. We used interviewer administered structured questionnaires to collect socio-demographic data. We also recorded gestational age, newborn weight, and newborn gender. We assessed maternal diet using a 22-item non-validated, and non-quantitative food frequency questionnaire to determine intake frequency of VK rich food [27]. Participants stated daily, weekly and monthly frequency with which they ate VK-rich foods using an interviewer administered food frequency questionnaire. We defined a frequent VK rich food intake as five or more servings per week of green vegetables and or peas.

2.2. Blood Collection and Laboratory Procedures

Maternal venous blood from the brachial vein and newborn cord blood were collected immediately at birth in the delivery room. Serum was separated and stored at negative 70 degrees Celsius. At the conclusion of study procedures, samples were transported by courier on dry ice to the Centre for Haemostasis and Thrombosis, Guy's and St. Thomas' Hospital Foundation Trust in London for analysis. We measured undercarboxylated prothrombin (factor II) also known as Protein Induced by vitamin K Absence-II (PIVKA-II) serum concentrations using a conformation-specific PIVKA-II monoclonal antibody with a sandwich ELISA [22,28–30]. Concentrations of PIVKA-II were expressed as Arbitrary Units per mL (AU/mL) with 1 AU/mL being equivalent to 1 μg of multiple species of uncarboxylated or partially carboxylated prothrombin purified by electrophoresis [22,28–30]. Using this same immunoassay, PIVKA-II concentrations in healthy VK replete adults and infants are <0.20 AU/mL. Newborn babies with PIVKA-II values $\geqslant 0.20$ AU/mL are defined as having vitamin K insufficiency with values $\geqslant 5.0$ AU/mL approaching a state of overt VK deficiency that are likely to be associated with abnormal coagulation indices and which are clinically relevant to bleeding risk [22]. However, it was not possible to perform any coagulation tests (e.g., prothrombin time) in our study.

2.3. Statistical Analyses

Our primary outcome was VK insufficiency at birth as defined by PIVKA-II of greater than or equal to 0.2 AU/mL. Exposures of interest were newborn weight, gender, gestational age [31] and maternal intake of VK rich foods [25]. We fitted univariable and multivariable logistic regression models to estimate associations between the primary outcome of interest (raised PIVKA-II) and exposures of interest. All variables for which we had a priori reason to consider as potential confounders or correlates of vitamin K insufficiency were maintained in the multivariable model. A p-value of less than or equal to 0.05 was considered statistically significant [32]. Data analysis was performed with Stata Version 12 (Statcorp, College Station, TX, USA).

2.4. Ethics Statement

All participants gave signed informed consent. All babies received intramuscular prophylactic VK after blood sample collection. The study procedures were reviewed and approved by Mbarara University Faculty of Medicine Research and Ethics committee, the Institutional Review Committee at the Mbarara University of Science and Technology and the Uganda National Council for Science and Technology.

3. Results

We enrolled 141 mother-baby pairs over a period of 4 months (June–September). The median maternal age was 25 years (Interquartile range: 21–29 years). All mothers approached to participate in the study, gave their written consent. All samples analyzed yielded useable laboratory values. Sixty six percent (93/141) of mothers came from town/urban settings mainly from Mbarara town where MRRH is located. Ninety six (136/141) of the women were married, 57.5% had no secondary education, and 33.3% were primigravidae. Sixty four percent of babies (90/141) were male, 9% (13/141) were preterm (born before 37 completed weeks of amenorrhea) and 3% (4/141) had low birth weight (<2.5 kg). The median birth weight was 3.2 kg (IQR: 2.9–3.8 kg). Spontaneous vaginal delivery accounted for 75% (107/141) of deliveries, caesarian section, 23.4% (33/141) and only one baby was delivered by vacuum extraction. VK insufficiency defined by a detectable PIVKA-II of ⩾0.2 AU/mL was present in 33% (47/141) of mothers and 66% (93/141) of babies as shown in Table 1. Six sets of twins were enrolled in the study, there was no PIVKA-II value-category difference between twin siblings, therefore, for the purposes of this study, the PIVKA-II value of the first-born twin were used for analysis. Highly elevated, concentrations of PIVKA-II (⩾5.0 AU/mL) indicative of likely abnormal coagulation [22] were found in 22% (31/141) of newborns but in none of their mothers. No newborn babies had detectable postpartum bleeding before hospital discharge. However, all newborn babies received intramuscular vitamin K within one hour of delivery during the period of the study irrespective of study enrolment status.

Table 1. Maternal dietary habits and newborn characteristics at birth for the total cohort and by presence of vitamin K (VK) insufficiency.

Variable	Total Cohort (n = 282)	PIVKA-II ⩾ 0.2 AU/mL $^{\acute{\epsilon}}$ (n = 140)	PIVKA-II < 0.2 AU/mL $^{\pi}$ (n = 142)	p-Value
Mothers, % (n)	100 (141)	33 (47)	67 (94)	
Newborn babies, % (n)	100 (141)	66 (93)	34 (48)	
Female newborn, % (n)	36 (51)	57 (29)	43 (22)	0.086
Low birth weight (<2.5 kg), % (n)	3 (4)	75 (3)	25 (1)	0.699
Preterm, % (n)	9 (13)	62 (8)	38 (5)	0.724
Maternal VK-rich intake *, % (n)	40 (56)	32 (18)	68 (38)	0.808

* Vitamin K-rich intake as defined by intake of greens and or peas five or more times a week; $^{\acute{\epsilon}}$ PIVKA-II: Protein induced in vitamin K absence, with a level ⩾ 0.2 Arbitrary Units indicative of vitamin K insufficiency; $^{\pi}$ PIVKA-II level < 0.20 AU/mL indicative of normal vitamin K status. AU/mL: Arbitrary Units per mL.

We found no significant predictors of newborn VK insufficiency among newborn or maternal characteristics including: infant weight (AOR (adjusted odds ratio) 1.85, 95% CI (confidence interval) 0.15–22.49), gender (AOR 0.54, 95% CI 0.26–1.11), term birth (AOR 0.72, 95% CI 0.20–2.62), maternal VK-rich diet (AOR 1.13, 95% CI 0.55–2.35) and maternal VK insufficiency (AOR 0.99, 95% CI 0.47–2.10) as shown in Table 2.

Table 2. Univariate and multivariate logistic regression models of correlates of vitamin K (VK) insufficiency in newborns, as defined by a PIVKA II concentration ⩾ 0.2 AU/mL.

	Univariable Logistic Regression		Multivariable Logistic Regression	
Characteristic	**AOR (95% CI)**	***p*-Value**	**AOR (95% CI)**	***p*-Value**
Female newborn	0.54 (0.26–1.09)	0.088	0.54 (0.26–1.11)	0.093
Low birth weight (<2,500 g)	1.57 (0.16–15.48)	0.701	1.85 (0.15–22.49)	0.630
Preterm (<37 weeks of gestation)	0.81 (0.25–2.62)	0.725	0.72 (0.20–2.62)	0.619
Maternal VK insufficiency	1.00 (0.48–2.09)	1.000	0.99 (0.47–2.10)	0.983
Maternal VK-rich intake *	0.915 (045–1.88)	0.808	1.13 (0.55–2.35)	0.737

* Vitamin K rich intake as defined by intake of greens and or peas five or more times a week; PIVKA-II: Protein induced in vitamin K absence, with a level ⩾ 0.2 Arbitrary Units indicative of vitamin K insufficiency. AOR: adjusted odds ratio; CI: confidence interval.

Up to 61.5% (8/13) of all premature babies had detectable PIVKA-II and 23% (3/13) had highly elevated PIVKA-II values (⩾5 AU/mL).

4. Discussion

Among mothers delivering at a publicly-operated referral hospital in rural southwestern Uganda, VK insufficiency is very common in both mothers (33%) and their newborns (66%). Our study is the first to characterize the prevalence of VK insufficiency in a Sub-Saharan Africa setting using the gold standard measurement (PIVKA-II assay) for functional VK insufficiency with respect to its coagulation function. We found no maternal or infant clinical or dietary predictors of VK insufficiency, implying that routine, prophylactic VK administration should continue to be the standard of care for prevention of VKDB in newborns. Given the high prevalence of VK insufficiency and potential devastating effects of VKDB, availability of VK should be prioritized in resource-limited settings, and especially in health facilities that perform perinatal care.

The 33% prevalence of functional VK insufficiency among mothers in our study is notable and higher than other previous reports. For example, using the same PIVKA-II assay, Chuansumrit *et al.*, found a prevalence of VK insufficiency of 12% among mothers delivering at Ramathibodi hospital in Thailand [22], a country in which the incidence of VKDB was estimated to be 72 cases per 10^5 births before universal prophylaxis was introduced [3]. Lower dietary intakes of VK by Ugandan mothers compared to Thai mothers may explain the high prevalence of VK insufficiency in our study population. However, the two studies used different methods to measure VK intake, limiting direct comparability.

Similarly, the prevalence of detectable PIVKA-II of 66% in newborn babies in our study was much higher than the 16% prevalence in the Thai study [22] or the 23% prevalence in a study of preterm infants in England [29], all done with the same PIVKA-II assay. Another notable difference between this Ugandan and the Thai study was that 22.0% (31/141) of Ugandan babies had clinically significant PIVKA-II concentrations (⩾5.0 AU/mL) compared to 1.5% (10/683) of Thai babies despite the fact that both cohorts were comparable in their birth characteristics. PIVKA-II concentrations greater than 5 AU/mL are likely associated with abnormal coagulopathy and an increased risk for spontaneous bleeding [22].

We found no consistent correlation between the presence or absence of detectable PIVKA-II in cord blood with its presence or absence in the respective paired sample from the mother. In other words, the concentration of PIVKA-II in the mother was not predictive of the concentration in her newborn baby. We should emphasize however that while highly raised PIVKA-II concentrations (⩾5.0 AU/mL) were found in 22% of newborns, none of their mothers showed evidence of such a similarly severe degree of VK insufficiency. In addition, the frequency of intakes of VK-rich foods in mothers was not predictive of the functional VK status of their newborns. This lack of correlation between maternal and newborn vitamin K status has been reported previously in a much smaller European study of PIVKA-II measurements in 22 infant-mother pairs [33], but the reasons for this disparity remain unexplained. Certainly, case reports have linked severe maternal dietary VK deficiency to intracranial bleeding in fetal life showing the importance of maintaining adequate maternal intakes of vitamin K during pregnancy [34,35]. Importantly, the lack of clear predictors or correlates of VKD in women or their babies reinforce the need for routine VK administration to newborn babies independent of maternal or newborn factors to help prevent VKDB.

We acknowledge limitations to our study, most importantly the use of a non-standardized dietary questionnaire for determination of VK intake. It should also be noted that our sample size and confidence intervals did not exclude the possibility of a type II error. For example, our estimated adjusted odds of VK insufficiency for each kilogram of birth weight was 1.85 (95% CI 0.15–22.49), suggesting that a significant effect of birth weight on VK insufficiency might have been detected with a larger sample size. To address these shortcomings and further explore these relationships, we intend to conduct a multicenter clinical study to measure VK intakes using a more accurate dietary assessment method (e.g., weighed dietary records) and the prevalence of VK insufficiency in pregnant women and their newborn babies in Sub-Saharan Africa. This additional data will broaden our understanding of the epidemiology of VK intake and deficiency, and help guide recommendations for VK requirements and administration in the region. The study also is characterized by a convenience sampling method in a regional referral Hospital located in an urban area in southwestern Uganda, which might affect generalizability to mothers in rural areas or those without means to reach a referral hospital.

5. Conclusions

Functional VK insufficiency evidenced by raised PIVKA-II is common among mothers and newborn babies in southwestern Uganda. Worryingly, 22% of babies had highly elevated PIVKA-II concentrations that are likely to be associated with an increased risk of bleeding. We found no predictors of newborn VK insufficiency, supporting a strategy of universal administration of newborn vitamin K prophylaxis to prevent VKDB.

Acknowledgments: We would like to thank Mbarara University of Science and Technology, The German Academic Exchange Service and the Centre for Haemostasis and Thrombosis, St. Thomas' Hospital, London for funding different aspects of this study either directly or indirectly. Additionally, we wish to thank Kieran Voong of the Centre for Haemostasis and Thrombosis, St Thomas' Hospital for performing the PIVKA-II assays.

Author Contributions: Santorino Data: Data took the lead in study conception and design, data and sample collection and analysis, led data analysis, wrote the first draft of the manuscript, and participated in editing of subsequent drafts. Unni Wariyar: Wariyar assisted in study conception, editing of manuscript drafts and approved the final version for submission. Martin Shearer: Shearer advised on study methodology, supervised analysis and interpretation of PIVKA-II measurements, edited manuscript drafts and approved the final version for submission. Juliet Mwanga-Amumpaire: Mwanga-Amumpaire helped in supervision and quality control during data collection, edited manuscript drafts and approved the final version for submission. Mark Siedner: Siedner assisted in data analysis, interpretation, edited manuscript drafts and approved the final version for submission. Dominic Harrington: Harrington assisted in sample analysis, edited manuscript drafts and approved the final version for submission.

References

1. Lane, P.A.; Hathaway, W.E. Vitamin K in infancy. *J. Pediatr.* **1985**, *106*, 351–359. [CrossRef]
2. Loughnan, P.M.; McDougall, P.N. Epidemiology of late onset haemorrhagic disease: A pooled data analysis. *J. Paediatr. Child Health* **1993**, *29*, 177–181. [CrossRef] [PubMed]
3. Chuansumrit, A.; Isarangkura, P.; Hathirat, P. Vitamin K deficiency bleeding in Thailand: A 32-year history. *Southeast Asian J. Trop. Med. Public Health* **1998**, *29*, 649–654. [PubMed]
4. Danielsson, N.; Hoa, D.P.; Thang, N.V.; Vos, T.; Loughnan, P.M. Intracranial haemorrhage due to late onset vitamin K deficiency bleeding in Hanoi province, Vietnam. *Arch. Dis. Child Fetal Neonatal Ed.* **2004**, *89*, F546–F550. [CrossRef] [PubMed]

5. Elalfy, M.; Elagouza, I.; Ibrahim, F.; Abdelmessieh, S.; Gadallah, M. Intracranial haemorrhage is linked to late onset vitamin K deficiency in infants aged 2–24 weeks. *Acta Paediatr.* **2014**, *17*, 12598. [CrossRef] [PubMed]
6. Sutherland, J.M.; Glueck, H.I.; Gleser, G. Hemorrhagic disease of the newborn: Breast feeding as a necessary factor in the pathogenesis. *Am. J. Dis. Child* **1967**, *113*, 524–533. [CrossRef] [PubMed]
7. Greer, F.R. Vitamin K status of lactating mothers and their infants. *Acta Paediatr. Suppl.* **1999**, *88*, 95–103. [CrossRef] [PubMed]
8. Lulseged, S. Haemorrhagic disease of the newborn: A review of 127 cases. *Ann. Trop. Paediatr.* **1993**, *13*, 331–336. [PubMed]
9. Shearer, M.J. Vitamin K deficiency bleeding (VKDB) in early infancy. *Blood Rev.* **2009**, *23*, 49–59. [CrossRef] [PubMed]
10. Von Kries, R.; Hanawa, Y. Neonatal vitamin K prophylaxis. Report of Scientific and Standardization Subcommittee on Perinatal Haemostasis. *Thromb. Haemost.* **1993**, *69*, 293–295. [PubMed]
11. Martin-Lopez, J.E.; Carlos-Gil, A.M.; Rodriguez-Lopez, R.; Villegas-Portero, R.; Luque-Romero, L.; Flores-Moreno, S. Prophylactic vitamin K for vitamin K deficiency bleeding of the newborn. *Farm Hosp.* **2011**, *35*, 148–155. [CrossRef] [PubMed]
12. Watson, R.R.; Grimble, G.; Preedy, V.R.; Zibaldi, S. *Nutrition in Infancy*; Springer Science: New York, NY, USA, 2013.
13. Plank, R.M.; Steinmetz, T.; Sokal, D.C.; Shearer, M.J.; Data, S. Vitamin K deficiency bleeding and early infant male circumcision in Africa. *Obstet. Gynecol.* **2013**, *122*, 503–505. [CrossRef] [PubMed]
14. Shearer, M.J.; Fu, X.; Booth, S.L. Vitamin K nutrition, metabolism, and requirements: Current concepts and future research. *Adv. Nutr.* **2012**, *3*, 182–195. [CrossRef] [PubMed]
15. McNinch, A.W.; Tripp, J.H. Haemorrhagic disease of the newborn in the British Isles: Two year prospective study. *BMJ* **1991**, *303*, 1105–1109. [CrossRef] [PubMed]
16. Choo, K.E.; Tan, K.K.; Chuah, S.P.; Ariffin, W.A.; Gururaj, A. Haemorrhagic disease in newborn and older infants: A study in hospitalized children in Kelantan, Malaysia. *Ann. Trop. Paediatr.* **1994**, *14*, 231–237. [PubMed]
17. Van Hasselt, P.M.; Kok, K.; Vorselaars, A.D.; van Vlerken, L.; Nieuwenhuys, E.; de Koning, T.J.; de Vries, R.A.; Houwen, R.H. Vitamin K deficiency bleeding in cholestatic infants with alpha-1-antitrypsin deficiency. *Arch. Dis. Child Fetal Neonatal Ed.* **2009**, *94*, 3. [CrossRef] [PubMed]
18. Miyao, M.; Abiru, H.; Ozeki, M.; Kotani, H.; Tsuruyama, T.; Kobayashi, N.; Omae, T.; Osamura, T.; Tamaki, K. Subdural hemorrhage: A unique case involving secondary vitamin K deficiency bleeding due to biliary atresia. *Forensic Sci. Int.* **2012**, *221*, 16. [CrossRef] [PubMed]
19. Haroon, Y.; Shearer, M.J.; Rahim, S.; Gunn, W.G.; McEnery, G.; Barkhan, P. The content of phylloquinone (vitamin K1) in human milk, cows' milk and infant formula foods determined by high-performance liquid chromatography. *J. Nutr.* **1982**, *112*, 1105–1117. [PubMed]
20. Von Kries, R.; Shearer, M.; McCarthy, P.T.; Haug, M.; Harzer, G.; Gobel, U. Vitamin K1 content of maternal milk: Influence of the stage of lactation, lipid composition, and vitamin K1 supplements given to the mother. *Pediatr. Res.* **1987**, *22*, 513–517. [CrossRef] [PubMed]
21. Greer, F.R.; Marshall, S.; Cherry, J.; Suttie, J.W. Vitamin K status of lactating mothers, human milk, and breast-feeding infants. *Pediatrics* **1991**, *88*, 751–756. [PubMed]
22. Chuansumrit, A.; Plueksacheeva, T.; Hanpinitsak, S.; Sangwarn, S.; Chatvutinun, S.; Suthutvoravut, U.; Herabutya, Y.; Shearer, M.J. Prevalence of subclinical vitamin K deficiency in Thai newborns: Relationship to maternal phylloquinone intakes and delivery risk. *Arch. Dis. Child Fetal Neonatal Ed.* **2010**, *95*, 11. [CrossRef] [PubMed]
23. Suttie, J.W. Vitamin K and human nutrition. *J. Am. Diet. Assoc.* **1992**, *92*, 585–590. [PubMed]
24. Clarke, P.; Mitchell, S.J.; Sundaram, S.; Sharma, V.; Wynn, R.; Shearer, M.J. Vitamin K status of preterm infants with a prolonged prothrombin time. *Acta Paediatr.* **2005**, *94*, 1822–1824. [CrossRef] [PubMed]
25. Booth, S.L.; Centurelli, M.A. Vitamin K: A practical guide to the dietary management of patients on warfarin. *Nutr. Rev.* **1999**, *57*, 288–296. [CrossRef] [PubMed]
26. Mager, D.R.; McGee, P.L.; Furuya, K.N.; Roberts, E.A. Prevalence of vitamin K deficiency in children with mild to moderate chronic liver disease. *J. Pediatr. Gastroenterol. Nutr.* **2006**, *42*, 71–76. [CrossRef] [PubMed]
27. Kowalkowska, J.; Slowinska, M.A.; Slowinski, D.; Dlugosz, A.; Niedzwiedzka, E.; Wadolowska, L. Comparison of a full food-frequency questionnaire with the three-day unweighted food records in young

Polish adult women: Implications for dietary assessment. *Nutrients* **2013**, *5*, 2747–2776. [CrossRef] [PubMed]

28. Belle, M.; Brebant, R.; Guinet, R.; Leclercq, M. Production of a new monoclonal antibody specific to human des-gamma-carboxyprothrombin in the presence of calcium ions. Application to the development of a sensitive ELISA-test. *J. Immunoass.* **1995**, *16*, 213–229. [CrossRef]
29. Clarke, P.; Mitchell, S.J.; Wynn, R.; Sundaram, S.; Speed, V.; Gardener, E.; Roeves, D.; Shearer, M.J. Vitamin K prophylaxis for preterm infants: A randomized, controlled trial of 3 regimens. *Pediatrics* **2006**, *118*, 13. [CrossRef] [PubMed]
30. O'Shaughnessy, D.; Allen, C.; Woodcock, T.; Pearce, K.; Harvey, J.; Shearer, M. Echis time, under-carboxylated prothrombin and vitamin K status in intensive care patients. *Clin. Lab. Haematol.* **2003**, *25*, 397–404. [CrossRef] [PubMed]
31. Salonvaara, M.; Riikonen, P.; Kekomaki, R.; Vahtera, E.; Mahlamaki, E.; Kiekara, O.; Heinonen, K. Intraventricular haemorrhage in very-low-birthweight preterm infants: Association with low prothrombin activity at birth. *Acta Paediatr.* **2005**, *94*, 807–811. [CrossRef] [PubMed]
32. Hosmer, D.W.; Lemeshow, S. *Applied Logistic Regression*; Wiley: New York, NY, USA, 1989.
33. Von Kries, R.; Shearer, M.J.; Widdershoven, J.; Motohara, K.; Umbach, G.; Gobel, U. Des-gamma-carboxyprothrombin (PIVKA II) and plasma vitamin K1 in newborns and their mothers. *Thromb. Haemost.* **1992**, *68*, 383–387. [PubMed]
34. Kawamura, Y.; Kawamata, K.; Shinya, M.; Higashi, M.; Niiro, M.; Douchi, T. Vitamin K deficiency in hyperemesis gravidarum as a potential cause of fetal intracranial hemorrhage and hydrocephalus. *Prenat. Diagn.* **2008**, *28*, 59–61. [CrossRef] [PubMed]
35. Eventov-Friedman, S.; Klinger, G.; Shinwell, E.S. Third trimester fetal intracranial hemorrhage owing to vitamin K deficiency associated with hyperemesis gravidarum. *J. Pediatr. Hematol. Oncol.* **2009**, *31*, 985–988. [CrossRef] [PubMed]

15

Concepts and Controversies in Evaluating Vitamin K Status in Population-Based Studies

M. Kyla Shea and Sarah L. Booth *

USDA Human Nutrition Research Center on Aging, Tufts University, Boston, MA 02111, USA
* Correspondence: sarah.booth@tufts.edu

Abstract: A better understanding of vitamin K's role in health and disease requires the assessment of vitamin K nutritional status in population and clinical studies. This is primarily accomplished using dietary questionnaires and/or biomarkers. Because food composition databases in the US are most complete for phylloquinone (vitamin K1, the primary form in Western diets), emphasis has been on phylloquinone intakes and associations with chronic diseases. There is growing interest in menaquinone (vitamin K2) intakes for which the food composition databases need to be expanded. Phylloquinone is commonly measured in circulation, has robust quality control schemes and changes in response to phylloquinone intake. Conversely, menaquinones are generally not detected in circulation unless large quantities are consumed. The undercarboxylated fractions of three vitamin K-dependent proteins are measurable in circulation, change in response to vitamin K supplementation and are modestly correlated. Since different vitamin K dependent proteins are implicated in different diseases the appropriate vitamin K-dependent protein biomarker depends on the outcome under study. In contrast to other nutrients, there is no single biomarker that is considered a gold-standard measure of vitamin K status. Most studies have limited volume of specimens. Strategic decisions, guided by the research question, need to be made when deciding on choice of biomarkers.

Keywords: vitamin K; epidemiology; vitamin K intake; biomarkers; review

---

1. Introduction

Vitamin K is a class of structurally-similar compounds, all of which function as an enzymatic co-factor in the γ-carboxylation of vitamin K-dependent proteins [1]. While the best known vitamin K-dependent proteins are clotting proteins, vitamin K-dependent proteins are also present in many extra-hepatic tissues that have been implicated in many chronic diseases [2]. As new roles for vitamin K in health and disease emerge, so has interest in measuring vitamin K status in population-based studies. The purpose of this review is to evaluate the methods currently available to assess vitamin K status in human studies.

2. Vitamin K Intakes

A seemingly straightforward approach to estimate nutrient status is to estimate how much of the nutrient is being consumed [3]. Dietary forms of vitamin K fall into two general categories: Phylloquinone (vitamin K1) and menaquinones (collectively referred to as vitamin K2), which are comprised of at least 10 compounds (menaquinone-4 to menaquinone-13) that differ from phylloquinone in the length and saturation of their side-chain (Figure 1).

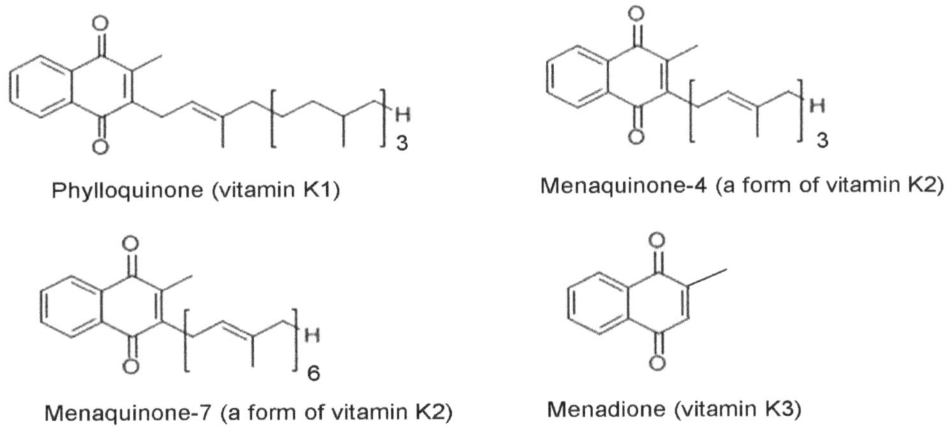

Figure 1. Forms of vitamin K.

Phylloquinone is plant-based, and concentrated in green leafy vegetables and certain plant oils (1). Longer chain menaquinones (menaquinone-7–menaquinone-13) have a bacterial origin, and are primarily concentrated in animal meats and fermented foods. Menaquinone-4, which is the most similar structurally to phylloquinone, is unique among the menaquinones in that it is not produced by bacteria, but instead is either formed from phylloquinone or a pro-vitamin menadione form used in animal feed. In the human diet, menaquinone-4 is concentrated in animal meats and dairy products.

The United States Institute of Medicine's Adequate Intake of vitamin K is set at 90 and 120 μg/day for adult women and men respectively [4]. These are based on median intakes reported in NHANES III [4]. Globally, dietary recommendations for vitamin K vary from 50 to 120 μg/day [5]. These recommendations do not differentiate phylloquinone intake from menaquinone intake. However, at the time the recommendations were set, the food composition databases from which they are based only contained the phylloquinone content of foods. Hence, the current vitamin K recommendations are based on phylloquinone, which is the primary form in Western diets [6–10]. As reviewed elsewhere, there is insufficient scientific knowledge at this time to determine an independent dietary recommendation for menaquinones [11].

Assessment of dietary intakes of vitamin K in population studies has relied on the use of the food frequency questionnaire (FFQ). There are many types of dietary questionnaires, which have been reviewed extensively [12,13]. In epidemiological studies, the FFQ is most commonly used because it is efficient in terms of cost and time, and imposes minimal burden on the study participant [3]. The FFQ appears to be suitable to rank individuals in terms of micronutrient intakes, but its ability to estimate absolute intakes of single nutrients is limited. The FFQ (similar to most diet questionnaires) is subjective and relies on individuals' recall ability and perceptions, which can bias the estimates of nutrient intake [14]. Nonetheless, the FFQ has been used to estimate phylloquinone and/or menaquinone intakes as measures of vitamin K status in several studies [9,14–18].

The findings of population-based studies that have related phylloquinone intake to chronic disease are inconsistent (Table 1).

Table 1. Population-based studies of vitamin K intake and disease.

Population	Region/Cohort	Vitamin K Form and Reported Intakes	Outcome	Results	References
1836 men and 2971 women, >55 years	Rotterdam, The Netherlands (Rotterdam Study)	PK: 257 ± 116 µg/day (men); 244 µg/day (women); MK (total): 31 ± 19 µg/day (men); 33 ± 16 µg/day (women)	CHD	Highest MK tertile had lower CHD risk; PK intake not associated with CHD	[9]
807 army personnel, 39–45 years, 82% male	United States	PK: 115 ± 79 µg/day	CAC	No association	[19]
564 post-menopausal women	Utrecht, The Netherlands (PROSPECT-EPIC)	PK: 217 ± 92 µg/day; MK: 32 ± 12 µg/day	CAC	Highest MK quartile (34 ± 3 µg/day) had lower prevalence CAC; PK intake not associated with CAC prevalence	[15]
16,057 post-menopausal women	Utrecht, The Netherlands (PROSPECT-EPIC)	PK: 212 ± 100 µg/day; MK: 29 ± 13 µg/day	CHD	Higher MK intake associated with lower CHD risk; PK intake not associated with CHD	[17]
72,874 women, 38–65 years	United States (Nurse's Health Study)	PK: 184 ± 106 µg/day	CHD	PK intake not associated with CHD once adjusted for healthy lifestyle characteristics	[20]
40,087 men, 40–75 years	United States (Physicians Health Study)	PK: 165 (67–383) µg/day (median, 5%–95%ile)	CHD	PK intake not associated with CHD once adjusted for healthy lifestyle characteristics	[8]
1112 men and 1479 women, 58 ± 9 years	Framingham, MA, United States (Framingham Offspring)	PK: 153 ± 115 µg/day (men); 171 ± 103 µg/day (women)	BMD	Higher PK intake associated with higher BMD in women, but not in men	[21]
898 women, 45–54 years	Scotland	PK: 109 ± 54 µg/day	BMD	Higher PK intake associated with higher BMD and less bone resorption	[22]
335 men and 553 women, 75 ± 5 years	Framingham, MA, United States (Framingham Heart Study)	PK: 143 ± 97 µg/day (men); 163 ± 115 µg/day (women)	BMD and hip fracture	Higher PK intake associated with lower fracture risk; not associated with BMD	[16]
72,327 women aged 38–63 years	United States (Nurse's Health Study)	PK: 169 (41–604) µg/day (median, 1%–99%ile)	Hip fracture	Higher quintiles PK intake (⩾109 µg/day) associated with lower hip fracture risk (RR: 0.70; 95% CI: 0.53, 0.93)	[23]
1605 men, 1339 women	Hong Kong	PK: 254 (157–362) µg/day (median (range), men); 239 (162–408) µg/day (median (range), women)	Hip and non-vertebral fracture	PK intake not associated with any fracture outcome	[24]
1800 women, peri-menopausal, 43–58 years	Denmark (Danish Osteoporosis Prevention Study)	PK: baseline: 67 (45–105) µg/day (median, 25%–75%iles); 5 year followup: 60 (37–99) µg/day (median, 25%–75%iles	BMD and fracture	PK intake not associated with BMD or fracture	[25]
1238 men, 1569 women, 71–75 years	Norway (Hordaland)	PK: 69 (67) µg/day (median (IQR), women); 75(62) µg/day (men); MK: 10 (7) µg/day (women); 12 (8) µg/day (men)	Hip fracture	Higher PK intake associated with lower fracture risk; no association between MK intake and fracture	[26]

Table 1. *Cont.*

Population	Region/Cohort	Vitamin K Form and Reported Intakes	Outcome	Results	References
625 men and women, 40–80 years	The Netherlands (PROSPECT-EPIC)	PK: 210 ± 127 µg/day; MK: 31 ± 13 µg/day	Metabolic Syndrome	Higher MK intake associated with lower prevalence MetSyn; PK intake not associated with MetSyn	[27]
510 men and women, diabetic and/or at risk for CHD, 67 ± 6 years	Spain (PREDIMED)	PK: 398 ± 201 µg/day	Insulin resistance and inflammation	Higher PK intake associated with improvements in IR and inflammation	[28]
662 men and women, 62 ± 10 years	United States (MESA)	PK: 93 ± 107 µg/day	Inflammation	No association between PK intake and inflammation	[29]
1247 men and 1472 women, 26–81 years	Framingham, MA, United States (Framingham Offspring)	PK: 139 (10 to 1975) µg/day (median (range))	Insulin resistance, sensitivity, glycemic status	Higher PK intake associated with better insulin sensitivity and glucose tolerance	[30]
11,319 men 40–64 years	Europe (EPIC-Heidelberg)	PK: 94 (71–124) µg/day (median (25%–75%ile); MK4-14: 35 (25–76) µg/day (median (25%–75%ile)	Prostate cancer	MK intake inversely associated with prostate cancer (p-trend = 0.06) and advanced prostate cancer (p-trend = 0.02)	[18]
24,340 men and women, 40–64 years	Europe (EPIC-Heidelberg)	PK 35 µg/day (median, men); MK 35 µg/day (median, men); PK 32 µg/day (median, women); MK 32 µg/day (median, women)	Cancer—lung, colorectal, breast, prostate	MK intake inversely associated with cancer incidence in men and mortality in men and women	[31]
7216 men and women, diabetic and/or at risk for CHD, 67 ± 6 years	Spain (PREDIMED)	PK: mean 356 µg/day; MK: mean 36 µg/day	Cardiovascular, cancer, all-cause mortality	Higher PK intake associated with lower cancer and all-cause mortality; MK intake not associated with mortality	[32]

Some found higher phylloquinone intake to be associated with higher BMD and lower fracture risk [16,26], lower cardiovascular disease (CVD) risk [8,20], improved insulin sensitivity [28,30], and lower mortality risk [32,33]. Others found phylloquinone intake was not associated with BMD [21,25], fracture [24], metabolic syndrome [27], or CVD [15,17,19,34]. The use of phylloquinone intake as the sole indicator of vitamin K status needs to be interpreted cautiously because phylloquinone intake also reflects healthy diets and lifestyles, given its concentration in green leafy vegetables and plant oils [8,20,35]. This residual confounding may not be completely eliminated when adjustments for healthy diet and/or lifestyle characteristics are made. When phylloquinone intake was estimated using the FFQ and a 5-day diet record, FFQ estimates were consistently higher, which may be due to over-reporting of vegetables [36,37]. In addition, the ability of the FFQ to accurately capture phylloquinone intakes greater than 200 µg/day is of concern. In the Framingham Offspring Study, which used the Harvard FFQ to estimate phylloquinone intake, plasma phylloquinone positively correlated with intakes up to 200 µg/d, above which the association between plasma phylloquinone and phylloquinone intake plateaued [38]. A similar pattern was observed in a separate cohort of older community-dwelling men and women in the U.S. participating in a phylloquinone supplementation trial when analyzed at baseline [39] (Figure 2).

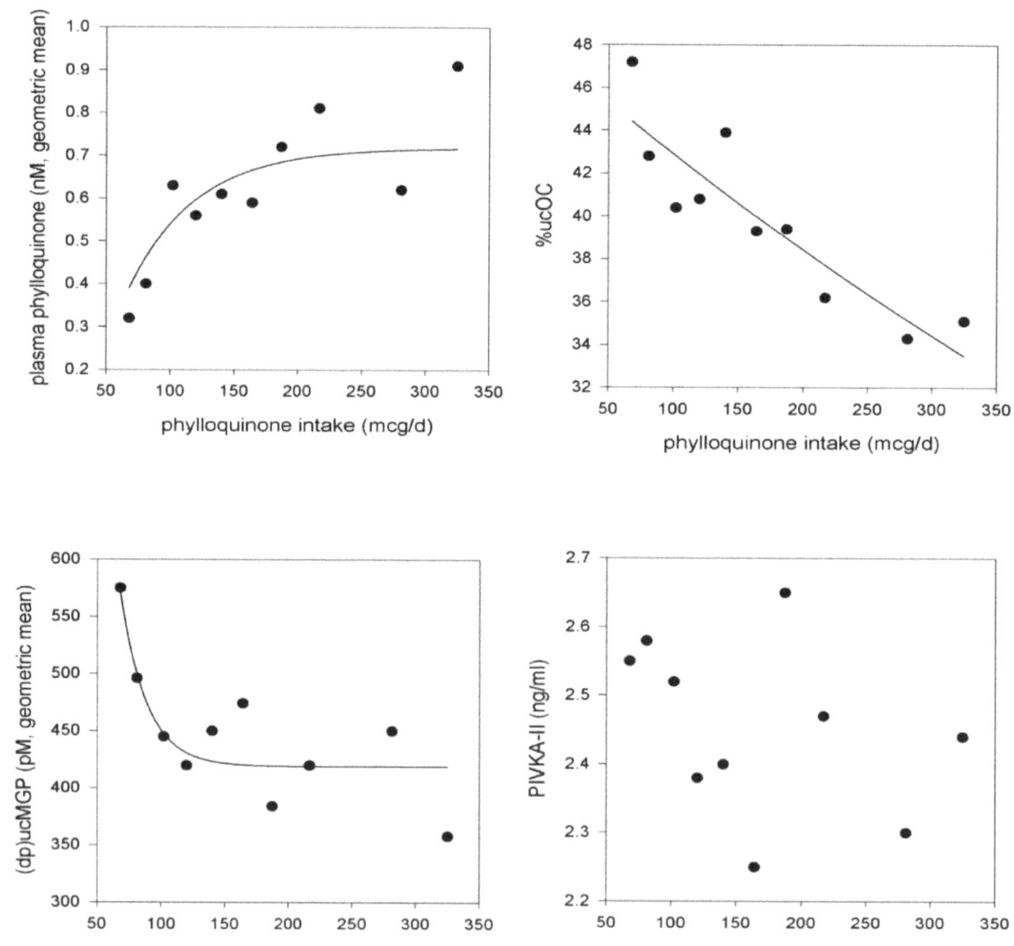

Figure 2. Association between food frequency questionnaire (FFQ)-estimated phylloquinone intake and circulating biomarkers of vitamin K status (at baseline) in community-dwelling older men and women participating in a phylloquinone supplementation trial [39,40]. The geometric mean of each biomarker is plotted at the median intake within each decile category. Adjustment was made for age, sex, BMI, energy intake (kcals/day), season, and triglycerides (for plasma phylloquinone).

While this plateau could reflect a saturation at the intakes >200 μg/day, circulating phylloquinone concentrations have been shown to increase to >2.0 nM in response to 500 μg/day and to >20 nM in response to 5000 μg/day of phylloquinone supplementation [39,41]. Therefore, it appears the FFQ may not be an appropriate method to estimate intakes in populations where phylloquinone intakes typically exceed 200 μg/day and results of studies doing so need to be interpreted accordingly.

Higher intakes of menaquinones were reported to be associated with less subclinical and clinical CVD, metabolic syndrome and some forms of cancer [9,15,17,18,27,31]. These associations may not be prone to confounding by a healthy diet because menaquinones are not found in foods that are typically characteristic of a healthy diet. However, the difference in total menaquinone intake between the highest and lowest categories of intake has been reported to be as narrow as ~20 μg/day [9,15,17,27]. The potential protective influence of a difference of 20 μg/day of total menaquinone is uncertain, and merits further research. It is also important to consider the food sources of menaquinones. Some cheeses rich in long-chain menaquinones are consumed in European countries more than in the US [42,43], and cheese intake itself has been associated with lower risk for type 2 diabetes, CVD, and mortality [44–47]. It is plausible menaquinone intake tracks intake of other nutrients and/or fatty acids found in cheese that have also been associated with cardiovascular disease [44,48].

The contribution of menaquinones, both in terms of forms and amounts to overall vitamin K intake varies regionally. In Western diets the relative contribution of menaquinones is thought to be much less than that of phylloquinone. However, food composition databases used in most countries do not quantify menaquinones specifically [11,49]. The most recent release of the USDA National Nutrient Database contains menaquinone-4 contents of a limited number of dairy and meat products [49]. Databases used in the Netherlands quantify individual menaquinones (menaquinone 4–10) in a limited number of foods, but are being updated [11,50]. Reported intakes of long-chain menaquinones are high in eastern Japan because *natto*, a bacterially-fermented soy food rich in menaquinone-7, is commonly eaten in that region [51]. Some have also suggested consumption of bacterially-fermented cheese, which is rich in long-chain menaquinones, is higher in the Netherlands, which may account for the long-chain menaquinone content of their diets [11]. However, a comparison of dairy intakes across EPIC study locations does not confirm this assertion [52].

Some have proposed dietary menaquinones to be more beneficial to cardiovascular and metabolic health than dietary phylloquinone [9,15,17,27]. However, the relative validity of the FFQ used in these studies was better for menaquinone than for phylloquinone [9,15,17,27]. Validity was assessed in reference to twelve 24-h recalls, but menaquinone intake validity has not yet been assessed in reference to any biomarkers. In contrast, the validity of the FFQ used to assess phylloquinone intake in these studies was poor, as acknowledged by the investigators, and the reported phylloquinone intakes were double what the current US recommendations are (means ranged from 212 to 257 μg/day) [9,17,27]. This may have blunted any ability to detect associations with dietary phylloquinone given the observed plateau effect. Furthermore, adjustment for intakes of cheese and/or other nutritional components of cheese associated with reduced CVD risk could be important but has not yet been done. Given the limitations inherent to using self-reported methods to estimate dietary intakes [3,53,54], population-based studies relating vitamin K status to chronic disease could be strengthened by the addition of vitamin K status biomarkers to dietary intake estimates.

3. Vitamin K Status Biomarkers

Nutritional biomarkers are biochemical measures measured in blood, urine, feces, adipose tissue or other tissues that reflect nutrient status [55]. Nutritional biomarkers are not limited by incomplete food composition databases, and are independent of recall, interviewer and social acceptance biases [55]. In contrast to dietary questionnaires which only estimate intake and generally do not account for relative bioavailability, biomarkers reflect intake, absorption and metabolism [55]. However, a thorough understanding of the biomarker's underlying biology is required in order to consider all the physiological factors that may influence its relationship to the intake of a specific nutrient. For a comprehensive review of vitamin K bioavailability, refer to Shearer *et al.* [5]. Biomarkers can be affected by health status, including the disease outcome of interest, which can lead to misclassification and erroneous conclusions in studies that aim to identify nutritional risk factors for disease. Temporal variability needs to be considered, since many biomarkers can vary post-prandially and/or diurnally [3]. Biomarkers represent nutrient status at one point in time, which may limit extrapolation to long-term status unless repeated measures are made. In addition, biomarker analyses require rigorous laboratory standardization and quality control procedures to reduce measurement error and misclassification [56]. Nonetheless biomarkers can provide valuable estimates of nutrient status in population studies when the studies' results are interpreted in the context of the strengths and limitations of the biomarker measured.

3.1. Circulating Vitamin K

Phylloquinone is the primary circulating form of vitamin K, and has been successfully measured to rank individuals' vitamin K status in population-based and clinic-based studies worldwide (Table 2). These studies also demonstrate the large variability in circulating vitamin K in most populations.

Table 2. Reported circulating concentrations of vitamin K in population- or clinic-based individuals not taking vitamin K supplements (Data are mean ± SD, unless otherwise indicated.).

Participants	Region	Phylloquinone	Menaquinone	Fasted	References
Post-menopausal women: generally healthy, 52–93 years (*n* = 23)	Japan	0.22 ± 0.32 nM [d]	MK4: 0.02 ± 0.001 nM [d]; MK7: 0.54 ± 1.00 nM [d]	not specified	[57]
with hip or vertebral fracture history, 66–93 years (*n* = 51)	Japan	0.21 ± 0.18 nM [d]	MK4: non-detectable [d]; MK7: 0.66 ± 1.00 nM [d]	not specified	
Pre-menopausal women generally healthy, 30–49 years (*n* = 52)	Nagano, Japan	0.68 ± 0.45 nM [d]	MK4: 0.03 ± 0.06 nM [d]; MK7: 2.23 ± 3.12 nM [d]	yes	[58]
Post-menopausal women generally healthy, 50–80 years (*n* = 344)		0.70 ± 0.53 nM [d]	MK4: 0.05 ± 0.08 nM [d]; MK7: 3.04 ± 4.32 nM [d]	yes	
Post-menopausal women: normal BMD, 54 ± 0.8 years (*n* = 52)	Osaka, Japan	0.29 ± 0.03 nM [d]	MK7: 2.44 ± 0.15 nM [d]	yes	[59]
low BMD, 55 ± 1.3 years, (*n* = 19)		0.18 ± 0.02 nM [d]	MK7 1.67 ± 0.07 nM [d]	yes	
Post-menopausal women	Tokyo, Japan (*n* = 49; 50–84 years)	0.33 ± 0.21 nM [d]	MK7: 2.37 ± 2.75 nM [d]	yes	[51]
	Hiroshima, Japan (*n* = 25; 51–66 years)	0.33 ± 0.26 nM [d]	MK7: 0.55 ± 0.83 nM [d]	yes	
	London & Nottingham, United Kingdom (*n* = 31; 48–84 years)	0.23 ± 0.24 nM [d]	MK7: 0.17 ± 0.09 nM [d]	yes	
Older men, nursing home residents: normal BMD, 74 ± 10 years (*n* = 15)	Japan	0.85 ± 0.73 nM	MK7: 1.44 ± 0.85 nM		[60]
low BMD, 74 ± 11 years (*n* = 12)		0.60 ± 0.73 nM	MK7: 0.71 ± 0.35 nM		
Free living older adults: men, ⩾65 years (*n* = 385)	Great Britain	0.34 (0.06–1.84) nM [a]	NR	yes	[61]
women, ⩾65 years (*n* = 493)		0.37(0.06–2.06) nM [a]	NR		
Institution-living older adults; men, ⩾65 years (*n* = 60)		0.26 (0.06–1.73) nM [a]	NR		
women, ⩾65 years (*n* = 165)		0.23 (0.06–0.89) nM [a]	NR		
Free living older adults: men, 19–64 years (*n* = 530)	Great Britain	1.13 (0.20–8.80) nM [a]	NR	yes	[62]
women, 19–64 years (*n* = 624)		0.81 (0.02–8.71) nM [a]	NR		
Free living older adults: men, 65–75 years (*n* = 86)	Shenyang, China	1.88 ± 2.19 nM	NR	yes	[63]
women, 65–75 years (*n* = 92)		2.48 ± 2.88 nM	NR		
men, 60–83 years (*n* = 67)	Cambridge, United Kingdom	0.66 ± 0.75 nM	NR		
women, 60–83 years (*n* = 67)		0.73 ± 0.84 nM	NR		

Table 2. *Cont.*

Participants	Region	Phylloquinone	Menaquinone	Fasted	References
Free-living women: Pre-menopausal, 31 ± 11 years (n = 11)	Shenyang, China	0.28 ± 0.04 nM [b,d]	NR	yes	[64]
Post-menopausal, 68 ± 3 years (n = 23)		0.45 ± 0.06 nM [b,d]	NR		
Pre-menopausal, 36 ± 11 years (n = 11)	Cambridge, United Kingdom	0.14 ± 0.02 nM [b,d]	NR		
Post-menopausal, 67 ± 7 years (n = 31)		0.14 ± 0.01 nM [b,d]	NR		
Pre-menopausal, 37 ± 4 years (n = 11)	Keneba, Gambia	0.27 ± 0.05 nM [b,d]	NR		
Post-menopausal, 68 ± 8 years (n = 50)		0.16 ± 0.02 nM [b,d]	NR		
Post-menopausal women, 57 ± 5 years (n = 508)	Utrecht, The Netherlands	18% non-detectable; among detectable: 1.08 ± 1.03 nM	NR	no	[65]
Hemodialysis patients, 64 ± 14 years, 63% male (n = 387)	Italy	0.44 ± 0.44 nM [d]	MK4: 0.30 ± 0.33 nM [d]; MK5: 0.45 ± 0.35 nM [d]; MK6: 0.28 ± 0.45 nM [d]; MK7: 0.52 ± 0.45 nM [d]	yes	[66]
Healthy Controls, 57 ± 4 years, 70% male (n = 62)		0.61 ± 0.45 nM [d]	MK4: 0.41 ± 0.38 nM [d]; MK5: 0.58 ± 0.50 nM [d]; MK6: 0.50 ± 0.51 nM [d]; MK7: 0.88 ± 0.62 nM [d]		
Patients with stage 3–5 CKD, 61 ± 14 years, 61% male (n = 162)	Kingston Ontario, Canada	2.1 ± 2.4 nM	NR		[67]
Patients with ESKD, 64 ± 15 years, 66% male (n = 44)	Kingston Ontario, Canada	1.25 ± 1.17 nM	NR		[68]
Free-living men and women: Men, 59 ± 9 years (n = 741)	Framingham, MA, United States	1.54 ± 2.00 nM	NR	yes	[69]
Premenopausal women, 47 ± 7 years, (n = 170)		1.05 ± 1.04 nM			
Postmenopausal women: Current estrogen use, 58 ± 7 years (n = 269)		1.46 ± 1.25 nM			
No current estrogen use, 63 ± 8 years (n = 424)		1.41 ± 1.54 nM			
Free-living adults: White, 62 ± 10 years, 45% male (n = 262)	6 communities across United States	1.3 ± 0.1 nM	NR	yes	[70]
African American, 63 ± 10 years, 47% male (n = 180)		1.5 ± 0.1 nM			
Hispanic, 60 ± 10 years, 51% male (n = 169)		1.2 ± 0.1 nM			
Chinese-American, 62 ± 10 years, 45% male (n = 93)		2.4 ± 0.2 nM			
Older free-living adults, 70–79 years, 38% male, 46% black (n = 791)	Memphis TN and Pittsburgh PA, United States	0.8 ± 0.9 nM [c]	NR		[71]

[a] geometric mean (inner 95% range); [b] geometric mean ± SEM; [c] median ± interquartile range; [d] reported as ng/mL, converted to nmol/L by multiplying ng/mL by 2.22; NR: Not reported.

However, the number of studies that have evaluated circulating phylloquinone in relation to chronic disease is relatively few compared to the studies that assessed dietary vitamin K intake. Higher circulating phylloquinone has been associated with less bone loss and fracture [66,69,72], less osteoarthritis [71,73,74], and less coronary calcium progression is some [75] but not all [65] cohorts. Circulating concentrations of phylloquinone are 50 to 25,000 times lower than other fat-soluble nutrients, which has historically presented technological challenges in its measurement [76]. Sensitive HPLC and mass spectrometry assays have been developed to measure phylloquinone in blood but there is considerable variability in the separation techniques and assay standards used, some of which leads to erroneous reporting. However external quality assurance programs are now available to standardize assays used from one laboratory to the next and monitor inter-laboratory variation, and any study measuring circulating phylloquinone should be an active member of these programs to verify accuracy of the measures reported [76].

Phylloquinone is transported on triglyceride-rich lipoproteins in circulation, with smaller fractions carried on HDL and LDL cholesterol [77] (Figure 3).

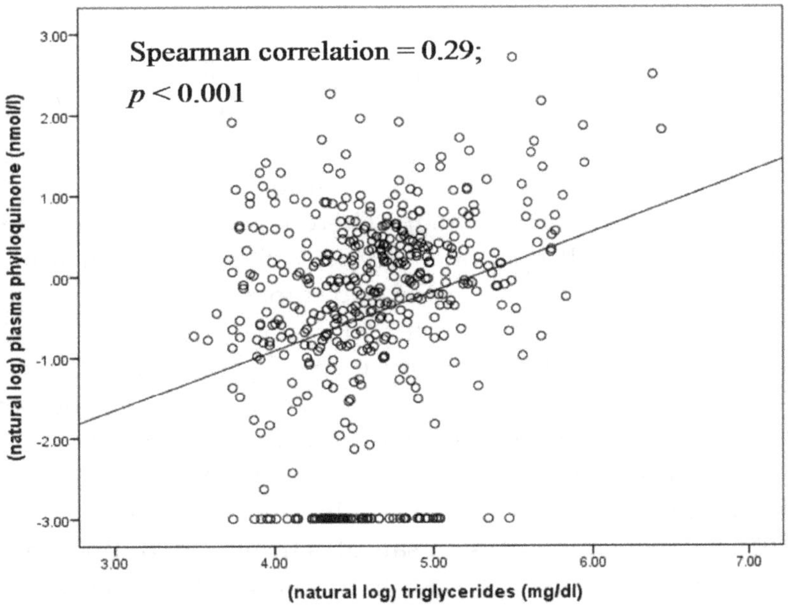

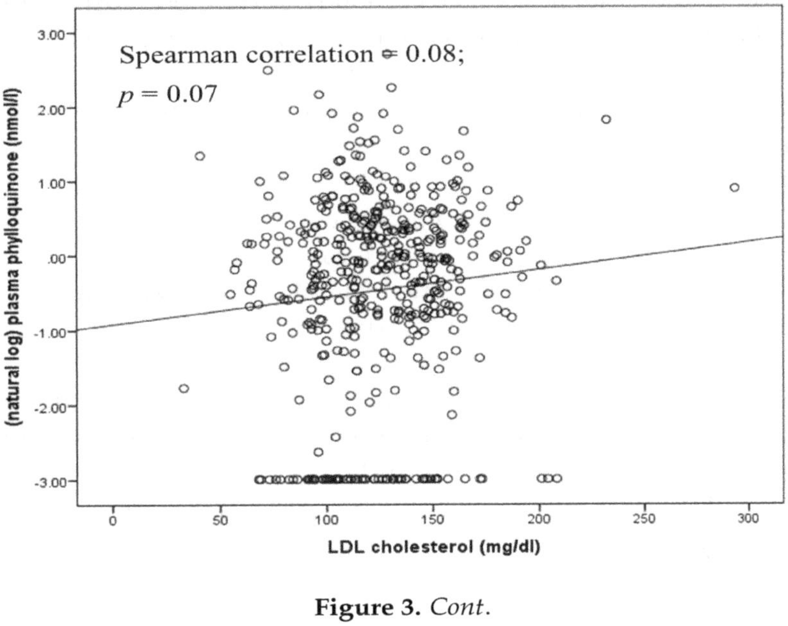

Figure 3. *Cont.*

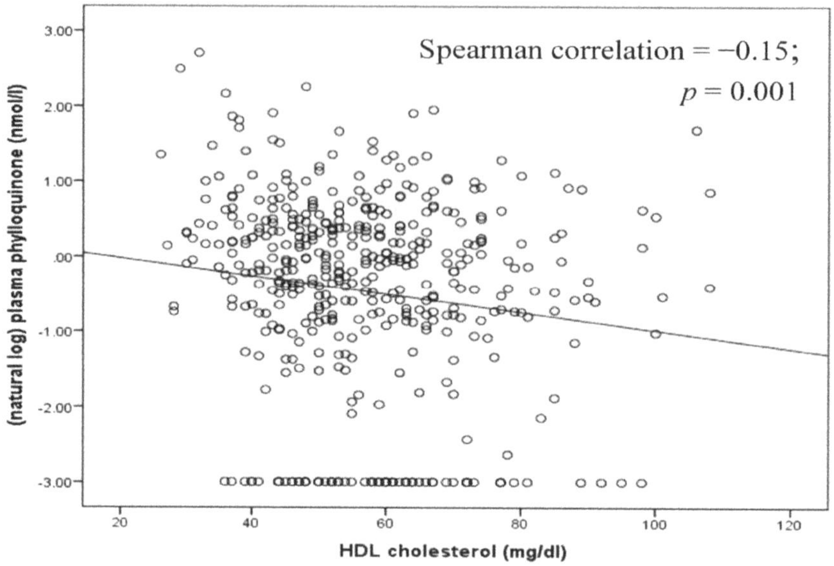

Figure 3. Correlation between circulating phylloquinone and lipids at baseline in community-dwelling older men and women participating in a phylloquinone supplementation trial [39,40].

Circulating phylloquinone responds to changes in dietary phylloquinone intake [78,79], and concentrations peak 6–10 h post-prandially [80]. There is also some indication that the response of circulating concentrations of phylloquinone vary with the type of meal pattern [81]. Given the physiology underlying phylloquinone absorption and transport, circulating phylloquinone should be measured in fasting samples and corrected for triglycerides to better reflect overall nutritional status. In population-based studies, adjustment for triglycerides strengthened associations between circulating phylloquinone and bone mineral density [69] and coronary calcium progression [75]. In studies that have not adjusted plasma phylloquinone for triglycerides, the data are more difficult to interpret. For example, in a sub-study of the Dutch Prospect cohort, post-menopausal women with the higher plasma phylloquinone had a higher prevalence of coronary calcium (CAC, an indicator of subclinical CVD) [65]. However, the plasma samples from which phylloquinone was measured were not obtained in a fasted state and triglyceride measures were unavailable. The investigators adjusted for cholesterol instead, but cholesterol is weakly correlated with circulating phylloquinone (Figure 3), and does not reflect its absorption. Since hypertriglyceridemia is a risk factor for CVD [82], it is plausible the phylloquinone tracked elevated triglycerides.

There is currently no established threshold of plasma/serum phylloquinone that indicates insufficiency or deficiency. When the Adequate Intake is met in controlled feeding studies, circulating phylloquinone concentrations approximate 1.0 nM [83]. However, it is not currently known if the Adequate Intake is sufficient to meet all physiological needs, especially health outcomes not related to coagulation [2]. As a corollary, it is not known if 1.0 nM of circulating phylloquinone is similarly sufficient. As such, low circulating phylloquinone has not been consistently defined in the scientific literature [71–75], making it difficult to clarify a threshold for insufficiency. Additional research in this area is needed.

Circulating phylloquinone appears to be influenced by more than dietary vitamin K intake and triglycerides [38,70,84], and much of the variability remains to be explained. In a multi-ethnic US cohort, race-ethnicity was identified as a significant predictor of serum phylloquinone with Chinese-Americans and African-Americans having higher concentrations than Caucasians and Hispanics [70]. In a primarily Caucasian cohort, plasma phylloquinone was not found to be significantly heritable [84]. However, a subsequent GWAS analysis of Caucasian participants in three US cohorts identified multiple candidate genes as potential determinants of circulating phylloquinone [85]. Since none of the variants achieved significance at the GWA level of $<1 \times 10^8$ larger studies are needed to confirm these findings, and more diverse cohorts are needed to expand these findings to include other race/ethnic groups. This requires more studies that measure plasma/serum phylloquinone, which to date has not been a common biomarker in large-scale population studies.

Studies reporting circulating menaquinones as a biomarker of vitamin K status are more limited (Table 2) because menaquinones are generally not detected in circulation unless supplements are taken or large quantities of menaquinone-rich foods are consumed. In women from Nagano Japan, circulating menaquinone-7 is reported to exceed 10 nM, which likely reflects natto consumption in that region. In these same women, the average concentration of menaquinone-4 was 0.2 nM, although >50% had non-detectable concentrations despite use of highly sensitive instrumentation [58]. In two studies using less sensitive HPLC methods with post-column reduction and fluorescence detection (lower limit of detection ~0.1 ng/mL), menaquinone-4 was detected in only 10% of 105 postmenopausal women from Japan or the United Kingdom [51] and in none of 440 postmenopausal Canadian women with osteopenia, half of whom were consuming daily doses of 5 mg of phylloquinone [41] (Booth *et al.*, unpublished data). These observational data are also consistent with a recent intervention study that showed single or consecutive oral administration of menaquinone-4 failed to increase serum menaquinone-4 concentrations [86]. At odds to the collective observations of others, in a study conducted in Italy, Fusaro *et al.* reported relatively high plasma concentrations of menaquinones 4–7 in chronic kidney disease patients and healthy controls not taking supplements, with chronic kidney disease patients having lower average menaquinone and phylloquinone concentrations [66]. In this same study, low concentrations of menaquinone-4 and menaquinone-7 were associated with significantly higher odds of aortic artery and iliac artery calcification respectively, and low menaquinone-5 concentrations were found to be associated with lower odds for abdominal aorta calcification. The concentration of menaquinone-5 was reported to be relatively equal to that of circulating phylloquinone, even though menaquinone-5 is not found in many foods and is rarely synthesized by bacteria [49]. No other study has reported such high concentrations of circulating menaquinone concentrations among individuals not taking menaquinone supplements and there are no other studies that have reported detectable menaquinone-5 concentrations in circulation despite concerted efforts to find circulating menaquinones using very sensitive mass spectrometry instrumentation [87]. Given the contradictory associations of menaquinone-5 with aortic calcification does not fit our current understanding of the role of vitamin K-dependent proteins in calcification, there are sufficient doubts regarding the validity of these findings. Until the findings of the study by Fusaro *et al.* [66] are independently replicated, use of circulating menaquinones as a measure of vitamin K status in population studies is uncertain.

3.2. *Undercarboxylated Vitamin K-Dependent Proteins*

When there is insufficient vitamin K due to low vitamin K intake or vitamin K antagonism with oral anticoagulants such as warfarin, the post-translational carboxylation of vitamin K dependent proteins is reduced, which means the undercarboxylated (inactive) fractions of these proteins increases. Of the known vitamin K-dependent proteins, clotting proteins are the most recognized [1]. As reviewed elsewhere [88] prothrombin time, also expressed as international normalized ratio, is a routine clinical assay that can reflect clinical deficiency of vitamin K. However, these tests are non-specific, have low sensitivity for detecting low vitamin K status [89] and do not reflect intakes in generally healthy adults (Figure 2), so are not used in population studies as a measure of vitamin K status. Undercarboxylated prothrombin, known as PIVKA-II (proteins induced in vitamin K absence or antagonism-factor II), is measurable in circulation, and PIVKA-II concentrations change in response to dietary vitamin K depletion [83] and warfarin use [90]. Commercially-available PIVKA-II assays have low sensitivity for detecting variation in normal vitamin K intakes, which limits its utility in ranking individuals in population studies. One exception is in patients with chronic kidney disease, given the high prevalence of vitamin K deficiency in this patient population. PIVKA-II is not affected by reduced kidney function so circulating concentrations should not be influenced by the disease itself [68].

Osteocalcin (OC) is a vitamin K-dependent protein synthesized exclusively in bone during bone formation. OC is also detectable in serum and is used as a bone formation biomarker [91–93]. During dietary vitamin K depletion, the undercarboxylated fraction of OC (ucOC) increases whereas it decreases in response to vitamin K supplementation [83,94]. UcOC is detectable in circulation even when vitamin K intakes are sufficient to maintain coagulation, suggesting the storage of vitamin K in extra-hepatic organs is secondary to hepatic storage, as demonstrated in animal models [95,96]. For this reason, ucOC reflects vitamin K intake more so than PIVKA-II and is thought to be a more sensitive indicator of vitamin K status in community-based individuals (Figure 2). There are two immunoassay methods available to measure undercarboxylated OC: the hydroxyapatite binding assay or a commercially available immunoassay, which measures fully undercarboxylated OC directly (Takara Inc., Kyoto, Japan) [91,97]. More recently, a mass spectrometric immunoassay was developed that can provide qualitative and relative percent abundance information on the molecular variants of OC present in serum [94]. The absolute concentration of ucOC is positively correlated with total OC ($r = 0.78$) (Table 3). Because of this, when serum ucOC is used as a measure of vitamin K status it should be expressed as a% of total OC (%ucOC; when measured using a hydroxyapatite binding assay) or as a ratio to the carboxylated OC when measured directly (using immunoassay) [91], but not all studies have done so [98].

Table 3. Correlations among phylloquinone intake and biomarkers of vitamin K status in community-dwelling primarily Caucasian older adults ($n = 443$). Data are presented as Pearson correlation coefficients (p-value).

	Phylloquinone Intake (μg/Day) [a,b]	Plasma Phylloquinone (nM) [a,c]	PIVKA (ng/mL) [d]	%ucOC [e]	ucOC (ng/mL) [e]	Total OC (ng/mL) [e]	(dp)ucMGP (pM) [a,f]
plasma phylloquinone (nM) [a,c]	0.17 (<0.001) [h,i]						
PIVKA (ng/mL) [d]	−0.05 (0.30) [h]	−0.17 (<0.001) [i]					
%ucOC [e]	−0.14 (0.003) [h]	−0.23 (<0.001) [i]	0.08 (0.11)				
ucOC (ng/mL) [e]	−0.06 (0.19) [h]	−0.18 (<0.001) [i]	0.04 (0.42)	0.78 (<0.001)			
Total OC (ng/mL) [e]	0.02 (0.64) [h]	−0.08 (0.09) [i]	−0.02 (0.74)	0.41 (<0.001)	0.84 (<0.001)		
(dp)ucMGP (pM) [af]	−0.14 (<0.001) [h]	−0.32 (<0.001)	−0.06 (0.24)	0.26 (<0.001)	0.22 (<0.001)	0.08 (0.08)	
Total MGP (ng/mL) [g]	0.08 (0.10) [h]	0.04 (0.46) [i]	−0.06 (0.24)	−0.10 (0.03)	−0.03 (0.52)	0.05 (0.29)	0.29 (<0.001)

[a] natural log transformed to reduce skewness; [b] estimated using the Harvard Food Frequency Questionaire [39]; [c] measured using reverse-phase HPLC [39]; [d] measured using enzyme-linked immunoassay (ELISA) (Diagnostica Stago) [99]; [e] measured using radioimmunoassay [39,91]; [f] measured using sandwich ELISA [100,101]; [g] measured using radioimmunoassay [40,102]; [h] $n = 438$; [i] adjusted for triglycerides.

Because osteocalcin is synthesized in bone, the early studies of %ucOC as a functional indicator of vitamin K status focused on bone. Observational evidence suggested lower %ucOC to be associated with higher bone mineral density and reduced hip fracture risk [69,103–106], leading to the hypothesis that reducing %ucOC with vitamin K supplementation would decrease age-related bone loss. While some randomized trials reported a beneficial effect of vitamin K on bone health [41,107,108], others did not, even though vitamin K supplementation effectively reduced %ucOC [39,109–112]. Hence, the relevance of %ucOC to bone health is equivocal, as previously reviewed [97].

There has been recent interest in ucOC and its putative role in regulating glucose homeostasis. This theory was developed based on animal models which found injection of ucOC reduced blood glucose and improved insulin sensitivity in mice [113,114]. Several [115–120], but not all [117,121], studies that sought to extrapolate this finding to humans, found circulating ucOC to be inversely correlated to measures of insulin resistance. This could suggest a protective role for ucOC and therefore infer a detrimental role for vitamin K in metabolic disease because vitamin K promotes OC carboxylation. Since the primary dietary sources of vitamin K are green leafy vegetables and vegetable oils, this would represent a paradigm shift with respect to health benefits of vitamin K-rich foods. However, these studies did not correct for total osteocalcin, hence did not differentiate between an overall bone effect, as indicated by changes in the osteocalcin molecule, and a vitamin K effect, which would have been isolated if expressed as %ucOC. The limitations of these earlier population studies have been reinforced by the results of a recent meta-analysis, which found total OC and ucOC to be similarly inversely associated with fasting plasma glucose and glycosylated hemoglobin. Collectively, these suggest that the OC, but not its carboxylation status, hence vitamin K status, may be relevant to insulin resistance [122].

Matrix gla protein (MGP) is a vitamin K-dependent protein that functions as a calcification inhibitor in vascular tissue and cartilage [123]. In addition to being post-translationally carboxylated, MGP is also phosphorylated [124]. Assays that measure different forms of MGP in plasma are available [100], and the different circulating species appear to be differentially associated with health outcomes related to calcification (Supplementary Table S1). Only the dephosphorylated undercarboxylated form ((dp)ucMGP) responds to vitamin K supplementation [100,101,125,126]. When plotted against FFQ-estimated vitamin K intake, (dp)ucMGP decreased up an intake of 100–150 μg/day at which point the association plateaued (Figure 2), which may reflect the limitations of estimating vitamin K intake using FFQs previously discussed. (Dp)ucMGP has been suggested to be a functional indicator of vitamin K status in tissues that utilize MGP [100,127], such that higher amounts of (dp)ucMGP reflect lower vitamin K status. Several [128–134], but not all [135,136] population-based studies found higher plasma (dp)ucMGP was associated with more arterial calcification, arterial stiffness (which is positively associated with calcification) and CVD. In a post hoc analysis of a randomized controlled trial that found phylloquinone supplementation reduced CAC progression over 3 years in older men and women, dp-ucMGP was reduced by phylloquinone supplementation, but the change in (dp)ucMGP did not correlate with change in CAC [101]. Recently menaquinone-7 was reported to reduce plasma (dp)ucMGP and have a beneficial effect on arterial stiffness in post-menopausal women. At baseline (dp)ucMGP was positively correlated with stiffness, but the investigators did not report if changes in (dp)ucMGP correlated with changes in stiffness [137]. Because the majority of studies that measured (dp)ucMGP were done in primarily Caucasian groups (Supplementary Table S1), the relevance of (dp)ucMGP to vitamin K status and health outcomes in non-Caucasian groups merits investigation.

Similar to the situation with osteocalcin, the amount of (dp)ucMGP in circulation also depends on the total amount of MGP available [91,101]. It may be inappropriate, therefore, to extrapolate the association of higher (dp)ucMGP with more adverse health outcomes as being related to vitamin K insufficiency because the associations may be related to overall MGP status. For example, total MGP increases with age, independent of vitamin K intake [102], and given that age is an independent predictor of CVD and other chronic diseases, MGP may simply be a strong biomarker for age. It is also plausible that diseases characterized by calcification and/or cardiac dysfunction affect the synthesis of MGP because calcium as well as cardiac overload can promote MGP expression [138–140]. This could suggest elevated MGP is a consequence of CVD rather than causal. Much remains to be understood about the physiology underlying MGPs role in health and disease, which cannot be ascertained using observational studies. It is premature to conclude increasing MGP carboxylation with vitamin K will reduce risk for CVD and other outcomes related to calcification until this is tested using well-designed clinical trials.

3.3. Urinary Biomarkers

In addition to the blood measures, methods have been developed to measure urinary biomarkers of vitamin K metabolism. Y-Carboxyglutamic acid (gla) is an indicator of the turnover of all vitamin K-dependent proteins. Some [83,141], but not all [79,142] studies found urinary gla decreased when vitamin K intake is decreased. As vitamin K is catabolized, 5 carbon and 7 carbon aglycone metabolites are produced, which are water soluble and excreted in urine. These metabolites increase in response to vitamin K supplementation [143] and repletion, with a concomitant decrease in response to vitamin K depletion [143]. Menadione (vitamin K3; Figure 1) is the naphthoquinone ring metabolite of vitamin K that is thought to be an intermediary in the tissue-specific conversion of phylloquinone to menaquinone-4. Menadione is detectable in urine [144] and was found to change in response to vitamin K depletion and repletion more than urinary gla [141]. Because these urinary measures ideally require 24 h urine collection, their utility in clinic-based or in large-scale population-based studies is very limited. To the best of our knowledge, there are no studies that have examined the association of any of these measures with health outcomes for which a role for vitamin K has been suggested.

3.4. Interrelatedness of Vitamin K Status Biomarkers

Although there are multiple biomarkers available to estimate vitamin K status, it is apparent that no single biomarker is valid for use across all population-based studies. Since most population-based studies have limited volume of specimens, strategic decisions need to be made when deciding on choice of biomarkers.

After three years of supplementation with 500 μg/day of phylloquinone, plasma phylloquinone increased by >100% and %ucOC (and ucOC ng/mL) and (dp)ucMGP decreased by 50%–80% (Figure 4) [39,40]. The total MGP decreased 3.5% in the placebo group and increased 3.5% in the phylloquinone supplemented group, and the between group difference in this change reached statistical significance. However, the biological relevance of this difference is uncertain.

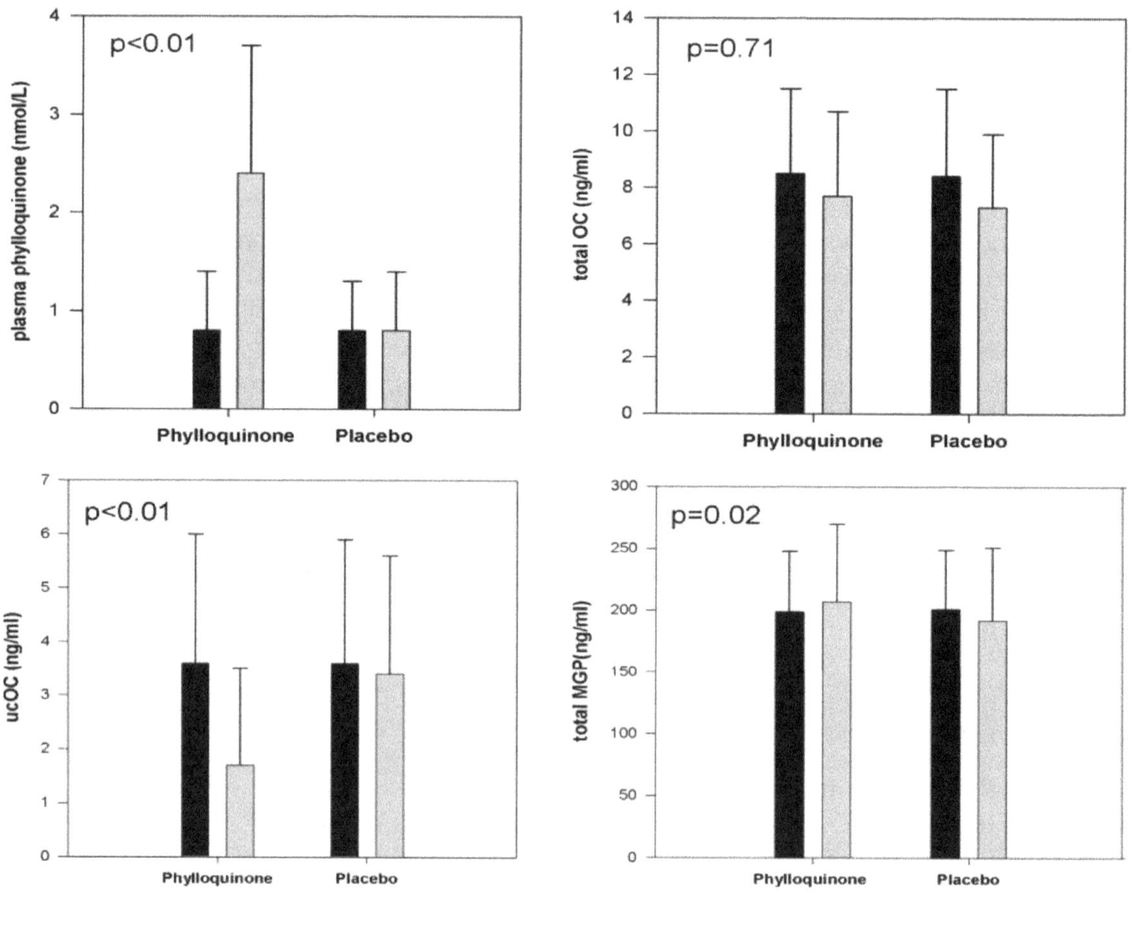

Figure 4. *Cont.*

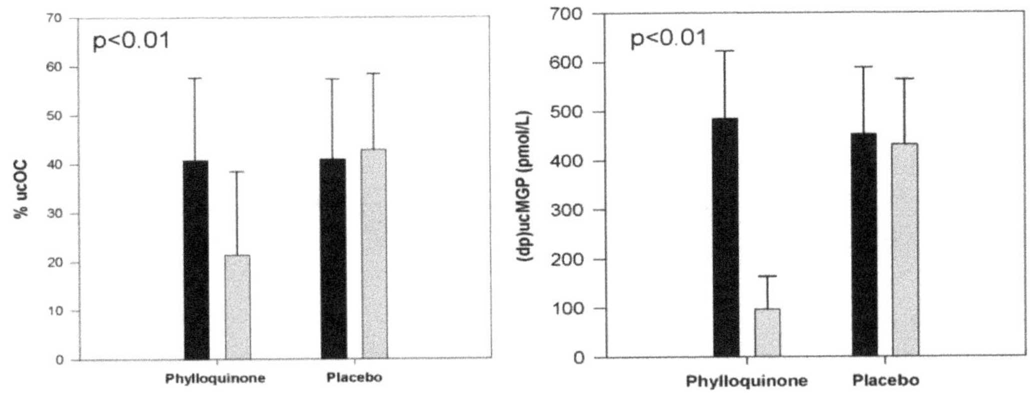

Figure 4. Circulating biomarkers at baseline (■) and after 3 years (□) of supplementation with 500 μg/day phylloquinone (n = 229) or placebo (n = 223) in primarily Caucasian community-dwelling men and women 65–80 years old. (Because of skewed distributions, plasma phylloquinone and (dp)ucMgp are presented as median values with error bars representing inter-quartile ranges. Otherwise data are presented as means with error bars representing standard deviations. p-values reflect the between-group difference for change in the biomarker in response to phylloquinone supplementation *versus* placebo).

PIVKA-II amounts were overall within the normal range at baseline [99], hence were not examined in response to supplementation given the low sensitivity of PIVKA-II to vitamin K supplementation in healthy individuals. Relative changes of urinary gla were more subtle compared to changes in circulating phylloquinone or undercarboxylated vitamin K-dependent proteins [83,141]. In this same cohort [39,40] observed at baseline, with the exception of PIVKA-II, circulating biomarkers of vitamin K significantly correlated with phylloquinone intake and with one another, but the correlations were overall not strong (Table 3). Unfortunately there are no urinary measures of vitamin K status available for comparison in population studies. Interestingly, in a racially diverse cohort, (dp)ucMGP was significantly correlated with plasma phylloquinone in whites but not in blacks (Figure 5) [145].

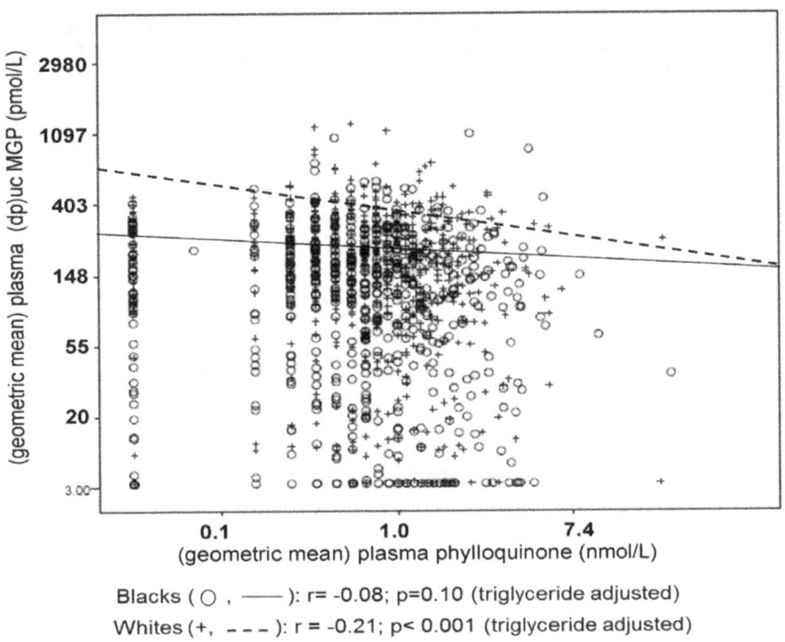

Figure 5. Correlation between circulating phylloquinone and (dp)ucMGP in black (n = 507) and white (n = 570) men and women 70–79 years old.

This may suggest the different measures of vitamin K status are influenced by physiological factors in addition to vitamin K. At this time, a combination of circulating concentrations of phylloquinone (and menaquinones when detectable), preferably corrected for circulating triglycerides, with an undercarboxylated non-coagulation protein, such as %ucOC (which can be corrected for the non-dietary influences on total protein concentrations), or (dp)ucMGP, would provide the most comprehensive approach to measure vitamin K status in population-based studies at this time, and allow for suitable ranking.

4. Conclusions

In summary, despite the multiple measures available, population- and clinic-based studies of vitamin K status are challenged by the lack of a single gold-standard measure. Dietary intake assessment by FFQ is convenient and easily implemented. Food composition databases are being expanded to include multiple menaquinone forms, so dietary questionnaires will no longer be limited to phylloquinone intake. Because menaquinones are generally not detected in circulation unless very large amounts are consumed, correlating menaquinone intake to circulating levels is problematic. While the use of biomarkers to estimate vitamin K status is not subject to the same limitations as the use dietary intake measures [3,53,54], there are limitations to each of the available biomarkers that need to be considered when studies are designed and interpreted. Circulating phylloquinone is carried on triglyceride-rich lipoproteins, which necessitates the use of fasting samples and concomitant measurement of triglycerides to reduce confounding. The amount of undercarboxylated vitamin K-dependent proteins in circulation depends on the total amount of protein, in addition to vitamin K availability. If these measures are not corrected for the total amount of the protein under study, they may reflect total protein status as well as vitamin K status which can confound the interpretation of the results. At this time, none of the urinary measures have been applied large cohorts so their utility epidemiologically is uncertain. Given the strengths and limitations of the available measures, and their modest inter-relatedness, vitamin K status may be estimated more accurately if multiple biomarkers, or biomarkers in combination with dietary intake are used.

Acknowledgments: This study was supported in part by the U.S. Department of Agriculture, Agricultural Research Service under Cooperative Agreement No. 58-1950-7-707, the National Institute of Aging (R01AG14759), the National Heart Lung and Blood Institute (R01HL69272), the National Institute of Arthritis Musculoskeletal and Skin Diseases (R21AR062284 and K01AR063167), and a New Investigator Grant from the Arthritis Foundation.

Author Contributions: M.K.S. and S.L.B. generated the concept of the review. M.K.S. drafted the manuscript and S.L.B. reviewed and edited the manuscript.

Abbreviations

BMD: bone mineral density, **CAC**: coronary artery calcium, **CHD**: coronary heart disease, **(dp)ucMGP**: dephosphorylated undercarboxylated matrix gla protein, **ELISA**: enzyme-linked immunoassay, **EPIC**: European Prospective Investigation into Cancer and Nutrition Study, **FFQ**: food frequency questionnaire, **HPLC**: high performance liquid chromatography, **IR**: insulin resistance, **MESA**: Multi-ethnic Study of Atherosclerosis, **MGP**: matrix gla protein, **MK**: menaquinone, **PIVKA-II**: proteins induced in vitamin K absence or antagonism-factor II, **PK**: phylloquinone, **ucOC** undercarboxylated osteocalcin, **%ucOC**: percent undercarboxylated osteocalcin.

References

1. Suttie, J.W. *Vitamin K in Health and Disease*; CRC Press: Boca Raton, FL, USA, 2009.
2. McCann, J.C.; Ames, B.N. Vitamin K, an example of triage theory: Is micronutrient inadequacy linked to diseases of aging? *Am. J. Clin. Nutr.* **2009**, *90*, 889–907. [CrossRef] [PubMed]

3. Willett, W.C. *Nutritional Epidemiology*, 3rd ed.; Oxford University Press: Oxford, UK, 2013.
4. Food and Nutrition Board, Insititue of Medicne. *Dietary Reference Intakes for Vitamin A, Vitamin K, Arsenic, Boron, Chromium, Copper, Iodine, Iron, Manganese, Molybdenum, Nickel, Silicon, Vanadium, and Zinc*; National Academy Press: Washington, DC, USA, 2002.
5. Shearer, M.J.; Fu, X.; Booth, S.L. Vitamin K nutrition, metabolism, and requirements: Current concepts and future research. *Adv. Nutr.* **2012**, *3*, 182–195. [CrossRef] [PubMed]
6. Booth, S.L.; Pennington, J.A.; Sadowski, J.A. Food sources and dietary intakes of vitamin K-1 (phylloquinone) in the American diet: Data from the FDA Total Diet Study. *J. Am. Diet. Assoc.* **1996**, *96*, 149–154. [CrossRef]
7. Duggan, P.; Cashman, K.D.; Flynn, A.; Bolton-Smith, C.; Kiely, M. Phylloquinone (vitamin K1) intakes and food sources in 18–64-year-old Irish adults. *Br. J. Nutr.* **2004**, *92*, 151–158. [CrossRef] [PubMed]
8. Erkkila, A.T.; Booth, S.L.; Hu, F.B.; Jacques, P.F.; Lichtenstein, A.H. Phylloquinone intake and risk of cardiovascular diseases in men. *Nutr. Metab. Cardiovasc. Dis.* **2007**, *17*, 58–62. [CrossRef] [PubMed]
9. Geleijnse, J.M.; Vermeer, C.; Grobbee, D.E.; Schurgers, L.J.; Knapen, M.H.; van der Meer, I.M.; Hofman, A.; Witteman, J.C. Dietary intake of menaquinone is associated with a reduced risk of coronary heart disease: The Rotterdam Study. *J. Nutr.* **2004**, *134*, 3100–3105. [PubMed]
10. Thane, C.W.; Bolton-Smith, C.; Coward, W.A. Comparative dietary intake and sources of phylloquinone (vitamin K1) among British adults in 1986–1987 and 2000–2001. *Br. J. Nutr.* **2006**, *96*, 1105–1115. [CrossRef] [PubMed]
11. Beulens, J.W.; Booth, S.L.; van den Heuvel, E.G.; Stoecklin, E.; Baka, A.; Vermeer, C. The role of menaquinones (vitamin K2) in human health. *Br. J. Nutr.* **2013**, *110*, 1357–1368. [CrossRef] [PubMed]
12. Tucker, K.L.; Smith, C.E.; Lai, C.Q.; Ordovas, J.M. Quantifying diet for nutrigenomic studies. *Annu. Rev. Nutr.* **2013**, *33*, 349–371. [CrossRef] [PubMed]
13. Barrett-Connor, E. Nutrition epidemiology: How do we know what they ate? *Am. J. Clin. Nutr.* **1991**, *54* (Suppl. S1), 182S–187S. [CrossRef]
14. Westerterp, K.R.; Goris, A.H. Validity of the assessment of dietary intake: Problems of misreporting. *Curr. Opin. Clin. Nutr. Metab. Care* **2002**, *5*, 489–493. [CrossRef] [PubMed]
15. Beulens, J.W.; Bots, M.L.; Atsma, F.; Bartelink, M.L.; Prokop, M.; Geleijnse, J.M.; Witteman, J.C.; Grobbee, D.E.; van der Schouw, Y.T. High dietary menaquinone intake is associated with reduced coronary calcification. *Atherosclerosis* **2009**, *203*, 489–493. [CrossRef] [PubMed]
16. Booth, S.L.; Tucker, K.L.; Chen, H.; Hannan, M.T.; Gagnon, D.R.; Cupples, L.A.; Wilson, P.W.; Ordovas, J.; Schaefer, E.J.; Dawson-Hughes, B.; *et al.* Dietary vitamin K intakes are associated with hip fracture but not with bone mineral density in elderly men and women. *Am. J. Clin. Nutr.* **2000**, *71*, 1201–1208. [PubMed]
17. Gast, G.C.; de Roos, N.M.; Sluijs, I.; Bots, M.L.; Beulens, J.W.; Geleijnse, J.M.; Witteman, J.C.; Grobbee, D.E.; Peeters, P.H.; van der Schouw, Y.T. A high menaquinone intake reduces the incidence of coronary heart disease. *Nutr. Metab. Cardiovasc. Dis.* **2009**, *19*, 504–510. [CrossRef] [PubMed]
18. Nimptsch, K.; Rohrmann, S.; Linseisen, J. Dietary intake of vitamin K and risk of prostate cancer in the Heidelberg cohort of the European Prospective Investigation into Cancer and Nutrition (EPIC-Heidelberg). *Am. J. Clin. Nutr.* **2008**, *87*, 985–992. [PubMed]
19. Villines, T.C.; Hatzigeorgiou, C.; Feuerstein, I.M.; O'Malley, P.G.; Taylor, A.J. Vitamin K1 intake and coronary calcification. *Coron. Artery Dis.* **2005**, *16*, 199–203. [CrossRef] [PubMed]
20. Erkkila, A.T.; Booth, S.L.; Hu, F.B.; Jacques, P.F.; Manson, J.E.; Rexrode, K.M.; Stampfer, M.J.; Lichtenstein, A.H. Phylloquinone intake as a marker for coronary heart disease risk but not stroke in women. *Eur. J. Clin. Nutr.* **2005**, *59*, 196–204. [CrossRef] [PubMed]
21. Booth, S.L.; Broe, K.E.; Gagnon, D.R.; Tucker, K.L.; Hannan, M.T.; McLean, R.R.; Dawson-Hughes, B.; Wilson, P.W.; Cupples, L.A.; Kiel, D.P. Vitamin K intake and bone mineral density in women and men. *Am. J. Clin. Nutr.* **2003**, *77*, 512–516. [PubMed]
22. Macdonald, H.M.; McGuigan, F.E.; Lanham-New, S.A.; Fraser, W.D.; Ralston, S.H.; Reid, D.M. Vitamin K1 intake is associated with higher bone mineral density and reduced bone resorption in early postmenopausal Scottish women: No evidence of gene-nutrient interaction with apolipoprotein E polymorphisms. *Am. J. Clin. Nutr.* **2008**, *87*, 1513–1520. [PubMed]
23. Feskanich, D.; Weber, P.; Willett, W.C.; Rockett, H.; Booth, S.L.; Colditz, G.A. Vitamin K intake and hip fractures in women: A prospective study. *Am. J. Clin. Nutr.* **1999**, *69*, 74–79. [PubMed]

24. Chan, R.; Leung, J.; Woo, J. No association between dietary vitamin K intake and fracture risk in chinese community-dwelling older men and women: A prospective study. *Calcif. Tissue Int.* **2012**, *90*, 396–403. [CrossRef] [PubMed]
25. Rejnmark, L.; Vestergaard, P.; Charles, P.; Hermann, A.P.; Brot, C.; Eiken, P.; Mosekilde, L. No effect of vitamin K1 intake on bone mineral density and fracture risk in perimenopausal women. *Osteoporos. Int.* **2006**, *17*, 1122–1132. [CrossRef] [PubMed]
26. Apalset, E.M.; Gjesdal, C.G.; Eide, G.E.; Tell, G.S. Intake of vitamin K1 and K2 and risk of hip fractures: The Hordaland Health Study. *Bone* **2011**, *49*, 990–995. [CrossRef] [PubMed]
27. Dam, V.; Dalmeijer, G.W.; Vermeer, C.; Drummen, N.E.; Knapen, M.H.; van der Schouw, Y.T.; Beulens, J.W. The association between vitamin K and the metabolic syndrome: A ten year follow-up study in adults. *J. Clin. Endocrinol. Metab.* **2015**, *100*, 2472–2479. [CrossRef] [PubMed]
28. Juanola-Falgarona, M.; Salas-Salvado, J.; Estruch, R.; Portillo, M.P.; Casas, R.; Miranda, J.; Martinez-Gonzalez, M.A.; Bullo, M. Association between dietary phylloquinone intake and peripheral metabolic risk markers related to insulin resistance and diabetes in elderly subjects at high cardiovascular risk. *Cardiovasc. Diabetol.* **2013**, *12*, 58–61. [CrossRef] [PubMed]
29. Shea, M.K.; Cushman, M.; Booth, S.L.; Burke, G.L.; Chen, H.; Kritchevsky, S.B. Associations between vitamin K status and haemostatic and inflammatory biomarkers in community-dwelling adults. The Multi-Ethnic Study of Atherosclerosis. *Thromb. Haemost.* **2014**, *112*, 438–444. [CrossRef] [PubMed]
30. Yoshida, M.; Booth, S.L.; Meigs, J.B.; Saltzman, E.; Jacques, P.F. Phylloquinone intake, insulin sensitivity, and glycemic status in men and women. *Am. J. Clin. Nutr.* **2008**, *88*, 210–215. [PubMed]
31. Nimptsch, K.; Rohrmann, S.; Kaaks, R.; Linseisen, J. Dietary vitamin K intake in relation to cancer incidence and mortality: Results from the Heidelberg cohort of the European Prospective Investigation into Cancer and Nutrition (EPIC-Heidelberg). *Am. J. Clin. Nutr.* **2010**, *91*, 1348–1358. [CrossRef] [PubMed]
32. Juanola-Falgarona, M.; Salas-Salvado, J.; Martinez-Gonzalez, M.A.; Corella, D.; Estruch, R.; Ros, E.; Fito, M.; Aros, F.; Gomez-Gracia, E.; Fiol, M.; *et al.* Dietary intake of vitamin K is inversely associated with mortality risk. *J. Nutr.* **2014**, *144*, 743–750. [CrossRef] [PubMed]
33. Cheung, C.L.; Sahni, S.; Cheung, B.M.; Sing, C.W.; Wong, I.C. Vitamin K intake and mortality in people with chronic kidney disease from NHANES III. *Clin. Nutr.* **2015**, *34*, 235–240. [CrossRef] [PubMed]
34. Geisen, C.; Watzka, M.; Sittinger, K.; Steffens, M.; Daugela, L.; Seifried, E.; Muller, C.R.; Wienker, T.F.; Oldenburg, J. VKORC1 haplotypes and their impact on the inter-individual and inter-ethnical variability of oral anticoagulation. *Thromb. Haemost.* **2005**, *94*, 773–779. [PubMed]
35. Braam, L.; McKeown, N.; Jacques, P.; Lichtenstein, A.; Vermeer, C.; Wilson, P.; Booth, S. Dietary phylloquinone intake as a potential marker for a heart-healthy dietary pattern in the Framingham Offspring cohort. *J. Am. Diet. Assoc.* **2004**, *104*, 1410–1414. [CrossRef] [PubMed]
36. Feskanich, D.; Rimm, E.B.; Giovannucci, E.L.; Colditz, G.A.; Stampfer, M.J.; Litin, L.B.; Willett, W.C. Reproducibility and validity of food intake measurements from a semiquantitative food frequency questionnaire. *J. Am. Diet. Assoc.* **1993**, *93*, 790–796. [CrossRef]
37. Presse, N.; Shatenstein, B.; Kergoat, M.J.; Ferland, G. Validation of a semi-quantitative food frequency questionnaire measuring dietary vitamin K intake in elderly people. *J. Am. Diet. Assoc.* **2009**, *109*, 1251–1255. [CrossRef] [PubMed]
38. McKeown, N.M.; Jacques, P.F.; Gundberg, C.M.; Peterson, J.W.; Tucker, K.L.; Kiel, D.P.; Wilson, P.W.; Booth, S.L. Dietary and nondietary determinants of vitamin K biochemical measures in men and women. *J. Nutr.* **2002**, *132*, 1329–1334. [PubMed]
39. Booth, S.L.; Dallal, G.; Shea, M.K.; Gundberg, C.; Peterson, J.W.; Dawson-Hughes, B. Effect of vitamin K supplementation on bone loss in elderly men and women. *J. Clin. Endocrinol. Metab.* **2008**, *93*, 1217–1223. [CrossRef] [PubMed]
40. Shea, M.K.; O'Donnell, C.J.; Hoffmann, U.; Dallal, G.E.; Dawson-Hughes, B.; Ordovas, J.M.; Price, P.A.; Williamson, M.K.; Booth, S.L. Vitamin K supplementation and progression of coronary artery calcium in older men and women. *Am. J. Clin. Nutr.* **2009**, *89*, 1799–1807. [CrossRef] [PubMed]
41. Cheung, A.M.; Tile, L.; Lee, Y.; Tomlinson, G.; Hawker, G.; Scher, J.; Hu, H.; Vieth, R.; Thompson, L.; Jamal, S.; *et al.* Vitamin K supplementation in postmenopausal women with osteopenia (ECKO trial): A randomized controlled trial. *PLoS Med.* **2008**, *5*, e196. [CrossRef] [PubMed]

42. Elder, S.J.; Haytowitz, D.B.; Howe, J.; Peterson, J.W.; Booth, S.L. Vitamin K contents of meat, dairy, and fast food in the U.S. Diet. *J. Agric. Food. Chem.* **2006**, *54*, 463–467. [CrossRef]

43. Manoury, E.; Jourdon, K.; Boyaval, P.; Fourcassie, P. Quantitative measurement of vitamin K2 (menaquinones) in various fermented dairy products using a reliable high-performance liquid chromatography method. *J. Dairy Sci.* **2013**, *96*, 1335–1346. [CrossRef] [PubMed]

44. Praagman, J.; Dalmeijer, G.W.; van der Schouw, Y.T.; Soedamah-Muthu, S.S.; Monique Verschuren, W.M.; Bas Bueno-de-Mesquita, H.; Geleijnse, J.M.; Beulens, J.W. The relationship between fermented food intake and mortality risk in the European Prospective Investigation into Cancer and Nutrition-Netherlands cohort. *Br. J. Nutr.* **2015**, *113*, 498–506. [CrossRef] [PubMed]

45. Sluijs, I.; Forouhi, N.G.; Beulens, J.W.; van der Schouw, Y.T.; Agnoli, C.; Arriola, L.; Balkau, B.; Barricarte, A.; Boeing, H.; Bueno-de-Mesquita, H.B.; *et al.* The amount and type of dairy product intake and incident type 2 diabetes: Results from the EPIC-InterAct Study. *Am. J. Clin. Nutr.* **2012**, *96*, 382–390. [CrossRef] [PubMed]

46. Aune, D.; Norat, T.; Romundstad, P.; Vatten, L.J. Dairy products and the risk of type 2 diabetes: A systematic review and dose-response meta-analysis of cohort studies. *Am. J. Clin. Nutr.* **2013**, *98*, 1066–1083. [CrossRef] [PubMed]

47. Sonestedt, E.; Wirfalt, E.; Wallstrom, P.; Gullberg, B.; Orho-Melander, M.; Hedblad, B. Dairy products and its association with incidence of cardiovascular disease: The Malmo diet and cancer cohort. *Eur. J. Epidemiol.* **2011**, *26*, 609–618. [CrossRef] [PubMed]

48. Farvid, M.S.; Ding, M.; Pan, A.; Sun, Q.; Chiuve, S.E.; Steffen, L.M.; Willett, W.C.; Hu, F.B. Dietary linoleic acid and risk of coronary heart disease: A systematic review and meta-analysis of prospective cohort studies. *Circulation* **2014**, *130*, 1568–1578. [CrossRef] [PubMed]

49. Walther, B.; Karl, J.P.; Booth, S.L.; Boyaval, P. Menaquinones, bacteria, and the food supply: The relevance of dairy and fermented food products to vitamin K requirements. *Adv. Nutr.* **2013**, *4*, 463–473. [CrossRef] [PubMed]

50. Schurgers, L.J.; Vermeer, C. Determination of phylloquinone and menaquinones in food. Effect of food matrix on circulating vitamin K concentrations. *Haemostasis* **2000**, *30*, 298–307. [PubMed]

51. Kaneki, M.; Hodges, S.J.; Hosoi, T.; Fujiwara, S.; Lyons, A.; Crean, S.J.; Ishida, N.; Nakagawa, M.; Takechi, M.; Sano, Y.; *et al.* Japanese fermented soybean food as the major determinant of the large geographic difference in circulating levels of vitamin K2: Possible implications for hip-fracture risk. *Nutrition* **2001**, *17*, 315–321. [CrossRef]

52. Hjartaker, A.; Lagiou, A.; Slimani, N.; Lund, E.; Chirlaque, M.D.; Vasilopoulou, E.; Zavitsanos, X.; Berrino, F.; Sacerdote, C.; Ocke, M.C.; *et al.* Consumption of dairy products in the European Prospective Investigation into Cancer and Nutrition (EPIC) cohort: Data from 35,955 24-h dietary recalls in 10 European countries. *Public Health Nutr.* **2002**, *5*, 1259–1271. [CrossRef] [PubMed]

53. Thompson, F.E.; Byers, T. Dietary assessment resource manual. *J. Nutr.* **1994**, *124* (Suppl. S11), 2245S–2317S. [PubMed]

54. Miller, T.M.; Abdel-Maksoud, M.F.; Crane, L.A.; Marcus, A.C.; Byers, T.E. Effects of social approval bias on self-reported fruit and vegetable consumption: A randomized controlled trial. *Nutr. J.* **2008**, *7*, 18588696. [CrossRef] [PubMed]

55. Potischman, N. Biologic and methodologic issues for nutritional biomarkers. *J. Nutr.* **2003**, *133* (Suppl. S3), 875S–880S. [PubMed]

56. Blanck, H.M.; Bowman, B.A.; Cooper, G.R.; Myers, G.L.; Miller, D.T. Laboratory issues: Use of nutritional biomarkers. *J. Nutr.* **2003**, *133* (Suppl. S3), 888S–894S. [PubMed]

57. Kawana, K.; Takahashi, M.; Hoshino, H.; Kushida, K. Circulating levels of vitamin K1, menaquinone-4, and menaquinone-7 in healthy elderly Japanese women and patients with vertebral fractures and patients with hip fractures. *Endocr. Res.* **2001**, *27*, 337–343. [CrossRef] [PubMed]

58. Tsugawa, N.; Shiraki, M.; Suhara, Y.; Kamao, M.; Tanaka, K.; Okano, T. Vitamin K status of healthy Japanese women: Age-related vitamin K requirement for gamma-carboxylation of osteocalcin. *Am. J. Clin. Nutr.* **2006**, *83*, 380–386. [PubMed]

59. Kanai, T.; Takagi, T.; Masuhiro, K.; Nakamura, M.; Iwata, M.; Saji, F. Serum vitamin K level and bone mineral density in post-menopausal women. *Int. J. Gynaecol. Obstet.* **1997**, *56*, 25–30. [CrossRef]

60. Tamatani, M.; Morimoto, S.; Nakajima, M.; Fukuo, K.; Onishi, T.; Kitano, S.; Niinobu, T.; Ogihara, T. Decreased circulating levels of vitamin K and 25-hydroxyvitamin D in osteopenic elderly men. *Metabolism* **1998**, *47*, 195–199. [CrossRef]
61. Thane, C.W.; Bates, C.J.; Shearer, M.J.; Unadkat, N.; Harrington, D.J.; Paul, A.A.; Prentice, A.; Bolton-Smith, C. Plasma phylloquinone (vitamin K1) concentration and its relationship to intake in a national sample of British elderly people. *Br. J. Nutr.* **2002**, *87*, 615–622. [CrossRef] [PubMed]
62. Thane, C.W.; Wang, L.Y.; Coward, W.A. Plasma phylloquinone (vitamin K1) concentration and its relationship to intake in British adults aged 19–64 years. *Br. J. Nutr.* **2006**, *96*, 1116–1124. [CrossRef] [PubMed]
63. Yan, L.; Zhou, B.; Greenberg, D.; Wang, L.; Nigdikar, S.; Prynne, C.; Prentice, A. Vitamin K status of older individuals in northern China is superior to that of older individuals in the UK. *Br. J. Nutr.* **2004**, *92*, 939–945. [CrossRef] [PubMed]
64. Beavan, S.R.; Prentice, A.; Stirling, D.M.; Dibba, B.; Yan, L.; Harrington, D.J.; Shearer, M.J. Ethnic differences in osteocalcin gamma-carboxylation, plasma phylloquinone (vitamin K1) and apolipoprotein E genotype. *Eur. J. Clin. Nutr.* **2005**, *59*, 72–81. [CrossRef] [PubMed]
65. Dalmeijer, G.W.; van der Schouw, Y.T.; Booth, S.L.; de Jong, P.A.; Beulens, J.W. Phylloquinone concentrations and the risk of vascular calcification in healthy women. *Arterioscler. Thromb. Vasc. Biol.* **2014**, *34*, 1587–1590. [CrossRef] [PubMed]
66. Fusaro, M.; Noale, M.; Viola, V.; Galli, F.; Tripepi, G.; Vajente, N.; Plebani, M.; Zaninotto, M.; Guglielmi, G.; Miotto, D.; *et al.* Vitamin K, vertebral fractures, vascular calcifications, and mortality: VItamin K Italian (VIKI) dialysis study. *J. Bone Miner. Res.* **2012**, *27*, 2271–2278. [CrossRef] [PubMed]
67. Holden, R.M.; Morton, A.R.; Garland, J.S.; Pavlov, A.; Day, A.G.; Booth, S.L. Vitamins K and D status in stages 3–5 chronic kidney disease. *Clin. J. Am. Soc. Nephrol.* **2010**, *5*, 590–597. [CrossRef] [PubMed]
68. Elliott, M.J.; Booth, S.L.; Hopman, W.M.; Holden, R.M. Assessment of potential biomarkers of subclinical vitamin K deficiency in patients with end-stage kidney disease. *Can. J. Kidney Health Dis.* **2014**, *1*. [CrossRef] [PubMed]
69. Booth, S.L.; Broe, K.E.; Peterson, J.W.; Cheng, D.M.; Dawson-Hughes, B.; Gundberg, C.M.; Cupples, L.A.; Wilson, P.W.; Kiel, D.P. Associations between vitamin K biochemical measures and bone mineral density in men and women. *J. Clin. Endocrinol. Metab.* **2004**, *89*, 4904–4909. [CrossRef] [PubMed]
70. Shea, M.K.; Booth, S.L.; Nettleton, J.A.; Burke, G.L.; Chen, H.; Kritchevsky, S.B. Circulating phylloquinone concentrations of adults in the United States differ according to race and ethnicity. *J. Nutr.* **2012**, *142*, 1060–1066. [CrossRef] [PubMed]
71. Shea, M.K.; Kritchevsky, S.B.; Hsu, F.C.; Nevitt, M.; Booth, S.L.; Kwoh, C.K.; McAlindon, T.E.; Vermeer, C.; Drummen, N.; Harris, T.B.; *et al.* The association between vitamin K status and knee osteoarthritis features in older adults: The Health, Aging and Body Composition Study. *Osteoarthr. Cartil.* **2015**, *23*, 370–378. [CrossRef] [PubMed]
72. Tsugawa, N.; Shiraki, M.; Suhara, Y.; Kamao, M.; Ozaki, R.; Tanaka, K.; Okano, T. Low plasma phylloquinone concentration is associated with high incidence of vertebral fracture in Japanese women. *J. Bone Miner. Metab.* **2008**, *26*, 79–85. [CrossRef] [PubMed]
73. Neogi, T.; Booth, S.L.; Zhang, Y.Q.; Jacques, P.F.; Terkeltaub, R.; Aliabadi, P.; Felson, D.T. Low vitamin K status is associated with osteoarthritis in the hand and knee. *Arthritis Rheum.* **2006**, *54*, 1255–1261. [CrossRef] [PubMed]
74. Misra, D.; Booth, S.L.; Tolstykh, I.; Felson, D.T.; Nevitt, M.C.; Lewis, C.E.; Torner, J.; Neogi, T. Vitamin K deficiency is associated with incident knee osteoarthritis. *Am. J. Med.* **2013**, *126*, 243–248. [CrossRef] [PubMed]
75. Shea, M.K.; Booth, S.L.; Miller, M.E.; Burke, G.L.; Chen, H.; Cushman, M.; Tracy, R.P.; Kritchevsky, S.B. Association between circulating vitamin K1 and coronary calcium progression in community-dwelling adults: The Multi-Ethnic Study of Atherosclerosis. *Am. J. Clin. Nutr.* **2013**, *98*, 197–208. [CrossRef] [PubMed]
76. Card, D.J.; Shearer, M.J.; Schurgers, L.J.; Harrington, D.J. The external quality assurance of phylloquinone (vitamin K(1)) analysis in human serum. *Biomed. Chromatogr.* **2009**, *23*, 1276–1282. [CrossRef] [PubMed]
77. Lamon-Fava, S.; Sadowski, J.A.; Davidson, K.W.; O'Brien, M.E.; McNamara, J.R.; Schaefer, E.J. Plasma lipoproteins as carriers of phylloquinone (vitamin K1) in humans. *Am. J. Clin. Nutr.* **1998**, *67*, 1226–1231. [PubMed]

78. Booth, S.L.; Tucker, K.L.; McKeown, N.M.; Davidson, K.W.; Dallal, G.E.; Sadowski, J.A. Relationships between dietary intakes and fasting plasma concentrations of fat-soluble vitamins in humans. *J. Nutr.* **1997**, *127*, 587–592. [PubMed]
79. Booth, S.L.; O'Brien-Morse, M.E.; Dallal, G.E.; Davidson, K.W.; Gundberg, C.M. Response of vitamin K status to different intakes and sources of phylloquinone-rich foods: Comparison of younger and older adults. *Am. J. Clin. Nutr.* **1999**, *70*, 368–377. [PubMed]
80. Novotny, J.A.; Kurilich, A.C.; Britz, S.J.; Baer, D.J.; Clevidence, B.A. Vitamin K absorption and kinetics in human subjects after consumption of 13C-labelled phylloquinone from kale. *Br. J. Nutr.* **2010**, *104*, 858–862. [CrossRef] [PubMed]
81. Jones, K.S.; Bluck, L.J.; Wang, L.Y.; Stephen, A.M.; Prynne, C.J.; Coward, W.A. The effect of different meals on the absorption of stable isotope-labelled phylloquinone. *Br. J. Nutr.* **2009**, *102*, 1195–1202. [CrossRef] [PubMed]
82. Nordestgaard, B.G.; Varbo, A. Triglycerides and cardiovascular disease. *Lancet* **2014**, *384*, 626–635. [CrossRef]
83. Booth, S.L.; Martini, L.; Peterson, J.W.; Saltzman, E.; Dallal, G.E.; Wood, R.J. Dietary phylloquinone depletion and repletion in older women. *J. Nutr.* **2003**, *133*, 2565–2569. [PubMed]
84. Shea, M.K.; Benjamin, E.J.; Dupuis, J.; Massaro, J.M.; Jacques, P.F.; D'Agostino, R.B., Sr.; Ordovas, J.M.; O'Donnell, C.J.; Dawson-Hughes, B.; *et al.* Genetic and non-genetic correlates of vitamins K and D. *Eur. J. Clin. Nutr.* **2009**, *63*, 458–464. [CrossRef] [PubMed]
85. Dashti, H.S.; Shea, M.K.; Smith, C.E.; Tanaka, T.; Hruby, A.; Richardson, K.; Wang, T.J.; Nalls, M.A.; Guo, X.; Liu, Y.; *et al.* Meta-analysis of genome-wide association studies for circulating phylloquinone concentrations. *Am. J. Clin. Nutr.* **2014**, *100*, 1462–1469. [CrossRef] [PubMed]
86. Sato, T.; Schurgers, L.J.; Uenishi, K. Comparison of menaquinone-4 and menaquinone-7 bioavailability in healthy women. *Nutr. J.* **2012**, *11*. [CrossRef] [PubMed]
87. Karl, J.P.; Fu, X.; Dolnikowski, G.G.; Saltzman, E.; Booth, S.L. Quantification of phylloquinone and menaquinones in feces, serum, and food by high-performance liquid chromatography-mass spectrometry. *J. Chromatogr. B Anal. Technol. Biomed. Life Sci.* **2014**, *963*, 128–133. [CrossRef] [PubMed]
88. Booth, S.L.; Al, R.A. Determinants of vitamin K status in humans. *Vitam. Horm.* **2008**, *78*, 1–22. [PubMed]
89. Suttie, J.W. Vitamin K and human nutrition. *J. Am. Diet. Assoc.* **1992**, *92*, 585–590. [PubMed]
90. Limdi, N.A.; Nolin, T.D.; Booth, S.L.; Centi, A.; Marques, M.B.; Crowley, M.R.; Allon, M.; Beasley, T.M. Influence of kidney function on risk of supratherapeutic international normalized ratio-related hemorrhage in warfarin users: A prospective cohort study. *Am. J. Kidney Dis.* **2015**, *65*, 701–709. [CrossRef] [PubMed]
91. Gundberg, C.M.; Nieman, S.D.; Abrams, S.; Rosen, H. Vitamin K status and bone health: An analysis of methods for determination of undercarboxylated osteocalcin. *J. Clin. Endocrinol. Metab.* **1998**, *83*, 3258–3266. [CrossRef] [PubMed]
92. Greenspan, S.L.; Resnick, N.M.; Parker, R.A. Early changes in biochemical markers of bone turnover are associated with long-term changes in bone mineral density in elderly women on alendronate, hormone replacement therapy, or combination therapy: A three-year, double-blind, placebo-controlled, randomized clinical trial. *J. Clin. Endocrinol. Metab.* **2005**, *90*, 2762–2767. [PubMed]
93. Rosen, C.J.; Chesnut, C.H., III; Mallinak, N.J. The predictive value of biochemical markers of bone turnover for bone mineral density in early postmenopausal women treated with hormone replacement or calcium supplementation. *J. Clin. Endocrinol. Metab.* **1997**, *82*, 1904–1910. [PubMed]
94. Rehder, D.S.; Gundberg, C.M.; Booth, S.L.; Borges, C.R. Gamma-carboxylation and fragmentation of osteocalcin in human serum defined by mass spectrometry. *Mol. Cell. Proteomics* **2015**, *14*, 1546–1555. [CrossRef] [PubMed]
95. Price, P.A.; Kaneda, Y. Vitamin K counteracts the effect of warfarin in liver but not in bone. *Thromb. Res.* **1987**, *46*, 121–131. [CrossRef]
96. Hara, K.; Kobayashi, M.; Akiyama, Y. Comparison of inhibitory effects of warfarin on gamma-carboxylation between bone and liver in rats. *J. Bone Miner. Metab.* **2005**, *23*, 366–372. [CrossRef] [PubMed]
97. Gundberg, C.M.; Lian, J.B.; Booth, S.L. Vitamin K-dependent carboxylation of osteocalcin: Friend or foe? *Adv. Nutr.* **2012**, *3*, 149–157. [CrossRef] [PubMed]
98. Theuwissen, E.; Magdeleyns, E.J.; Braam, L.A.; Teunissen, K.J.; Knapen, M.H.; Binnekamp, I.A.; van Summeren, M.J.; Vermeer, C. Vitamin K status in healthy volunteers. *Food Funct.* **2014**, *5*, 229–234. [CrossRef] [PubMed]

99. Shea, M.K.; Booth, S.L.; Gundberg, C.M.; Peterson, J.W.; Waddell, C.; Dawson-Hughes, B.; Saltzman, E. Adulthood obesity is positively associated with adipose tissue concentrations of vitamin K and inversely associated with circulating indicators of vitamin K status in men and women. *J. Nutr.* **2010**, *140*, 1029–1034. [CrossRef] [PubMed]
100. Cranenburg, E.C.; Koos, R.; Schurgers, L.J.; Magdeleyns, E.J.; Schoonbrood, T.H.; Landewe, R.B.; Brandenburg, V.M.; Bekers, O.; Vermeer, C. Characterisation and potential diagnostic value of circulating matrix Gla protein (MGP) species. *Thromb. Haemost.* **2010**, *104*, 811–822. [PubMed]
101. Shea, M.K.; O'Donnell, C.J.; Vermeer, C.; Magdeleyns, E.J.; Crosier, M.D.; Gundberg, C.M.; Ordovas, J.M.; Kritchevsky, S.B.; Booth, S.L. Circulating uncarboxylated matrix gla protein is associated with vitamin K nutritional status, but not coronary artery calcium, in older adults. *J. Nutr.* **2011**, *141*, 1529–1534. [CrossRef] [PubMed]
102. O'Donnell, C.J.; Shea, M.K.; Price, P.A.; Gagnon, D.R.; Wilson, P.W.; Larson, M.G.; Kiel, D.P.; Hoffmann, U.; Ferencik, M.; Clouse, M.E.; *et al.* Matrix Gla protein is associated with risk factors for atherosclerosis but not with coronary artery calcification. *Arterioscler. Thromb. Vasc. Biol.* **2006**, *26*, 2769–2774. [CrossRef] [PubMed]
103. Liu, G.; Peacock, M. Age-related changes in serum undercarboxylated osteocalcin and its relationships with bone density, bone quality, and hip fracture. *Calcif. Tissue Int.* **1998**, *62*, 286–289. [CrossRef] [PubMed]
104. Szulc, P.; Chapuy, M.C.; Meunier, P.J.; Delmas, P.D. Serum undercarboxylated osteocalcin is a marker of the risk of hip fracture in elderly women. *J. Clin. Invest.* **1993**, *91*, 1769–1774. [CrossRef] [PubMed]
105. Szulc, P.; Arlot, M.; Chapuy, M.C.; Duboeuf, F.; Meunier, P.J.; Delmas, P.D. Serum undercarboxylated osteocalcin correlates with hip bone mineral density in elderly women. *J. Bone Miner. Res.* **1994**, *9*, 1591–1595. [CrossRef] [PubMed]
106. Vergnaud, P.; Garnero, P.; Meunier, P.J.; Breart, G.; Kamihagi, K.; Delmas, P.D. Undercarboxylated osteocalcin measured with a specific immunoassay predicts hip fracture in elderly women: The EPIDOS Study. *J. Clin. Endocrinol. Metab.* **1997**, *82*, 719–724. [CrossRef] [PubMed]
107. Braam, L.A.; Knapen, M.H.; Geusens, P.; Brouns, F.; Hamulyak, K.; Gerichhausen, M.J.; Vermeer, C. Vitamin K1 supplementation retards bone loss in postmenopausal women between 50 and 60 years of age. *Calcif. Tissue Int.* **2003**, *73*, 21–26. [CrossRef] [PubMed]
108. Knapen, M.H.; Drummen, N.E.; Smit, E.; Vermeer, C.; Theuwissen, E. Three-year low-dose menaquinone-7 supplementation helps decrease bone loss in healthy postmenopausal women. *Osteoporos. Int.* **2013**, *24*, 2499–2507. [CrossRef] [PubMed]
109. Binkley, N.; Harke, J.; Krueger, D.; Engelke, J.; Vallarta-Ast, N.; Gemar, D.; Checovich, M.; Chappell, R.; Suttie, J. Vitamin K treatment reduces undercarboxylated osteocalcin but does not alter bone turnover, density, or geometry in healthy postmenopausal North American women. *J. Bone Miner. Res.* **2009**, *24*, 983–991. [CrossRef] [PubMed]
110. Bolton-Smith, C.; McMurdo, M.E.; Paterson, C.R.; Mole, P.A.; Harvey, J.M.; Fenton, S.T.; Prynne, C.J.; Mishra, G.D.; Shearer, M.J. Two-year randomized controlled trial of vitamin K1 (phylloquinone) and vitamin D3 plus calcium on the bone health of older women. *J. Bone Miner. Res.* **2007**, *22*, 509–519. [CrossRef] [PubMed]
111. O'Connor, E.M.; Grealy, G.; McCarthy, J.; Desmond, A.; Craig, O.; Shanahan, F.; Cashman, K.D. Effect of phylloquinone (vitamin K1) supplementation for 12 months on the indices of vitamin K status and bone health in adult patients with Crohn's disease. *Br. J. Nutr.* **2014**, *112*, 1163–1174. [CrossRef] [PubMed]
112. Emaus, N.; Gjesdal, C.G.; Almas, B.; Christensen, M.; Grimsgaard, A.S.; Berntsen, G.K.; Salomonsen, L.; Fonnebo, V. Vitamin K2 supplementation does not influence bone loss in early menopausal women: A randomised double-blind placebo-controlled trial. *Osteoporos. Int.* **2010**, *21*, 1731–1740. [CrossRef] [PubMed]
113. Ferron, M.; Hinoi, E.; Karsenty, G.; Ducy, P. Osteocalcin differentially regulates beta cell and adipocyte gene expression and affects the development of metabolic diseases in wild-type mice. *Proc. Natl. Acad. Sci. USA* **2008**, *105*, 5266–5270. [CrossRef] [PubMed]
114. Ferron, M.; McKee, M.D.; Levine, R.L.; Ducy, P.; Karsenty, G. Intermittent injections of osteocalcin improve glucose metabolism and prevent type 2 diabetes in mice. *Bone* **2012**, *50*, 568–575. [CrossRef] [PubMed]
115. Pollock, N.K.; Bernard, P.J.; Gower, B.A.; Gundberg, C.M.; Wenger, K.; Misra, S.; Bassali, R.W.; Davis, C.L. Lower uncarboxylated osteocalcin concentrations in children with prediabetes is associated with beta-cell function. *J. Clin. Endocrinol. Metab.* **2011**, *96*, E1092–E1099. [CrossRef] [PubMed]

116. Prats-Puig, A.; Mas-Parareda, M.; Riera-Perez, E.; Gonzalez-Forcadell, D.; Mier, C.; Mallol-Guisset, M.; Diaz, M.; Bassols, J.; de Zegher, F.; Ibanez, L.; *et al.* Carboxylation of osteocalcin affects its association with metabolic parameters in healthy children. *Diabetes Care* **2010**, *33*, 661–663. [CrossRef] [PubMed]
117. Lu, C.; Ivaska, K.K.; Alen, M.; Wang, Q.; Tormakangas, T.; Xu, L.; Wiklund, P.; Mikkola, T.M.; Pekkala, S.; Tian, H.; Vaananen, H.K.; *et al.* Serum osteocalcin is not associated with glucose but is inversely associated with leptin across generations of nondiabetic women. *J. Clin. Endocrinol. Metab.* **2012**, *97*, 4106–4114. [CrossRef] [PubMed]
118. Iki, M.; Tamaki, J.; Fujita, Y.; Kouda, K.; Yura, A.; Kadowaki, E.; Sato, Y.; Moon, J.S.; Tomioka, K.; Okamoto, N.; *et al.* Serum undercarboxylated osteocalcin levels are inversely associated with glycemic status and insulin resistance in an elderly Japanese male population: Fujiwara-kyo Osteoporosis Risk in Men (FORMEN) Study. *Osteoporos. Int.* **2012**, *23*, 761–770. [CrossRef] [PubMed]
119. Okuno, S.; Ishimura, E.; Tsuboniwa, N.; Norimine, K.; Yamakawa, K.; Yamakawa, T.; Shoji, S.; Mori, K.; Nishizawa, Y.; Inaba, M. Significant inverse relationship between serum undercarboxylated osteocalcin and glycemic control in maintenance hemodialysis patients. *Osteoporos. Int.* **2013**, *24*, 605–612. [CrossRef] [PubMed]
120. Yeap, B.B.; Alfonso, H.; Chubb, S.A.; Gauci, R.; Byrnes, E.; Beilby, J.P.; Ebeling, P.R.; Handelsman, D.J.; Allan, C.A.; Grossmann, M.; *et al.* Higher serum undercarboxylated osteocalcin and other bone turnover markers are associated with reduced diabetes risk and lower estradiol concentrations in older men. *J. Clin. Endocrinol. Metab.* **2015**, *100*, 63–71. [CrossRef] [PubMed]
121. Shea, M.K.; Gundberg, C.M.; Meigs, J.B.; Dallal, G.E.; Saltzman, E.; Yoshida, M.; Jacques, P.F.; Booth, S.L. Gamma-carboxylation of osteocalcin and insulin resistance in older men and women. *Am. J. Clin. Nutr.* **2009**, *90*, 1230–1235. [CrossRef] [PubMed]
122. Liu, D.M.; Guo, X.Z.; Tong, H.J.; Tao, B.; Sun, L.H.; Zhao, H.Y.; Ning, G.; Liu, J.M. Association between osteocalcin and glucose metabolism: A meta-analysis. *Osteoporos. Int.* **2015**, *26*, 2823–2833. [CrossRef] [PubMed]
123. Luo, G.; Ducy, P.; McKee, M.D.; Pinero, G.J.; Loyer, E.; Behringer, R.R.; Karsenty, G. Spontaneous calcification of arteries and cartilage in mice lacking matrix GLA protein. *Nature* **1997**, *386*, 78–81. [CrossRef] [PubMed]
124. Schurgers, L.J.; Spronk, H.M.; Skepper, J.N.; Hackeng, T.M.; Shanahan, C.M.; Vermeer, C.; Weissberg, P.L.; Proudfoot, D. Post-translational modifications regulate matrix Gla protein function: Importance for inhibition of vascular smooth muscle cell calcification. *J. Thromb. Haemost.* **2007**, *5*, 2503–2511. [CrossRef] [PubMed]
125. Dalmeijer, G.W.; van der Schouw, Y.T.; Magdeleyns, E.; Ahmed, N.; Vermeer, C.; Beulens, J.W. The effect of menaquinone-7 supplementation on circulating species of matrix Gla protein. *Atherosclerosis* **2012**, *225*, 397–402. [CrossRef] [PubMed]
126. Schlieper, G.; Westenfeld, R.; Kruger, T.; Cranenburg, E.C.; Magdeleyns, E.J.; Brandenburg, V.M.; Djuric, Z.; Damjanovic, T.; Ketteler, M.; Vermeer, C.; *et al.* Circulating nonphosphorylated carboxylated matrix gla protein predicts survival in ESRD. *J. Am. Soc. Nephrol.* **2011**, *22*, 387–395. [CrossRef] [PubMed]
127. Westenfeld, R.; Krueger, T.; Schlieper, G.; Cranenburg, E.C.; Magdeleyns, E.J.; Heidenreich, S.; Holzmann, S.; Vermeer, C.; Jahnen-Dechent, W.; Ketteler, M.; *et al.* Effect of vitamin K2 supplementation on functional vitamin K deficiency in hemodialysis patients: A randomized trial. *Am. J. Kidney Dis.* **2012**, *59*, 186–195. [CrossRef] [PubMed]
128. Dalmeijer, G.W.; van der Schouw, Y.T.; Magdeleyns, E.J.; Vermeer, C.; Verschuren, W.M.; Boer, J.M.; Beulens, J.W. Matrix Gla protein species and risk of cardiovascular events in type 2 diabetic patients. *Diabetes Care* **2013**, *36*, 3766–3771. [CrossRef] [PubMed]
129. Liu, Y.P.; Gu, Y.M.; Thijs, L.; Knapen, M.H.; Salvi, E.; Citterio, L.; Petit, T.; Carpini, S.D.; Zhang, Z.; Jacobs, L.; *et al.* Inactive matrix Gla protein is causally related to adverse health outcomes: A Mendelian randomization study in a Flemish population. *Hypertension* **2015**, *65*, 463–470. [CrossRef] [PubMed]
130. Mayer, O., Jr.; Seidlerova, J.; Bruthans, J.; Filipovsky, J.; Timoracka, K.; Vanek, J.; Cerna, L.; Wohlfahrt, P.; Cifkova, R.; Theuwissen, E.; *et al.* Desphospho-uncarboxylated matrix Gla-protein is associated with mortality risk in patients with chronic stable vascular disease. *Atherosclerosis* **2014**, *235*, 162–168. [CrossRef] [PubMed]
131. Mayer, O., Jr.; Seidlerova, J.; Wohlfahrt, P.; Filipovsky, J.; Vanek, J.; Cifkova, R.; Windrichova, J.; Topolcan, O.; Knapen, M.H.; Drummen, N.E.; *et al.* Desphospho-uncarboxylated matrix Gla protein is associated with increased aortic stiffness in a general population. *J. Hum. Hypertens.* **2015**. [CrossRef] [PubMed]

132. Pivin, E.; Ponte, B.; Pruijm, M.; Ackermann, D.; Guessous, I.; Ehret, G.; Liu, Y.P.; Drummen, N.E.; Knapen, M.H.; Pechere-Bertschi, A.; *et al.* Inactive matrix Gla-protein is associated with arterial stiffness in an adult population-based study. *Hypertension* **2015**, *66*, 85–92. [CrossRef] [PubMed]

133. Pivin, E.; Pruijm, M.; Ackermann, D.; Guessous, I.; Ehret, G.; Pechere-Bertschi, A.; Paccaud, F.; Mohaupt, M.; Vermeer, C.; Staessen, J.A.; *et al.* 1D.03: Inactive matrix gla protein is associated with renal resistive index in a population-based study. *J. Hypertens.* **2015**, *33* (Suppl. S1). [CrossRef] [PubMed]

134. van den Heuvel, E.G.; van Schoor, N.M.; Lips, P.; Magdeleyns, E.J.; Deeg, D.J.; Vermeer, C.; den, H.M. Circulating uncarboxylated matrix Gla protein, a marker of vitamin K status, as a risk factor of cardiovascular disease. *Maturitas* **2014**, *77*, 137–141. [CrossRef] [PubMed]

135. Dalmeijer, G.W.; van der Schouw, Y.T.; Vermeer, C.; Magdeleyns, E.J.; Schurgers, L.J.; Beulens, J.W. Circulating matrix Gla protein is associated with coronary artery calcification and vitamin K status in healthy women. *J. Nutr. Biochem.* **2013**, *24*, 624–628. [CrossRef] [PubMed]

136. Dalmeijer, G.W.; van der Schouw, Y.T.; Magdeleyns, E.J.; Vermeer, C.; Verschuren, W.M.; Boer, J.M.; Beulens, J.W. Circulating desphospho-uncarboxylated matrix gamma-carboxyglutamate protein and the risk of coronary heart disease and stroke. *J. Thromb. Haemost.* **2014**, *12*, 1028–1034. [CrossRef] [PubMed]

137. Knapen, M.H.; Braam, L.A.; Drummen, N.E.; Bekers, O.; Hoeks, A.P.; Vermeer, C. Menaquinone-7 supplementation improves arterial stiffness in healthy postmenopausal women: Double-blind randomised clinical trial. *Thromb. Haemost.* **2015**, *113*, 1135–1144. [CrossRef] [PubMed]

138. Farzaneh-Far, A.; Weissberg, P.L.; Proudfoot, D.; Shanahan, C.M. Transcriptional regulation of matrix gla protein. *Z. Kardiol.* **2001**, *90* (Suppl. S3), 38–42. [CrossRef] [PubMed]

139. Mustonen, E.; Pohjolainen, V.; Aro, J.; Pikkarainen, S.; Leskinen, H.; Ruskoaho, H.; Rysa, J. Upregulation of cardiac matrix Gla protein expression in response to hypertrophic stimuli. *Blood Press* **2009**, *18*, 286–293. [CrossRef] [PubMed]

140. Price, P.A.; Thomas, G.R.; Pardini, A.W.; Figueira, W.F.; Caputo, J.M.; Williamson, M.K. Discovery of a high molecular weight complex of calcium, phosphate, fetuin, and matrix gamma-carboxyglutamic acid protein in the serum of etidronate-treated rats. *J. Biol. Chem.* **2002**, *277*, 3926–3934. [CrossRef] [PubMed]

141. Truong, J.T.; Fu, X.; Saltzman, E.; Al, R.A.; Dallal, G.E.; Gundberg, C.M.; Booth, S.L. Age group and sex do not influence responses of vitamin K biomarkers to changes in dietary vitamin K. *J. Nutr.* **2012**, *142*, 936–941. [CrossRef] [PubMed]

142. Bugel, S.; Sorensen, A.D.; Hels, O.; Kristensen, M.; Vermeer, C.; Jakobsen, J.; Flynn, A.; Molgaard, C.; Cashman, K.D. Effect of phylloquinone supplementation on biochemical markers of vitamin K status and bone turnover in postmenopausal women. *Br. J. Nutr.* **2007**, *97*, 373–380. [CrossRef] [PubMed]

143. Harrington, D.J.; Soper, R.; Edwards, C.; Savidge, G.F.; Hodges, S.J.; Shearer, M.J. Determination of the urinary aglycone metabolites of vitamin K by HPLC with redox-mode electrochemical detection. *J. Lipid Res.* **2005**, *46*, 1053–1060. [CrossRef] [PubMed]

144. Al, R.A.; Peterson, J.; Choi, S.W.; Suttie, J.; Barakat, S.; Booth, S.L. Measurement of menadione in urine by HPLC. *J. Chromatogr. B Anal. Technol. Biomed. Life Sci.* **2010**, *878*, 2457–2460.

145. Shea, M.K.; Booth, S.L.; Brinkley, T.E.; Kritchevsky, S.B. Vitamin K status in black and white older adults and its relationship with cardiovascular disease risk. *FASEB J.* **2015**, *29* (Suppl. S1), 906.4.

Permissions

All chapters in this book were first published by MDPI; hereby published with permission under the Creative Commons Attribution License or equivalent. Every chapter published in this book has been scrutinized by our experts. Their significance has been extensively debated. The topics covered herein carry significant findings which will fuel the growth of the discipline. They may even be implemented as practical applications or may be referred to as a beginning point for another development.

The contributors of this book come from diverse backgrounds, making this book a truly international effort. This book will bring forth new frontiers with its revolutionizing research information and detailed analysis of the nascent developments around the world.

We would like to thank all the contributing authors for lending their expertise to make the book truly unique. They have played a crucial role in the development of this book. Without their invaluable contributions this book wouldn't have been possible. They have made vital efforts to compile up to date information on the varied aspects of this subject to make this book a valuable addition to the collection of many professionals and students.

This book was conceptualized with the vision of imparting up-to-date information and advanced data in this field. To ensure the same, a matchless editorial board was set up. Every individual on the board went through rigorous rounds of assessment to prove their worth. After which they invested a large part of their time researching and compiling the most relevant data for our readers.

The editorial board has been involved in producing this book since its inception. They have spent rigorous hours researching and exploring the diverse topics which have resulted in the successful publishing of this book. They have passed on their knowledge of decades through this book. To expedite this challenging task, the publisher supported the team at every step. A small team of assistant editors was also appointed to further simplify the editing procedure and attain best results for the readers.

Apart from the editorial board, the designing team has also invested a significant amount of their time in understanding the subject and creating the most relevant covers. They scrutinized every image to scout for the most suitable representation of the subject and create an appropriate cover for the book.

The publishing team has been an ardent support to the editorial, designing and production team. Their endless efforts to recruit the best for this project, has resulted in the accomplishment of this book. They are a veteran in the field of academics and their pool of knowledge is as vast as their experience in printing. Their expertise and guidance has proved useful at every step. Their uncompromising quality standards have made this book an exceptional effort. Their encouragement from time to time has been an inspiration for everyone.

The publisher and the editorial board hope that this book will prove to be a valuable piece of knowledge for researchers, students, practitioners and scholars across the globe.

List of Contributors

Wojciech Skrobot, Ewelina Perzanowska and Katarzyna Krasowska
Department of Functional Diagnostics and Kinesiology, Gdansk University of Physical Education and Sport, 80-336 Gdansk, Poland

Damian J. Flis, Katarzyna P. Dzik and Jan Jacek Kaczor
Department of Physiology and Biochemistry, Gdansk University of Physical Education and Sport, 80-336 Gdansk, Poland

Wojciech Kloc
Department of Neurosurgery, Copernicus Hospital, 80-803 Gdansk, Poland
Department of Neurology and Neurosurgery, University of Warmia and Mazury in Olsztyn, 10-719 Olsztyn, Poland

Jędrzej Antosiewicz
Department of Bioenergetics and Physiology of Exercise, Medical University of Gdansk, 80-211 Gdansk, Poland

Alexandra Povaliaeva, Ekaterina Pigarova, Artem Zhukov, Viktor Bogdanov, Larisa Dzeranova, Olga Mel'nikova, Elena Pekareva, Natalya Malysheva, Vitaliy Ioutsi, Larisa Nikankina and Liudmila Rozhinskaya
Endocrinology Research Centre, 117036 Moscow, Russia

Ian T. Zajac, Paul Cavuoto and Manny Noakes
Commonwealth Scientific and Industrial Research Organisation—Health and Biosecurity, Adelaide 5000, Australia

Mary Barnes
Centre for Epidemiology and Biostatistics, Flinders University, Adelaide 5001, Australia

Gary Wittert
Freemasons Foundation Centre for Men's Health, North Terrace, Adelaide 5000, Australia
Centre for Nutrition and Gastrointestinal Disease, South Australian Health and Medical Research Institute, Adelaide 5000, Australia

Chisato Saeki, Tomoya Kanai, Masanori Nakano and Yuichi Torisu
Division of Gastroenterology and Hepatology, Department of Internal Medicine, The Jikei University School of Medicine, 3-25-8 Nishi-shimbashi, Minatoku, Tokyo 105-8461, Japan
Division of Gastroenterology, Department of Internal Medicine, Fuji City General Hospital, 50 Takashimacho, Fuji-shi 417-8567, Shizuoka, Japan

Masayuki Saruta and Tsunekazu Oikawa
Division of Gastroenterology and Hepatology, Department of Internal Medicine, The Jikei University School of Medicine, 3-25-8 Nishi-shimbashi, Minatoku, Tokyo 105-8461, Japan

Akihito Tsubota
Core Research Facilities, Research Center for Medical Science, The Jikei University School of Medicine, 3-25-8 Nishi-shimbashi, Minato-ku, Tokyo 105-8461, Japan

Ran Uchitomi, Mamoru Oyabu and Yasutomi Kamei
Graduate School of Life and Environmental Sciences, Kyoto Prefectural University, Kyoto 606-8522, Japan

Rick H. van Gorp
Department of Biochemistry, Cardiovascular Research Institute Maastricht, Maastricht University, 6200 MD Maastricht, The Netherlands
Nattopharma ASA, 1363 Høvik, Norway

Leon J. Schurgers
Department of Biochemistry, Cardiovascular Research Institute Maastricht, Maastricht University, 6200 MD Maastricht, The Netherlands
Department of Biochemistry, Cardiovascular Research Institute Maastricht (CARIM), University of Maastricht, Maastricht 6229ER, The Netherlands

Laurent Mène-Saffrané
Department of Biology, University of Fribourg, Chemin du Musée, 10, 1700 Fribourg, Switzerland

Guylaine Ferland
Département de nutrition, Université de Montréal, Montréal, QC H3C 3J7, Canada
Centre de recherche, Institut Universitaire de Gériatrie de Montréal, Montréal, QC H3W 1W5, Canada

Isabelle Doucet
Département de nutrition, Université de Montréal, Montréal, QC H3C 3J7, Canada
Hôpital de la Cité-de-la-Santé, Laval, QC H7M 3L9, Canada

Steffi Fritsche and Christian Jung
Plant Breeding Institute, Christian-Albrechts-University of Kiel, 24118 Kiel, Germany

Dominique Mainville
Département de nutrition, Université de Montréal, Montréal, QC H3C 3J7, Canada
CIUSSS du Centre-Sud-de-l'Île-de-Montréal, Centre de réadaptation Lucie-Bruneau, Montréal, QC H2H 2N8, Canada

Xingxing Wang
Plant Breeding Institute, Christian-Albrechts-University of Kiel, 24118 Kiel, Germany
Institute of Cotton Research of Chinese Academy of Agricultural Sciences, Anyang 455000, China

Daniel Scheiber, Verena Veulemans, Patrick Horn and Ralf Westenfeld
Division of Cardiology, Pulmonology, and Vascular Medicine, Medical Faculty, University Duesseldorf, Duesseldorf 40225, Germany

Martijn L. Chatrou
Department of Biochemistry, Cardiovascular Research Institute Maastricht, Maastricht University, Maastricht 6229 ER, The Netherlands

Sebastian A. Potthoff
Department of Nephrology, University Duesseldorf, Medical Faculty, Duesseldorf 40225, Germany

Malte Kelm
Division of Cardiology, Pulmonology, and Vascular Medicine, Medical Faculty, University Duesseldorf, Duesseldorf 40225, Germany
Cardiovascular Research Institute Duesseldorf, University Duesseldorf, Medical Faculty, Duesseldorf 40225, Germany

Ossama Kodad
Département Arboriculture-Viticulture, École Nationale d'Agriculture de Meknès, Meknès BP S/40, Morocco

Rafel Socias i Company and José M. Alonso
Unidad de Hortofruticutura, Centro de Investigación y Tecnología Agroalimentaria de Aragón (CITA), Av. Montañana 930, 50059 Zaragoza, Spain

Paul Clarke
Neonatal Unit, Norfolk and Norwich University Hospitals NHS Foundation Trust, Colney Lane, Norwich, Norfolk NR4 7UY, UK

Martin J. Shearer and Dominic J. Harrington
Centre for Haemostasis and Thrombosis, St. Thomas' Hospital, Westminster Bridge Road, London SE1 7EH, UK

Simon J. Mitchell
Newborn Intensive Care, St Mary's Hospital, Oxford Road, Manchester M13 9WL, UK

Justine Chouet and Olivier Beauchet
Department of Neuroscience, Division of Geriatric Medicine, Angers University Hospital; Angers University Memory Clinic; UPRES EA 4638, University of Angers, UNAM, Angers F-49933, France

Nancy Presse and Kariane Boucher
Centre de recherche, Institut Universitaire de Gériatrie de Montréal, Montréal, QC H3W 1W5, Canada

Catherine Féart and Pascale Barberger-Gateau
Université Bordeaux, ISPED, Centre INSERM U897-Epidemiologie-Biostatistique, Bordeaux F-33000, France
INSERM, ISPED, INSERM U897-Epidemiologie-Biostatistique, Bordeaux F-33000, France

Yves Rolland
Department of Geriatric Medicine, Institut du Vieillissement, University Hospital; INSERM U1027, Toulouse F-31400, France

Cedric Annweiler
Department of Neuroscience, Division of Geriatric Medicine, Angers University Hospital; Angers University Memory Clinic; UPRES EA 4638, University of Angers, UNAM, Angers F-49933, France
Robarts Research Institute, Department of Medical Biophysics, Schulich School of Medicine and Dentistry, the University of Western Ontario, London, ON N6A 5B7, Canada

Guylaine Ferland
Département de nutrition, Université de Montréal, Montréal, QC H3C 3J7, Canada
Centre de recherche, Institut Universitaire de Gériatrie de Montréal, Montréal, QC H3W 1W5, Canada

Data Santorino, Juliet Mwanga-Amumpaire and Unni Wariyar
Department of Pediatrics and Child Health, Mbarara University of Science and Technology, Plot 8-18 Mbarara-Kabale Road, Mbarara, Uganda

Mark J. Siedner
Department of Medicine and Infectious Diseases, Massachusetts General Hospital and Harvard Medical School, 125 Nashua Street, Boston, MA 02114, USA

M. Kyla Shea and Sarah L. Booth
USDA Human Nutrition Research Center on Aging, Tufts University, Boston, MA 02111, USA

Index

www.ingramcontent.com/pod-product-compliance
Lightning Source LLC
LaVergne TN
LVHW060540210926
848485LV00005B/1230
9781639276691